Eye Movement Disorders

Eye Movement Disorders

Agnes M.F. Wong, MD, PhD, FRCSC

Associate Professor of Ophthalmology and Vision Sciences, Neurology, and Otolaryngology—Head and Neck Surgery

University of Toronto

Adjunct Associate Professor of Ophthalmology and Visual Sciences

Washington University in St. Louis

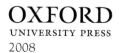

OXFORD
UNIVERSITY PRESS
2008

OXFORD
UNIVERSITY PRESS

Oxford University Press, Inc., publishes works that further
Oxford University's objective of excellence
in research, scholarship, and education.

Oxford New York
Auckland Cape Town Dar es Salaam Hong Kong Karachi
Kuala Lumpur Madrid Melbourne Mexico City Nairobi
New Delhi Shanghai Taipei Toronto

With offices in
Argentina Austria Brazil Chile Czech Republic France Greece
Guatemala Hungary Italy Japan Poland Portugal Singapore
South Korea Switzerland Thailand Turkey Ukraine Vietnam

Published by Oxford University Press, Inc.
198 Madison Avenue, New York, New York 10016

www.oup.com

Oxford is a registered trademark of Oxford University Press

Library of Congress Cataloging-in-Publication Data
Wong, Agnes M.F., 1968–
Eye movement disorders / Agnes M.F. Wong.
p. cm.
Includes bibliographical references and index.
ISBN 978-0-19-532426-6
1. Eye—Movement disorders.   I. Title.
[DNLM: 1. Ocular Motility Disorders. WW 410 W872e 2007]
RE731.W66 2007
617.7'62—dc22   2006037210

22 21 20 19 18 17 16 15 14
Printed in Canada
on acid-free paper

To my parents, Esther and Joseph,

and William, James, and Stephen

Preface

Eye movement disorders are commonly encountered in clinical practice. They are often the initial manifestation of diseases affecting the central nervous system. Understanding eye movement disorders remains challenging, partly because it requires knowledge of the underlying anatomy and physiology. Although there are a number of excellent texts covering this subject, few present the information in a clear and concise manner with accompanying anatomic diagrams to elucidate the intricate relationships among clinical phenomena, basic neuroanatomy, and neurophysiology. With this book, I have attempted to fill this gap: text and illustrations are combined to provide a coherent and easy-to-assimilate description and explanation of different eye movement disorders.

The text is divided into four parts. The first part consists of chapters for each of the eye movement subsystems. Readers will find a description of thematic "concepts" on the left-hand pages, with accompanying figures, a synopsis of the pertinent points, and important clinical points (green boxes) on the right-hand pages. My aim is to present the material that appears on the left-hand pages as succinct, accessible information for easy review on the right-hand pages.

Parts II through IV describe different eye movement disorders in detail. Bulleted and numbered lists have been used to reduce the overall volume of the text without compromising the clarity of the information. Each chapter contains color-coded sections to allow ready review. The clinical features of different disorders are summarized in yellow boxes, etiology in green boxes, and differential diagnosis in orange boxes. Main eye movement abnormalities characteristic of different diseases are summarized in blue boxes, and the anatomic and physiological basis for the observed abnormal eye movements are explained separately, as footnotes. Throughout the text, readers will also find this icon ▸▸, which indicates that a video clip of the corresponding eye movement disorder is available in the book's accompanying CD-ROM. In addition, the book is amply illustrated with schematic diagrams of relevant anatomy and brain pathways. Tables have also been used liberally to provide a readily accessible overview of information.

The book is comprehensive, though not exhaustive; I have aimed at a clear and understandable presentation of what I think are the most important aspects of eye movement disorders. I encourage readers to consult other excellent texts and the references provided for more detail on particular subjects of interest, particularly Leigh and Zee, *The Neurology of Eye Movements*, Fourth Edition, and Miller et al., *Walsh and Hoyt's Clinical Neuro-Ophthalmology*, Sixth Edition. Readers who would like to view additional videos of different eye movement disorders can visit a number of web pages that are accessible to the public, such as the resourceful NOVEL website of the North American Neuro-Ophthalmology Society (http://library.med.utah.edu/NOVEL/), and the eTextbook of Eye Movements on the Canadian

Neuro-Ophthalmology Group website (www.neuroophthalmology.ca/textbook/ NOeyemovt.html).

It is my hope that this book will serve as a resource for residents, fellows, and clinicians in different specialties: ophthalmology, neurology, neuro-ophthalmology, and neurosurgery. Neuro-otologists, orthoptists, medical students, as well as undergraduate and graduate students in behavioral neurosciences, should also find useful information here.

Acknowledgments

A number of individuals provided encouragement throughout this project and reviewed the manuscript critically. I would particularly like to thank Martin ten Hove, Barry Skarf, Lawrence Tychsen, Nancy Newman, Martin Steinbach, Carol Westall, Raymond Buncic, James Sharpe, Susan Culican, Daniel Weisbrod, Megumi Iizuka, Michael Richards, Peter Karagiannis, and Alan Blakeman. I would also like to express my gratitude to John Leigh and David Zee for writing an outstanding reference book on the neurology of eye movements; some information and many tables, particularly in Part III, included in this textbook are modified from their book, *The Neurology of Eye Movements*, Third Edition.

I am grateful to the past and present ophthalmology and neurology residents at the University of Toronto and Washington University in St. Louis for their feedback on my lectures notes, on which this book is based. I am also thankful to the PGY1 ophthalmology residents from across Canada who attended the Toronto Ophthalmology Residency Introductory Course for their support and suggestions. I am indebted to Mano Chandrakumar, who spent many hours helping me prepare the figures and the manuscript and who provided excellent technical support. Finally, I would like to thank the Canadian Institutes for Health Research, the E.A. Baker Foundation of the Canadian National Institute for the Blind, the Ontario Ministry of Research and Innovation, the Ophthalmology Practice Plan of the Toronto Western Hospital, the Department of Ophthalmology and Vision Sciences at the University of Toronto, and the Hospital for Sick Children in Toronto for their continued support of my work.

Contents

Abbreviations

AC	Anterior canal		FEF	Frontal eye field
A_g	Gravitational acceleration vector		FEFsac	Saccade subregion of the frontal eye field
A_i	Inertial (or linear translational) acceleration vector		FEFsem	Pursuit subregion of the frontal eye field
ANA	Antinuclear antibody		FL/VPF	Flocculus and ventral paraflocculus
ATD	Ascending tract of Deiters		FOR	Fastigial oculomotor region
BC	Brachium conjunctivum		FTN	Flocculus target neurons
BPPV	Benign paroxysmal positioning vertigo		GEN	Gaze-evoked nystagmus
CCN	Central caudal nucleus		GIA	Gravitoinertial acceleration vector
CFEOM1	Congenital fibrosis of the extraocular muscles type 1		GPi	Globus pallidus internal segment
CFEOM2	Congenital fibrosis of the extraocular muscles type 2		HAART	Highly active antiretroviral therapy
CFEOM3	Congenital fibrosis of the extraocular muscles type 3		HC	Horizontal canal
CHAMPS	Controlled High Risk Avonex Multiple Sclerosis Trial		HGPPS	Horizontal gaze palsy and progressive scoliosis
CJD	Creutzfeldt-Jakob Disease		HT	Hypertropia
CMAPs	Compound muscle action potentials		IBN	Inhibitory burst neurons
cMRF	Central mesencephalic reticular formation		IML	Internal medullary lamina
CNS	Central nervous system		INC	Interstitial nucleus of Cajal
CPEO	Chronic progressive external ophthalmoplegia		INO	Internuclear ophthalmoplegia
CSF	Cerebrospinal fluid		IO	Inferior oblique
DLPC	Dorsolateral prefrontal cortex		IR	Inferior rectus
DLPN	Dorsolateral pontine nuclei		IVIG	Intravenous immunoglobulin
DVD	Dissociated vertical deviation		LGN	Lateral geniculate nucleus
EA-2	Episodic ataxia type 2		LIP	Lateral interparietal area
EBN	Excitatory burst neurons		LP	Lumbar puncture
EEG	Electroencephalography		LR	Lateral rectus
EKG	Electrocardiogram		LS	Lateral suprasylvian area
EMG	Electromyography		MBP	Myelin basic protein
ERG	Electroretinogram		mepps	Miniature endplate potentials
ESR	Erythrocyte sedimentation rate		Med RF	Medullary reticular formation
EWN	Edinger-Westphal nucleus		MIF	Multiply innervated fibers
			MLF	Medial longitudinal fasciculus
			MOG	Myelin oligodendrocyte glycoprotein
			MR	Medial rectus

MRF	Mesencephalic reticular formation		PIVC	Parieto-insular-vestibular cortex
MSA-C	Multiple system atrophy dominated by cerebellar ataxia		PLP	Proteolipid protein
			PMT	Cell groups of the paramedian tracts
MSA-P	Multiple system atrophy dominated by parkinsonism		PPRF	Paramedian pontine reticular formation
MST	Medial superior temporal visual area		PrP^c	Cellular proteinaceous infectious particle
MT	Middle temporal visual area		PrP^{Sc}	Scrapie proteinaceous infectious particle
MuSK	Muscle specific kinase			
MVH-NPH	Medial vestibular nucleus - nucleus prepositus hypoglossi		PSP	Progressive supranuclear palsy
			PVN	Post-rotatory vestibular nystagmus
MVN	Medial vestibular nucleus		RAPD	Relative afferent pupillary defect
NMDA	N-methyl-D-aspartate		riMLF	Rostral interstitial nucleus of the medial longitudinal fasciculus
NOT	Nucleus of the optic tract			
NPC	Near point of convergence		rip	Nucleus raphe interpositus
nPC	Nucleus of the posterior commissure		SC	Superior colliculus
			SCA2	Spinocerebellar ataxia type 2
NPH	Nucleus prepositus hypoglossi		SCA6	Spinocerebellar ataxia type 6
NPH-MVN	Nucleus prepositus hypoglossi and medial vestibular nucleus complex		SEF	Supplementary eye field
			SIF	Singly innervated fibers
NRPC	Nucleus reticularis pontis caudalis		SNpc	Substantia nigra pars compacta
NRTP	Nucleus reticularis tegmenti pontis		SNpr	Substantia nigra pars reticulata
OFR	Ocular following response		SO	Superior oblique
OKAN	Optokinetic after-nystagmus		SR	Superior rectus
OKN	Optokinetic nystagmus		SVN	Superior vestibular nucleus
ONTT	Optic Neuritis Treatment Trial		SWJ	Square wave jerks
OPCA	Olivopontocerebellar atrophy		TMP-SMX	Trimethoprim-sulfamethoxazole
OTR	Ocular tilt reaction		V_1	Ophthalmic division of the trigeminal nerve
PC	Posterior canal			
PoC	Posterior commissure		V_2	Maxillary division of the trigeminal nerve
PCR	Polymerase chain reaction			
PD	Prism diopters		VN	Vestibular nystagmus
PEF	Parietal eye field		VOR	Vestibulo-ocular reflex
PGD	Nucleus paragigantocellularis dorsalis		VPF	Ventral paraflocculus
PhyH	Phytanoyl-CoA hydroxyl-ase			

Eye Movement Disorders

Part I   *The Six Eye Movement Systems*

Chapter 1 — *Eye Rotations, the Extraocular Muscles, and Strabismus Terminology*

To understand how eye muscles move the eyeball, it is necessary to understand the geometry of the eye and the functions of the muscles. The eyeball rotates about three axes: horizontal, vertical, and torsional. These axes intersect at the center of the eyeball. Eye rotations are achieved by coordinated contraction and relaxation of six extraocular muscles—four rectus and two oblique—attached to each eye. The action of the muscles on the globe is determined by the point of rotation of the globe, as well as the origin and insertion of each muscle. Recent evidence suggests that the muscles also exert their effects on the globe via the extraocular muscle pulleys.

Considering that we make at least 100,000 saccades alone each day, it is not surprising that many extraocular muscles are very resistant to fatigue. Extraocular muscles are also different from other skeletal muscles in many respects. For example, eye muscle fibers are richly innervated, and each motoneuron innervates only 10–20 muscle fibers, the smallest motor unit known in the body. Extraocular muscles also have more mitochondria and a higher metabolic rate than other skeletal muscles. Thus, extraocular muscles are one of the fastest contracting muscles. This property allows animals to shift gaze swiftly, so that they can avoid approaching predators or detect prey in the vicinity. The unique immunologic and physiologic properties of extraocular muscles may also explain why they are more susceptible to certain disease processes, such as Grave's disease and chronic progressive external ophthalmoplegia, but more resistant to others such as Duchenne's dystrophy, which mainly affects skeletal muscles in the rest of the body.

1.1 Three Axes of Eye Rotations

The eyeball rotates about three axes: x-axis (naso-occipital or roll axis), y-axis (earth-horizontal or pitch axis), and z-axis (earth-vertical or yaw axis).

Ductions refer to monocular movements of each eye. They include abduction, adduction, elevation (sursumduction), depression (deorsumduction), incycloduction or incyclotorsion, and excycloduction or excyclotorsion (see table on opposite page).

Versions refer to binocular conjugate movements of both eyes, such that the visual axes of the eyes move in the same direction. They include dextroversion, levoversion, elevation (sursumversion), depression (deorsumversion), dextrocycloversion, and levocycloversion (see table).

Vergences refer to binocular disjunctive movements, such that the visual axes of the eyes move in opposite directions. They include convergence, divergence, incyclovergence, and excyclovergence (see table).

Eye rotations are achieved by coordinated contraction of six extraocular muscles in each eye: the medial rectus, lateral rectus, superior rectus, inferior rectus, superior oblique, and inferior oblique. The action of the muscles on the globe is determined by the point of rotation of the globe, as well as by the origin and insertion of each muscle. The tendons of the rectus muscles pass through sleevelike pulleys located several millimeters posterior to the equator of the globe and approximately 10 mm posterior to the insertion sites of the muscles. These pulleys, consisting of fibrous tissue and smooth muscle, limit side-slip movement of the rectus muscles during eye rotations and act as the functional origins of the rectus muscles.

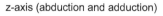

z-axis (abduction and adduction)

y-axis (elevation and depression)

x-axis (incyclotorsion and excyclotorsion)

Term	Definition
Ductions	Ductions refer to **monocular** movements of each eye • **Abduction** occurs about the z-axis and is away from the median plane • **Adduction** occurs about the z-axis and is toward the median plane • **Elevation** occurs about the y-axis and is an upward rotation of the eye • **Depression** occurs about the y-axis and is a downward rotation of the eye • **Incycloduction** (incyclotorsion) occurs about the x-axis so that the upper pole of the eye rotates toward the median plane • **Excycloduction** (excyclotorsion) occurs about the x-axis so that the upper pole of the eye rotates away from the median plane
Versions	Versions refer to binocular **conjugate** movements of both eyes, such that the visual axes of the eyes move in the same direction • **Dextroversion**: both eyes rotating about their z-axes to the right • **Levoversion**: both eyes rotating about their z-axes to the left • **Elevation**: both eyes rotating about their y-axes to look upward • **Depression**: both eyes rotating about their y-axes to look downward • **Dextrocycloversion**: both eyes rotating about their x-axes so that the upper pole of both eyes rotates to the subject's right • **Levocycloversion**: both eyes rotating about their x-axes so that the upper pole of both eyes rotates to the subject's left
Vergences	Vergences refer to binocular **disjunctive** movements, such that the visual axes of the eyes move in opposite directions • **Convergence**: both eyes rotating about their z-axes toward the median plane • **Divergence**: both eyes rotating about their z-axes away from the median plane • **Incyclovergence**: rotation of both eyes about their x-axes so that the upper pole of both eyes rotates toward the median plane • **Excyclovergence**: rotation of both eyes about their x-axes so that the upper pole of both eyes rotates away from the median plane

The primary position of the eye is defined clinically as the position in which the eye is directed straight ahead with the body and head erect. The primary action of a muscle is its major rotational effect on the eye while the eye is in primary position. The secondary and tertiary actions of a muscle are additional rotational effects on the eye while it is in primary position.

The four rectus muscles arise from the annulus of Zinn at the apex of the orbit. The **medial rectus** inserts onto the medial side of the globe at approximately 5.3 ($\pm$0.7) mm from the corneoscleral limbus, whereas the **lateral rectus** inserts onto the lateral side of the globe at approximately 6.9 ($\pm$0.7) mm from the limbus. Because the origins and insertions of the horizontal rectus muscles are symmetric and lie in the horizontal meridian of the globe, their functions are relatively simple and are antagonistic; contraction of the medial rectus adducts the globe, whereas contraction of the lateral rectus abducts the globe.

The superior and inferior recti also originate from the annulus of Zinn. The **superior rectus** inserts onto the globe superiorly at approximately 7.9 ($\pm$0.6) mm from the limbus, and the **inferior rectus** inserts inferiorly at approximately 6.8 ($\pm$0.8) mm from the limbus. In addition, their insertions onto the globe subtend a 23° angle with the visual axis when the eye is in primary position, straddling the vertical meridian of the globe. Thus, in addition to its primary action of elevation, the superior rectus has a secondary action of incyclotorsion and a tertiary action of adduction. The primary action of the inferior rectus is depression, its secondary action is excyclotorsion, and its tertiary action is adduction. The relative importance of the primary and secondary actions depends on the direction of the visual axis. When the eye is abducted 23°, the superior rectus acts solely as an elevator, and the inferior rectus acts solely as a depressor. When the eye is adducted 67°, the superior rectus acts solely to incyclotort the globe, and the inferior rectus acts solely to excyclotort the globe.

The **superior oblique** also arises from the annulus of Zinn; however, its functional origin is the trochlea in the superomedial orbit. The superior oblique is tendinous after it passes through the trochlea. This tendon then assumes a posterolateral direction and inserts onto the superior posterotemporal quadrant of the globe behind the center of rotation. This vector plane subtends a 54° angle with the visual axis when the eye is in primary position. Thus, in addition to its primary action of incyclotorsion, the superior oblique also has a secondary action of depression and tertiary action of abduction. When the eye is adducted 54°, the superior oblique acts solely to depress the globe, and when the eye is abducted 36°, it acts solely to incyclotort the globe.

The **inferior oblique** arises from the anterior medial orbital floor, and thus it is the only extraocular muscle that does not arise from the annulus of Zinn. It inserts onto the inferior posterotemporal quadrant of the globe behind the center of rotation and subtends a 51° angle with the visual axis when the eye is in primary position. Thus, in addition to its primary action of excyclotorsion, the inferior oblique has a secondary action of elevation and a tertiary action of abduction. When the eye is adducted 51°, the inferior oblique acts solely to elevate the globe, and when the eye is abducted 39°, it acts solely to excyclotort the globe.

	Eye in primary position	Eye abducted	Eye adducted
Superior rectus (Top view)	Combined elevation & incyclotorsion when the eye is in primary position	Elevation when the eye is in 23° abducted position	Incyclotorsion when the eye is in 67° adducted position
Inferior rectus (Bottom view)	Combined depression & excyclotorsion when the eye is in primary position	Depression when the eye is in 23° abducted position	Excyclotorsion when the eye is in 67° adducted position
Superior oblique (Top view)	Combined incyclotorsion and depression when the eye is in primary position	Incyclotorsion when the eye is in 36° abducted position	Depression when the eye is in 54° adducted position
Inferior oblique (Bottom view)	Combined excyclotorsion and elevation when the eye is in primary position	Excyclotorsion when the eye is in 39° abducted position	Elevation when the eye is in 51° adducted position

Extraocular Muscles	Primary Action	Secondary Action	Tertiary Action
Lateral rectus	Abduction	None	None
Medial rectus	Adduction	None	None
Superior rectus	Elevation	Incyclotorsion	Adduction
Inferior rectus	Depression	Excyclotorsion	Adduction
Superior Oblique	Incyclotorsion	Depression	Abduction
Inferior oblique	Excyclotorsion	Elevation	Abduction

Agonist muscle moves the eye toward the desired direction, whereas antagonist muscle moves the eye away from the desired direction. **Sherrington's law of reciprocal innervation** states that, whenever an agonist muscle (e.g., the medial rectus of the right eye during adduction) receives an excitatory signal to contract, an equivalent inhibitory signal is sent to the antagonist muscle (e.g., the right lateral rectus) of the same eye. This reciprocal innervation is mainly due to central connections in the brainstem.

A yoked muscle pair consists of one muscle from each eye and moves both eyes toward the same direction. For example, the right lateral rectus and the left medial rectus contract simultaneously when looking to the right. **Hering's law of equal innervation** (or law of motor correspondence) states that, during conjugate eye movements, the yoked muscle pair receives equal innervation so that the eyes move together. Vertically acting muscles are also conceptualized as being arranged as yoked pairs (e.g., the right superior rectus and left inferior oblique form a pair, and the right inferior rectus and the left superior oblique form another pair). However, the way in which extraocular muscles interact is very complex, and all muscles probably contribute, even during a simple horizontal movement.

During clinical examination, the **primary position** refers to the position when the eyes look straight ahead. Secondary positions are right gaze, left gaze, straight up, and straight down. Tertiary positions are up and right, down and right, up and left, and down and left.

The **six cardinal positions** include right gaze, left gaze, and the four tertiary positions. These eye positions provide the most information about the horizontal function of the horizontal rectus muscles (lateral and medial rectus) and the vertical function of the cyclovertical muscles (superior rectus, inferior rectus, superior oblique, and inferior oblique). For example, on right and up gaze, the prime elevators are the superior rectus in the right eye and the inferior oblique in the left eye. In this gaze position, the right superior rectus is the prime elevator when the right eye is abducted (by the action of the lateral rectus) because it inserts at a 23° angle to the visual axis. Similarly, the left inferior oblique is the prime elevator when the left eye is adducted (by the action of the medial rectus) because it inserts at a 51° angle to the visual axis.

It is important to emphasize that the cardinal positions of gaze do not correspond to the primary, secondary, or tertiary actions of the muscles. For example, when the right eye looks right and up, the right superior rectus is not responsible for *both* elevation *and* abduction; in fact, the tertiary action of the superior rectus is adduction, not abduction. In other words, when the right eye looks right and up, elevation comes mainly from contraction of the superior rectus, whereas abduction comes mainly from contraction of the lateral rectus.

Sherrington's law of reciprocal innervation

Whenever an agonist muscle (e.g., the medial rectus of the right eye during adduction) receives an excitatory signal to contract, an equivalent inhibitory signal is sent to the antagonist muscle (e.g., the right lateral rectus) of the same eye.

Hering's law of equal innervation

During conjugate eye movements, the yoked muscle pair receives equal innervation so that the eyes move together.

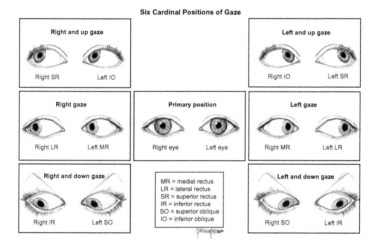

Six Cardinal Positions of Gaze

Clinical Points

The six cardinal positions of gaze are the eye positions that provide the most information about:

- The horizontal function of the horizontal muscles (lateral and medial rectus)
- The vertical function of the cyclovertical muscles (superior rectus, inferior rectus, superior oblique, and inferior oblique).

For example, on right and upgaze:

- The right superior rectus (SR) is most responsible for elevation when the right eye is *abducted* because the SR inserts at a 23° angle to the visual axis when the eye is in primary position. Note that the tertiary action of the superior rectus is *adduction*, not abduction. Thus, the cardinal position does not correspond to the action of the muscle; rather, it corresponds to the position of the eye that gives the most information about the vertical function of the cyclovertical muscle.
- The left inferior oblique (IO) is most responsible for elevation when the left eye is *adducted* because the IO inserts at a 51° angle to the visual axis when the eye is in primary position. Note that the tertiary action of the inferior oblique is *abduction*, not adduction.

The rectus and oblique muscles consist of two distinct layers: an outer **orbital layer** adjacent to the periorbita and orbital bone, and an inner **global layer** adjacent to the eye and the optic nerve. Whereas the global layer extends the full muscle length, inserting via a well-defined tendon, the orbital layer ends before the muscle becomes tendinous. Each layer contains fibers more suited for sustained contraction or for brief, rapid contraction. Six types of fibers have been identified in the extraocular muscles.

In the orbital layer, about 80% of the fibers are **singly innervated fibers** (SIF). Not only do these fibers exhibit the fast type of myofibrillar ATPase and high oxidative activity, but they also appear to be capable of anaerobic activity. They have twitch capacity and are the most fatigue-resistant fibers. They are the only fiber type that shows long-term effects after injection of botulinum toxin. The remaining 20% of orbital fibers are **multiply innervated fibers** (MIF). They have twitch capacity near the center of the fiber and non-twitch activity proximal and distal to the endplate band.

In the global layer, about 33% of fibers are **red SIFs**, which are fast twitch and highly fatigue resistant. Another 32% are **white (pale) SIFs** with fast-twitch properties but low fatigue resistance. **Intermediate SIFs** constitute about another 25% of fibers. They have fast-twitch properties and an intermediate level of fatigue resistance. The remaining 10% are **MIFs**, with synaptic endplate along their entire length, as well as at the myotendinous junction, where there are palisade organ proprioceptors. These fibers show tonic properties, with slow, graded, nonpropagated responses to neural or pharmacological activation.

The **levator palpebrae** muscle contains the three singly innervated muscle types found in the global layer of the extraocular muscles and a true slow-twitch fiber type. The MIF type and the fatigue-resistant SIF type seen in the orbital layer of the extraocular muscles are absent in the levator.

The functional arrangement of muscle fiber types is related to the threshold at which motor units are recruited. During saccades and quick phases of nystagmus, all fiber types are recruited synchronously. In contrast, during slow eye movements and fixation (gaze holding), there is a differential recruitment of fiber types that is dependent on eye position. Orbital SIFs and global red SIFs are recruited first, when eye position is still in the direction opposite to the muscle action. Multiply innervated fiber types are recruited next, probably near straight-ahead position, where their fine increments of force would be of value for fixation. The increasingly faster but fatigable fibers are recruited last, at eye position well into the direction of muscle action.

The **palisade tendon organs** are the primary proprioceptors in human extraocular muscles. They are found in the distal myotendinous junctions of global MIFs. Afferents from these proprioceptors project, via the ophthalmic branch of the trigeminal nerve and the Gasserian ganglion, to the spinal trigeminal nucleus. They may also project centrally via the ocular motor nerves. From the trigeminal nucleus, proprioceptive information is sent to structures involved in ocular motor control, including the superior colliculus, vestibular nuclei, nucleus prepositus hypoglossi, cerebellum, and frontal eye fields. Proprioceptive information is also sent to structures involved in visual processing, including the lateral geniculate body, pulvinar, and visual cortex.

	Orbital layer		Global layer			
	Orbital SIF	Orbital MIF	Global Red SIF	Global White SIF	Global Intermediate SIF	Global MIF
% of layer	80	20	33	32	25	10
Contraction mode	Twitch	Mixed	Twitch	Twitch	Twitch	Non-twitch
Contraction speed	Fast	Fast/slow	Fast	Fast	Fast	Slow
Fatigue resistance	High	Variable	High	Low	Intermediate	High
Recruitment order *Slow eye movements and fixation*	1st	3rd	2nd	6th	5th	4th
Saccades and quick phases of nystagmus	All fiber types recruited simultaneously					

SIF, singly innervated fibers; MIF, multiply innervated fibers. (Modified from Porter et al. Extraocular muscles: Basic and clinical aspects of structure and function. Surv Ophthelmol. 1995; 39: 451–84.)

The **palisade tendon organs**

- Primary proprioceptors in human extraocular muscles
- Found in the distal myotendinous junctions of global multiply innervated fibers
- Project to the spinal trigeminal nucleus via the ophthalmic branch of the trigeminal nerve and the Gasserian ganglion, or via the ocular motor nerves
- From the spinal trigeminal nucleus, proprioceptive information is sent to

  1. Structures involved in ocular motor control (e.g., superior colliculus, vestibular nuclei, nucleus prepositus hypoglossi, cerebellum, frontal eye fields)
  2. Structures involved in visual processing (e.g., lateral geniculate body, pulvinar, visual cortex).

1.5 Strabismus Terminology

The line connecting the object of fixation to the fovea is the **visual axis**. **Strabismus** is defined as a misalignment of the visual axes between the two eyes.

Orthophoria is the ideal condition of eye alignment. In reality, it is seldom encountered because the majority of people have a latent misalignment. By definition, orthophoria indicates that the oculomotor apparatus is in perfect equilibrium so that both eyes remain aligned in all positions of gaze and at all distances of fixation during viewing with one eye (monocular viewing). **Orthotropia** refers to perfect alignment of the eyes during viewing with both eyes (binocular viewing).

Heterodeviation refers to ocular alignment that differs from orthophoria. It includes both **heterophoria** and **heterotropia**. Heterophoria is a latent deviation controlled by binocular fixation, such that, during viewing with both eyes, the eyes remain aligned. In contrast, heterotropia is a deviation present during viewing with both eyes (i.e., manifest deviation).

There are a variety of heterophoric and heterotropic deviations. If the visual axes converge, the condition is called **esophoria** (for latent deviation) or **esotropia** (for manifest deviation). If the visual axes diverge, the condition is known as **exophoria** or **exotropia**. **Uncrossed diplopia** is double vision caused by esotropia. The false image is displaced on the same side as the deviated eye. **Crossed diplopia** is double vision caused by exotropia. The false image is displaced to the side opposite the deviated eye.

Hyperphoria (for latent deviation) or **hypertropia** (for manifest deviation) occurs if the visual axis of the nonfixating eye is higher than that of the fixating eye. For example, a right hyperphoria or hypertropia is a deviation in which the visual axis of the nonfixating right eye is higher than that of the left. **Cyclodeviation** is a torsional misalignment of the eyes, causing a cyclodisparity. **Incyclodeviation** refers to a relative incyclotorsion of the eyes (decreased separation of upper poles of eyes), whereas **excyclodeviation** refers to a relative excyclotorsion of the eyes (increased separation of upper poles of eyes).

Strabismus may be comitant or incomitant. In **concomitant** or comitant strabismus, the magnitude of deviation is the same in all directions of gaze and does not depend on the eye used for fixation. In **incomitant** or noncomitant strabismus, the deviation varies in different directions of gaze. Most incomitant strabismus is caused by a paralytic or a mechanical restrictive process. The deviation is largest when the eyes turn in the direction of the paralytic or underacting muscle. The deviation in incomitant strabismus also varies with the eye used for fixation. When the normal eye is fixating, the amount of misalignment is called **primary deviation**. When the paretic eye is fixating, the amount of misalignment is called **secondary deviation**. Secondary deviation is larger than primary deviation in incomitant strabismus because an increase in innervation is needed for a paretic eye to fixate a target. By Hering's law, the contralateral yoked muscle also receives more innervation, resulting in a larger deviation.

Weakness of a muscle can be classified as a paralysis or paresis. If the action of a muscle is completely abolished, the condition is a paralysis or palsy; if the action of a muscle is weakened but not abolished, it is called a paresis. The terms palsy and paresis are often used interchangeably in clinical settings and in neurologic practice. In this book, the term palsy is used to denote a partial or a complete impairment of muscle action.

Term	Definition
Visual axis	The line connecting the object of fixation to the fovea
Strabismus	A misalignment or deviation of the visual axes
Orthophoria	Alignment of the visual axes while viewing with one eye
Orthotropia	Alignment of the visual axes while viewing with both eyes
Heterophoria	A latent misalignment of the visual axes while viewing with one eye
Heterotropia	A manifest misalignment of the visual axes while viewing with both eyes
Esophoria/esotropia	Convergence of visual axes (i.e., crossed eyes) during viewing with one eye (esophoria) or during viewing with both eyes (esotropia)
Exophoria/exotropia	Divergence of visual axes (i.e., walled eyes) during viewing with one eye (exophoria) or during viewing with both eyes (exotropia)
Hyperphoria/hypertropia	Vertical misalignment of the visual axes with the nonfixating eye higher than the fixating eye during viewing with one eye (hyperphoria) or during viewing with both eyes (hypertropia)
Hypophoria/hypotropia	Vertical misalignment of the visual axes with the nonfixating eye lower than the fixating eye during viewing with one eye (hypophoria) or during viewing with both eyes (hypotropia)
Cyclodeviation	Torsional misalignment of the eyes, causing a cyclodisparity
Incyclodeviation	Relative incyclotorsion of the eyes (decreased separation of upper poles of eyes)
Excyclodeviation	Relative excyclotorsion of the eyes (increased separation of upper poles of eyes)
Uncrossed diplopia	Double vision caused by esotropia; the false image is displaced on the same side as the deviated eye
Crossed diplopia	Double vision caused by exotropia; the false image is displaced to the side opposite to the deviated eye
Concomitant deviation	Misalignment of the visual axes that does not change with gaze direction during fixation with either eye
Incomitant deviation	Misalignment of the visual axes that changes with gaze direction and depends on which eye is fixating; causes include mechanical restriction or muscle palsy
Primary deviation	The deviation of the paretic eye while the normal eye is fixating
Secondary deviation	The deviation of the normal eye while the paretic eye is fixating; secondary deviation is larger than primary deviation in incomitant strabismus

Chapter 2

Introduction to the Six Eye Movement Systems and the Visual Fixation System

One main reason that we make eye movements is to solve a problem of information overload. A large field of vision allows an animal to survey the environment for food and to avoid predators, thus increasing its survival rate. Similarly, a high visual acuity also increases survival rates by allowing an animal to aim at a target more accurately, leading to higher killing rates and more food. However, there are simply not enough neurons in the brain to support a visual system that has high resolution over the entire field of vision. Faced with the competing evolutionary demands for high visual acuity and a large field of vision, an effective strategy is needed so that the brain will not be overwhelmed by a large amount of visual input. Some animals, such as rabbits, give up high resolution in favor of a larger field of vision (rabbits can see nearly 360°), whereas others, such as hawks, restrict their field of vision in return for a high visual acuity (hawks have vision as good as 20/2, about 10 times better than humans). In humans, rather than using one strategy over the other, the retina develops a very high spatial resolution in the center (i.e., the fovea), and a much lower resolution in the periphery. Although this "foveal compromise" strategy solves the problem of information overload, one result is that unless the image of an object of interest happens to fall on the fovea, the image is relegated to the low-resolution retinal periphery.

The evolution of a mechanism to move the eyes is therefore necessary to complement this foveal compromise strategy by ensuring that an object of interest is maintained or brought to the fovea. To maintain the image of an object on the fovea, the vestibulo-ocular (VOR) and optokinetic systems generate eye movements to compensate for head motions. Likewise, the saccadic, smooth pursuit, and vergence systems generate eye movements to bring the image of an object of interest on the fovea. These different eye movements have different characteristics and involve different parts of the brain. In this chapter, the fixation system is discussed; the VOR and optokinetic systems, saccades, smooth pursuit, and vergence systems are discussed in subsequent chapters.

2.1 Introduction to the Six Eye Movement Systems

The six eye movement systems can be functionally divided into those that hold images of a target steady on the retina and those that direct the fovea onto an object of interest. The former category includes (1) the **fixation** system, which holds the image of a stationary object on the fovea when the head is immobile; (2) the **vestibular** system (or the vestibulo-ocular reflex), which holds the image of a target steady on the retina during brief head movements; and (3) the **optokinetic** system, which holds the image of a target steady on the retina during sustained head movements.

The latter category, systems that direct the fovea onto an object of interest, includes (1) the **saccadic** system, which brings the image of an object of interest rapidly onto the fovea; (2) the **smooth pursuit** system, which holds the image of a small, moving target on the fovea; and (3) the **vergence** system, which moves the eyes in an opposite direction (i.e., convergence or divergence) so that images of a single object are held simultaneously on both foveae.

Clinically, to localize a lesion, it is important to assess whether one or more eye movement systems are affected. For example, a discrete lesion in the paramedian pontine reticular formation affects ipsilesional horizontal saccades only, whereas a lesion in the abducens nucleus affects all ipsilesional horizontal eye movements, including saccades, smooth pursuit, and the VOR (see sections 9.3.1 and 9.3.2).

Hold images steady on the retina

Fixation: holds the image of a stationary object on the fovea when the head is immobile

Vestibular (VOR): holds image steady on the retina during brief head movements

Optokinetic: holds image steady on the retina during sustained head movements

Direct the fovea to an object of interest

Saccades: bring the image of an object of interest rapidly onto the fovea

Smooth pursuit: holds the image of a small moving target on the fovea

Vergence: moves the eyes in an opposite direction (i.e., convergence or divergence) so that images of a single object are held simultaneously on both foveae

---

Clinical Point

To localize a lesion, it is important to assess whether one or more eye movement systems are affected. For example, a discrete lesion in the paramedian pontine reticular formation affects ipsilesional horizontal saccades only, whereas a lesion in the abducens nucleus affects all ipsilesional horizontal eye movements, including saccades, smooth pursuit, and VOR (see sections 9.3.1 and 9.3.2).

2.2 The Visual Fixation System

The fixation system holds the image of a stationary object on the fovea when the head is immobile. Steady fixation is actually an illusion. Normal fixation consists of three distinct types of physiological miniature movements that are not detectable by the naked eye: microsaccades, microdrift, and microtremor.

Microsaccades are miniature saccades that have an amplitude of less than 26 min of arc, with an average amplitude of 6 min of arc. They occur at a mean frequency of approximately 120 Hz. Microsaccades have no known function and are considered superfluous to visual perception.

Microdrift consists of smooth eye movements that occur at a velocity of less than 20 min of arc per second. They are necessary to prevent the image of a stable object from fading.

Microtremor is continuous, high-frequency ocular motor activity that underlies both microdrift and microsaccades. Microtremor occurs at a frequency of 50–100 Hz. Its average amplitude is <1 min of arc (usually 5–30 sec of arc) and is much smaller than the amplitude of microsaccades.

Visual fixation is an active process, not merely an absence of visible eye movements. Several cerebral areas participate in visual fixation. They include the parietal eye field (lateral interparietal area [LIP] and area 7a in monkeys), V5 and V5A (middle temporal [MT] and medial superior temporal [MST] areas in monkeys), supplementary eye field, and dorsolateral prefrontal cortex. Brainstem structures, including substantia nigra pars reticulata in the basal ganglia and the rostral pole of the superior colliculus, are also involved in fixation.

Involuntary disruption of normal fixation may cause **oscillopsia**, an illusion of movement of the stationary environment. Oscillopsia can be caused by ocular oscillations, which include (1) nystagmus, *sustained* oscillation initiated by *slow* eye movements; (2) saccadic intrusion, *intermittent* oscillation initiated by *fast* eye movements; and (3) saccadic oscillation, *sustained* oscillation initiated by *fast* eye movements. Oscillopsia can also occur in patients with peripheral or central vestibular dysfunction, as well as in patients with central lesion, such as seizure or occipital lobe infarct. Nystagmus and saccadic dyskinesia are discussed further in part II.

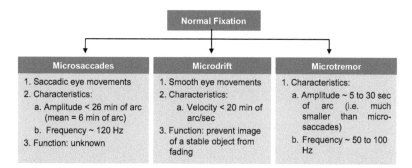

Microsaccades	Microdrift	Microtremor

1. Saccadic eye movements
2. Characteristics:
  a. Amplitude < 26 min of arc (mean = 6 min of arc)
  b. Frequency ~ 120 Hz
3. Function: unknown
	1. Smooth eye movements
	2. Characteristics:
	  a. Velocity < 20 min of arc/sec
	3. Function: prevent image of a stable object from fading
		1. Characteristics:
		  a. Amplitude ~ 5 to 30 sec of arc (i.e. much smaller than micro-saccades)
		  b. Frequency ~ 50 to 100 Hz

Fixation is an active process, not merely an absence of visible eye movements. The *cerebral structures* involved in fixation are:

- Parietal eye field (lateral interparietal area and area 7a in monkeys)
- V5 and V5A (MT and MST in monkeys)
- Supplementary eye field
- Dorsolateral prefrontal cortex

The *brainstem structures* involved in fixation are:

- Substantia nigra pars reticulata in the basal ganglia
- Rostral pole of the superior colliculus

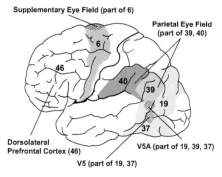

Supplementary Eye Field (part of 6)
Parietal Eye Field (part of 39, 40)
Dorsolateral Prefrontal Cortex (46)
V5A (part of 19, 39, 37)
V5 (part of 19, 37)

* Numbered areas denote corresponding Brodmann areas

Clinical Points

Involuntary disruption of normal fixation may cause **oscillopsia**, an illusion of movement of the stationary environment. Oscillopsia can be caused by:

1. Nystagmus: *sustained* oscillation initiated by *slow* eye movements
2. Saccadic intrusions: *intermittent* oscillation initiated by *fast* eye movements
3. Saccadic oscillations: *sustained* oscillations initiated by *fast* eye movements
4. Peripheral or central vestibular dysfunction
5. Central lesions (e.g., seizure, occipital lobe infarct)

Chapter 3   *The Vestibular and Optokinetic Systems*

The vestibulo-ocular and optokinetic reflexes are the earliest eye movements to appear phylogenetically. The **vestibulo-ocular reflex (VOR)** stabilizes retinal images during head motion by counter-rotating the eyes at the same speed as the head but in the opposite direction. Information about head motion passes from the vestibular sensors in the inner ear to the VOR circuitry within the brainstem, which computes an appropriate eye velocity command. The eyes, confined in their bony orbits, normally do not change position, and their motion relative to the head is restricted to a change in orientation. However, the head can both change position and orientation relative to space. Thus, the function of the VOR is to generate eye orientation that best compensates for changes in position and orientation of the head. Because the drive for this reflex is vestibular rather than visual, it operates even in darkness.

To appreciate the benefits of having our eyes under vestibular and not just visual control, hold a page of text in front of you, and oscillate it back and forth horizontally at a rate of about two cycles per second. You will find that the text is blurred. However, if you hold the page still and instead oscillate your head at the same rate, you will be able to read the text clearly. This is because when the page moves, only visual information is available. Visual information normally takes about 100 msec to travel from the visual cortices, through a series of brain structures, to the ocular motoneurons that move the eyes. This delay is simply too long for the eyes to keep up with the oscillating page. However, when the head moves, both vestibular and visual information are available. Vestibular information takes only about 7–15 msec to travel from the vestibular sensors, through the brainstem, to the ocular motoneurons. With this short latency, the eyes can easily compensate for the rapid oscillation of the head. Thus, damages to the vestibular system often cause oscillopsia, an illusion of motion in the stationary environment, especially during head movements. Indeed, as described by a physician who lost his vestibular function from streptomycin ototoxicity; without a VOR, every movement, including his own carotid pulse, jarred his vision (*LIVING without a balancing mechanism, New England Journal of Medicine,* 1952).

Optokinetic eye movements stabilize the eyes during tracking of a large moving visual scene, which causes an illusionary sensation of self-rotation (circularvection) in the opposite direction. Optokinetic eye movements must be distinguished from smooth pursuit movements (discussed in chapter 5), which are used to keep the image of a small moving target on the fovea. If you sit inside a rotating drum painted on the inside with stripes or spots such that the entire visual field is perceived as rotating en bloc, your eyes will track the field rotation with a nystagmus pattern of slow phases in the direction of drum rotation and quick phases in the opposite direction. This response is called optokinetic nystagmus (OKN), and the neural system responsible for it is the optokinetic reflex (OKR). In nature, almost the only situation in which a large visual scene moves en bloc is when the animal itself is moving and its VOR is not compensating perfectly. Therefore, it is believed that the OKR serves as a visual backup for the VOR to generate compensatory eye movements. That the brain normally interprets en bloc motion of the visual field as evidence for self-motion is shown by the compelling motion illusions we experience while watching IMAX movies, or when the train beside the one you are on begins to move out of the station.

Clinically, damage to the vestibular sensors on one side, say, the left side, upsets the balance between vestibular signals generated from both sides. This leads to an illusory sensation of self-rotation (vertigo) to the right. In addition, because the brain mistakenly believes that the head is rotating to the right, it rotates the eyes slowly to the left to compensate. As the eyes reach their leftward orbital limits, they quickly snap back rightward toward the straight-ahead positions and then resume their leftward drift. This repetitive combination of slow phases that alternate with corrective quick phases is called **nystagmus**. Usually, the nystagmus and vertigo only last for a few days. This is because the abnormal vestibular sensation contradicts information from all other senses, including vision, sense of limb position, and sense of touch. Thus, with time, the brain makes an unconscious self-diagnosis by localizing the lesion to the left vestibular sensors and adapts by reestablishing the balance between the right and left inner ears. These adaptive and repair functions are performed by the cerebellum.

In this chapter, the characteristics of the VOR, as well as the anatomy, physiology, and functional organization of the vestibular sensors (the semicircular canals and the otoliths) are described. The role of the cerebellum in VOR adaptation and the concept of velocity storage, which explains disorders such as periodic alternating nystagmus, are discussed next. The optokinetic system, which serves as a visual backup for the VOR, is then discussed. Finally, some tests of vestibular functions that could be performed at bedside are described.

3.1 The Vestibulo-Ocular Reflex

The VOR stabilizes retinal images during brief head movements by counter-rotating the eyes at the same speed as the head but in the opposite direction. There are two types of head motion: **rotation** and **translation**. A change in orientation is called rotation, whereas a change in position is called translation.

Motion of the head is detected by the peripheral vestibular apparatus, or labyrinth, which is composed of two parts: (1) the three **semicircular canals** and (2) the **otolith** organs, which consist of the **utricle** and the **saccule.**

The three semicircular canals are oriented perpendicular to one another. This arrangement allows them to detect rotation (angular acceleration) of the head in three directions: horizontal (yaw, about the earth-vertical axis), vertical (pitch, about the earth-horizontal or interaural axis), and torsional (roll, about the naso-occipital axis). The otolith organs, in contrast, detect translation (linear acceleration) of the head in three directions: horizontal (heave, or side to side, along the interaural axis), vertical (bob, or up and down, along the dorsal–ventral axis) and fore and aft (surge, along the naso-occipital axis). The otolith organs also detect static head tilt (i.e., the position of the head with respect to gravity).

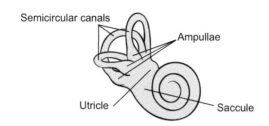

Semicircular canals — Ampullae

Utricle — Saccule

Rotation		
Yaw (horizontal rotation)	Pitch (vertical rotation)	Roll (torsional rotation)

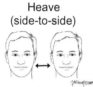
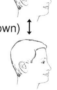
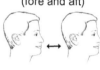

Translation

Heave (side-to-side)

Bob (up and down)

Surge (fore and aft)

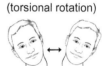

The Semicircular Canals	The Otolith Organs
Detect head rotation (rotational/ angular VOR) 1. Horizontal (yaw) 2. Vertical (pitch) 3. Torsional (roll)	Consist of the **utricle** and **saccule** Detect head translation (translational/linear VOR) 1. Side to side (heave) 2. Up and down (bob) 3. Fore and aft (surge) Detect static lateral head tilt (ocular counterroll)

Vestibulo-ocular reflex **gain** is defined as the ratio of the velocity of smooth eye movements in one direction to the velocity of head movements in the opposite direction. Vestibulo-ocular reflex gain varies with frequency of head motion, and it must approximate −1.0 to prevent retinal images from slipping. At frequencies that correspond to most natural head rotations (0.5–5 Hz), horizontal and vertical VOR gains approximate −0.9 in dark. In light, the gains are close to −1.0 due to visual enhancement, which is mediated by the optokinetic, smooth pursuit, or the fixation systems. If the gain is too much above or below its ideal value of unity, a target image remains off the fovea, although it may be transiently stable on the retina. The motion of the eyes and head must also be 180° out of phase. This normal **phase** difference is designated zero, by convention. If there is a phase lead of the eyes before the head or a phase lag behind it, the target image is never stationary on the retina. An abnormal gain or phase of the VOR causes **visual blur** and **oscillopsia**.

During dynamic head roll (i.e., tilting of the head alternately between the right and left shoulder), compensatory eye movements are generated by torsional VOR, which is mediated predominantly by the vertical semicircular canals (i.e., the anterior and posterior canals). The dynamic torsional VOR has a lower gain than horizontal or vertical VOR, typically ranging from −0.4 to −0.7, depending on the frequency of head roll. In contrast, static head roll evokes compensatory changes in torsional eye position, which are mediated by the otolith–ocular reflex from inputs of the utricles. Static torsional VOR (also known as **ocular counter-roll**) has a lower gain than its dynamic counterpart, ranging from −0.1 to −0.24, depending on target distance and target features.

Peripheral and central vestibular lesions cause static and dynamic imbalance of the VOR. Static imbalance of canal inputs or connections leads to spontaneous nystagmus, whereas dynamic imbalance affects the gain and phase of the VOR.

Function: The VOR stabilizes retinal image during brief head movement by generating eye movements that are equal in amplitude and opposite in direction to head movements

Quantified by: VOR gain and phase

Gain = Eye velocity/Head velocity
     = −1.0 (ideally)

Phase = Temporal difference between head and eye movements
      = 180° out of phase (i.e., zero phase shift) (ideally)

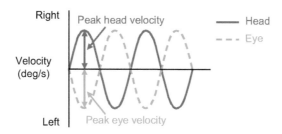

Normal values

1. Horizontal and vertical VOR

   - In dark, VOR gain approximates −0.9, and phase shift approximates zero.
   - In light, VOR gain approximates −1.0 (i.e., visual enhancement), and phase shift approximates zero.

2. Torsional VOR

   - Dynamic torsional VOR gain ranges from −0.4 to −0.7.
   - Static torsional VOR gain (ocular counter-roll) ranges from −0.1 to −0.24.

Clinical Points

VOR gain and phase

- If gain is too high or too low, a target image remains off the fovea, although it may be transiently stable on the retina.
- If there is a phase lead of the eyes before the head or a phase lag behind it, the target image is never stationary on the retina.
- Abnormal gain or phase causes **visual blur** and **oscillopsia**.

Peripheral and central vestibular lesions

- Cause static imbalance (i.e., nystagmus)
- Cause dynamic imbalance (i.e., abnormal VOR gain and phase)

The membranous labyrinth is filled with a fluid called **endolymph**. One end of each semicircular canal dilates to form the **ampulla**, the epithelium of which thickens in a region called the **ampullary crest**. The ampullary crest contains vestibular hair cells, which are innervated by bipolar sensory neurons of the vestibular nerve. The ampullary crest is covered by a gelatinous, diaphragmlike mass called the **cupula**. When the head changes its velocity of rotation (i.e., undergoes a net **angular acceleration**), endolymph is free to continue in its prior state of motion or lack of it (i.e., **inertia**), such that the endolymph flows relative to the canal wall, which is embedded in the skull. Whenever net endolymph motion is registered, the force exerted by the inertia of the endolymph distends the cupula in the opposite direction to the head rotation. This in turn displaces the cilia on the hair cells, elicits a receptor potential, and activates the vestibular nerve. Once the head attains a stable angular velocity (i.e., zero acceleration), the endolymph catches up through frictional forces to reach the same velocity as the head, so that no net movement occurs between the endolymph and the wall of the canal, causing the receptor potential to cease. Hence, net endolymph motion with respect to the canal wall is a function of angular acceleration, and the semicircular canals detect angular acceleration of the head.

The internal diameter of the semicircular canals is small relative to their radius of curvature. This geometry, together with the hydrodynamic properties of the endolymph, dictates that the motion of endolymph and the change in position of the cupula be proportional to head velocity. In other words, the semicircular canals mechanically integrate, in the mathematical sense, the angular head acceleration that they detect to yield a head velocity signal that is then encoded by the vestibular nerve.

A portion of the floor of the utricle and the medial wall of the saccule is also thickened to form the **macula**, which contains hair cells innervated by bipolar sensory neurons of the vestibular nerve. In contrast to the ampulla of the canals, the macula of the utricle and saccule is covered with a gelatinous substance that contains crystals of calcium carbonate called **otoconia**. The macula of the utricle lies approximately in the horizontal plane, whereas the macula of the saccule lies approximately in the vertical plane. When the head is tilted or undergoes linear acceleration, the otoliths deform the gelatinous mass, which in turn bends the protruding cilia on the hair cells, resulting in a receptor potential and altering the activity level of the vestibular nerve.

The cell bodies of the bipolar sensory neurons lie in the vestibular ganglion (**Scarpa's ganglion**) near the internal auditory meatus. The peripheral axons of bipolar sensory neurons form the vestibular nerve and enter the vestibular ganglion via two divisions: superior and inferior. The superior division of the vestibular nerve innervates the macula of the utricle, the anterior part of the macula of the saccule, and the ampullae of the horizontal and anterior semicircular canals. The inferior division innervates the posterior part of the macula of the saccule and the ampulla of the posterior canal. The vestibular nerve then joins the cochlear nerve to form the vestibulocochlear nerve (the eighth cranial nerve), which runs through the internal auditory meatus along with the facial nerve. The vestibulocochlear nerve then traverses the cerebellopontine angle to enter the brainstem between the inferior cerebellar peduncle and the spinal trigeminal tract to synapse in the vestibular nucleus.

One end of each semicircular canal dilates to form the ampulla, which contains hair cells that are innervated by bipolar sensory neurons of the vestibular nerve. The ampullary crest is covered by a gelatinous, diaphragm-like mass called the **cupula**.

Semicircular canals detect angular acceleration of the head

When the head changes its velocity of rotation (i.e., undergoes a net angular acceleration), the force exerted by the inertia of the endolymph distends the cupula in the opposite direction to the head rotation. This in turn displaces the cilia on the hair cells, elicits a receptor potential, and activates the vestibular nerve. Hence, the semicircular canals detect angular acceleration.

Semicircular canals mechanically integrate head acceleration to head velocity signal

The internal diameter of the semicircular canals is small relative to their radius of curvature. This geometry, together with the hydrodynamic properties of the endolymph, causes the motion of endolymph and the change in position of the cupula to be proportional to head velocity.

The semicircular canal and the ampulla

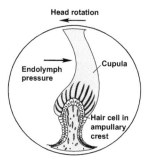

Redrawn from MacKay WA. Neuro 101: Neurophysiology Without Tears. 3rd ed. Toronto: Sefalotek; 1999. With permission of W. A. MacKay.

A portion of the floor of the utricle and the medial wall of the saccule is thickened to form the **macula**, which contains hair cells innervated by bipolar sensory neurons of the vestibular nerve. The macula is covered with a gelatinous substance that contains crystals of calcium carbonate called **otoconia**.

The otolith detects linear acceleration of the head

When the head is tilted or undergoes linear acceleration, the otoliths deform the gelatinous mass, which bends the cilia on the hair cells, elicits a receptor potential, and alters the activity of the vestibular nerve.

The Otolith and the Macula

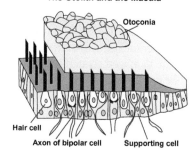

Redrawn from MacKay WA. Neuro 101: Neurophysiology Without Tears. 3rd ed. Toronto: Sefalotek; 1999. With permission of W.A. MacKay.

The free surface of each hair cell is differentiated into 40–70 stereocilia and a single kinocilium. The kinocilium is always found on one side of the hair bundle, giving each hair cell a morphological axis of polarity. The hair cells release transmitter tonically. Bending of the stereocilia toward the kinocilium leads to **depolarization** of the hair cell, an increase in the release of transmitter, and an increase in firing of the afferent fibers. Conversely, bending of the stereocilia away from the kinocilium leads to **hyperpolarization** of the hair cell, a decrease in the release of transmitter, and a decrease in firing of the afferent fibers.

For example, as the head rotates to the left, the endolymph fluid in the canals lags behind the movement of the head because of inertia. As a result, the fluid in the left canal deflects the stereocilia in the direction of their axes of polarity, leading to depolarization and excitation of the left vestibular nerve. At the same time, the fluid in the right canal deflects the stereocilia against their axes of polarity, leading to hyperpolarization and inhibition of the right vestibular nerve. The brain thus receives two inputs from a leftward head rotation: an increase in firing of vestibular nerve on the left side, and a decrease in firing on the right side.

The right and left horizontal canals work as a functional pair because they lie in approximately the same plane. However, the anterior canal on one side lies approximately in the same plane as the posterior canal on the opposite side, so the anterior and posterior canals of either side are functional pairs. For example, a chin-down (pitch) head rotation 45° to the right of the mid-sagittal plane will activate the right anterior canal and inhibit the left posterior canal.

This **push–pull arrangement** allows for functional recovery in the event of lesion on one side. The brain can continue to detect head rotation to the lesioned side by using information from the normal decrease in activity of the intact side. Thus, although acute unilateral lesion of the labyrinth causes nystagmus (see sections 3.5 and 3.6) and vertigo, these symptoms often subside within days because a central compensatory mechanism restores the balance between the right and left side. If the other labyrinth is damaged after recovery from a unilateral lesion, a new imbalance occurs as if the previously damaged labyrinth were left intact. This results in nystagmus and vertigo in the opposite direction from before, which gradually subside with central compensation. Notice that this second bout of nystagmus, called **Bechterew nystagmus,** only occurs if the labyrinths on both sides are damaged sequentially. If the labyrinths are damaged at the same time, there will be no imbalance between the right and left side and hence no nystagmus.

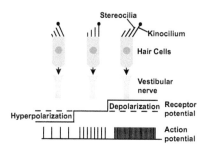

Redrawn from Leigh RJ, Zee DS. The Neurology of Eye Movements. 3rd ed. New York: Oxford University Press; 1999. With permission of Oxford University Press.

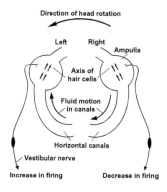

Redrawn from Kandel ER, Schwartz JH, Jessell TM. Principles of Neural Science. 3rd ed. Norwalk, CT: Appleton & Lange; 1991. With permission of McGraw-Hill.

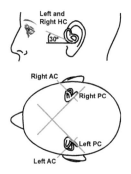

Redrawn from Kandel ER, Schwartz JH, Jessell TM. Principles of Neural Science. 3rd ed. Norwalk, CT: Appleton & Lange; 1991. With permission of McGraw-Hill.

Transduction of head motion by hair cells

- At rest, hair cells release transmitter tonically, leading to tonic firing of the vestibular nerve.

- Bending of the stereocilia toward the kinocilium leads to depolarization of the hair cells, an increase in transmitter release, and an increase in firing of the vestibular nerve.

- Bending of the stereocilia away from the kinocilium leads to hyperpolarization of the hair cells, a decrease in transmitter release, and firing of the vestibular nerve.

The right and left horizontal canals work as a functional pair (push–pull arrangement)

- Head rotation to the left causes the endolymph in the left canal to deflect the stereocilia in the direction of their axes of polarity, leading to depolarization and excitation of the left vestibular nerve.

- At the same time, the endolymph in the right canal deflects the stereocilia against their axes of polarity, leading to hyperpolarization and inhibition of the right vestibular nerve.

- When one side is lesioned, the brain can continue to detect head rotation to the lesioned side because it uses information from the normal decrease in activity of the intact side.

The right anterior and the left posterior canals work as a functional pair (and vice versa)

- The anterior canal on one side lies approximately in the same plane as the posterior canal on the opposite side, so the anterior and posterior canals of either side are functional pairs.

- For example, a chin-down (pitch) head rotation 45° to the right of the mid-sagittal plane will activate the right anterior canal (AC) and inhibit the left posterior canal (PC).

A three- to four-neuron arc connects the semicircular canals to the extraocular muscles. Primary afferents of the horizontal VOR pathway originate from the horizontal (lateral) canals. Stimulation of a horizontal canal by ipsilateral head acceleration results in slow movements of both eyes away from the side of the canal. For example, a head rotation to the right stimulates the right (ipsilateral) horizontal canal, which leads to activation of the left lateral rectus and right medial rectus, so that both eyes rotate to the left (i.e., contralateral slow phase). At the same time, inhibitory signals are sent to the left medial rectus and right lateral rectus (i.e., the antagonist muscles).

The horizontal angular VOR is served by two projections. The first is a direct excitatory projection from the horizontal canal to second-order neurons in the medial vestibular nucleus (MVN). Axons of these second-order neurons then project to the contralateral abducens nucleus. Two populations of neurons lie within the abducens nucleus: the **abducens motoneurons**, which innervate the lateral rectus on that side, forming a three-neuron arc, and the **abducens internuclear neurons**, the axons of which cross the midline and ascend within the medial longitudinal fasciculus (MLF) to innervate the medial rectus motoneurons in the oculomotor nucleus on the opposite side. This internuclear pathway to the medial rectus muscle forms a four-neuron arc and is thought to be the most important VOR pathway to the medial rectus. This arc also transmits saccadic and pursuit eye movement signals to the medial rectus. Thus, axons from the two populations of neurons within the abducens nucleus project simultaneously to the ipsilateral lateral rectus and contralateral medial rectus (a yoked muscle pair). This arrangement provides the anatomical and physiological basis for Hering's law.

A second direct excitatory pathway arises from the horizontal canals and projects to second-order neurons in the lateral vestibular nucleus. Axons of these second-order neurons project to the ipsilateral abducens nucleus without synapsing. They ascend through the ascending tract of Deiters (ATD) to the ipsilateral medial rectus subnucleus.

In addition to sending excitatory projections to the agonist muscles, the horizontal canal sends reciprocal inhibitory projections to the antagonist muscles—that is, the ipsilateral lateral rectus and contralateral medial rectus. This arrangement provides the anatomical and physiological basis for Sherrington's law.

The nystagmus caused by a unilateral peripheral vestibular lesion that involves the horizontal VOR pathway can be explained by the push–pull arrangement between the horizontal canals on each side. In the normal resting state (head immobile), the tonic discharge from the canals on each side is equal and balanced. If the left horizontal canal is damaged, discharge from the left horizontal canal is reduced, while the discharge from the right horizontal canal remains at the same tonic level. This creates a static imbalance between the canals such that the action of the right horizontal canal becomes unopposed, causing a tonic bias for the eyes to turn to the left. This results in a vestibular nystagmus with slow phases that move the eyes toward the left (ipsilesional) and corrective quick phases that move the eyes toward the right (contralesional).

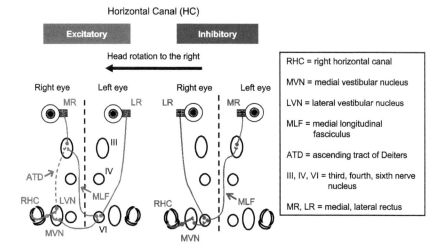

(Redrawn from Ito M. Nisimaru N, Yamamoto M. Pathways for the vestibulo-ocular reflex excitation arising from semicircular canals of rabbits. Exp Brain Res. 1976;24:257–71.)

Head rotation to the right stimulates the right (ipsilateral) horizontal canal (RHC), which leads to activation of the left lateral rectus (LR) and right medial rectus (MR), so that both eyes rotate to the left (i.e., contralateral slow phase). At the same time, inhibitory signals are sent to the antagonist muscles (i.e., the left MR and right LR).

Clinical Points

A lesion to left horizontal canal leads to unopposed action of the right horizontal canal, causing a tonic bias for the eyes to turn to the left. This results in a **vestibular nystagmus** with slow phases toward the left (ipsilesional) and corrective quick phases toward the right (contralesional).

Mnemonic for vestibular nystagmus quick phase: **COWS**

Cold (or lesion), eyes beat in Opposite direction to the side of lesion;

Warm (or stimulation), eyes beat in Same direction as the side of stimulation

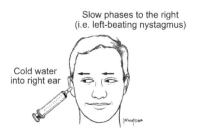

Slow phases to the right
(i.e. left-beating nystagmus)

Cold water
into right ear

Primary afferents of the vertical and torsional angular VOR pathway originate from the anterior and posterior canals. When one anterior (or posterior) canal is stimulated, the posterior (or anterior) canal in the opposite labyrinth is inhibited.

Primary afferents from the anterior canal project to second-order neurons in the superior vestibular nucleus (SVN). Axons of these second-order neurons project to the contralateral oculomotor nucleus, via the brachium conjunctivum, to excite the ipsilateral superior rectus and the contralateral inferior oblique (basis for Hering's law). Thus the anterior canal activates elevation and contralateral torsion of the upper poles of both eyes. At the same time, the anterior canal sends reciprocal inhibitory signals to the SVN, the axons of which ascend via the MLF to innervate the antagonist muscles; that is, the ipsilateral inferior rectus and contralateral superior oblique (basis for Sherrington's law).

Primary afferents from the posterior canal project to second-order neurons in the MVN, the axons of which project, via the MLF, to the contralateral oculomotor nucleus to excite the inferior rectus and to the contralateral trochlear nucleus to excite the superior oblique (basis for Hering's law). Thus, the posterior canal activates depression and contralateral torsion of the upper poles of both eyes. Reciprocal inhibition is conveyed from the posterior canal, via the SVN and MLF, to the antagonist muscles; that is, ipsilateral inferior oblique and contralateral superior rectus (basis for Sherrington's law).

Stimulation of both anterior canals by downward head acceleration activates the upward angular VOR, whereas stimulation of both posterior canals by upward head acceleration activates the downward angular VOR. Stimulation of the anterior and posterior canals on one side during ipsilateral head roll activates the torsional angular VOR, so that the upper poles of the eyes roll toward the contralateral shoulder.

The nystagmus caused by a central vestibular lesion that involves projections from both anterior canals (or both posterior canals) can be explained by the push–pull arrangement between the anterior and posterior canals that act as functional pairs (i.e., right anterior and left posterior canals as a pair, and left anterior and right posterior canals as another pair). In the normal resting state (head immobile), the tonic discharge from all four vertical canals is equal and balanced. If a central vestibular lesion causes disruption of posterior canal projections from both sides, the signal from the posterior canals is reduced, but the signal from the anterior canals remains at the same tonic level. This creates a static imbalance such that the action of the anterior canals becomes unopposed, causing a tonic bias for the eyes to rotate upward. This results in a **downbeat nystagmus** with upward slow phases.

Empirically, the vertical VOR is biased, favoring the upward VOR which is mediated by the anterior canals. To ensure that the resting tonic discharge from all four vertical canals is equal and balanced, such that no spontaneous nystagmus occurs during normal fixation, Purkinje cells in the flocculus and ventral paraflocculus of the cerebellum send more inhibitory projections to the anterior canal than to the posterior canal pathways in the vestibular nucleus. Lesion of the flocculus and ventral paraflocculus removes this asymmetric inhibition, uncovering the underlying anterior canal bias. Thus, **lesion of the flocculus and ventral paraflocculus** typically causes downbeat nystagmus.

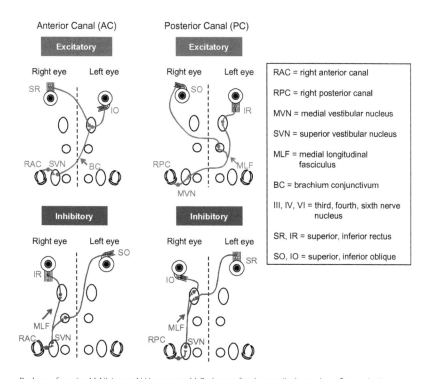

Redrawn from Ito M, Nisimaru N, Yamamoto M. Pathways for the vestibulo-ocular reflex excitation arising from semicircular canals of rabbits. Exp Brain Res. 1976; 24:257–71. With permission of Springer Science and Business Media and the authors.

- Downward head acceleration (chin down) stimulates both anterior canals (ACs) so that both eyes rotate upward.
- Upward head acceleration (chin up) stimulates both posterior canals (PCs) so that both eyes rotate downward.
- Head roll to the right stimulates both right AC and PC so that both eyes roll to opposite shoulder (upper pole of right eye incyclotorts and that of the left eye excyclotorts).

Clinical Points

1. A central vestibular lesion that disrupts bilateral PC projection leads to unopposed action of bilateral AC projection, resulting in a tonic bias for the eyes to rotate upward. This results in a **downbeat nystagmus** with upward slow phases.
2. Purkinje cells in the flocculus and ventral paraflocculus (FL/VPF) of the cerebellum send more inhibitory projections to the AC than to the PC pathways in the vestibular nucleus. Lesion of FL/VPF removes this asymmetric inhibition, uncovering an underlying AC bias. Thus, **lesion of the flocculus and ventral paraflocculus** typically causes downbeat nystagmus.

3.7 Eye Movements from Stimulation of Individual and Combinations of Semicircular Canals

Stimulation of a single canal produces slow-phase movements of both eyes in a plane parallel to one in which the canal lies (**Flourens' law**). For horizontal canals, stimulation of the right horizontal canal causes both eyes to turn to the left by activating the right medial rectus and left lateral rectus, whereas stimulation of the left horizontal canal causes both eyes to turn to the right by activating the right lateral rectus and left medial rectus. For anterior canals, stimulation of the right anterior canal causes both eyes to elevate and rotate counterclockwise from the patient's point of view (that is, right eye incyclotorts and left eye excyclotorts), by activating the right superior rectus and the left inferior oblique. Stimulation of the left anterior canal causes both eyes to elevate and rotate clockwise (that is, right eye excyclotorts and left eye incyclotorts), by activating the right inferior oblique and the left superior rectus. For posterior canals, stimulation of the right posterior canal causes both eyes to depress and rotate counterclockwise (that is, right eye incyclotorts and left eye excyclotorts), by activating the right superior oblique and the left inferior rectus. Stimulation of the left posterior canal causes both eyes to depress and rotate clockwise (that is, right eye excyclotorts and left eye incyclotorts), by activating the right inferior rectus and the left superior oblique.

The typical waveforms seen in peripheral versus central vestibular nystagmus can be explained by the combined effects of one or more canals on either side. Combined involvement of all three canals on one side, as is often seen in a unilateral **peripheral vestibular lesion**, causes a mixed horizontal–torsional nystagmus. For example, a combined lesion that affects all three canals on the left side (horizontal, anterior, and posterior) leads to a static imbalance such that the combined action of all three canals on the right side becomes unopposed, causing a tonic bias for the eyes to rotate to the left and counterclockwise (from the patient's viewpoint). This results in a **mixed horizontal and torsional nystagmus** that beats to the right and clockwise.

In contrast, a **central vestibular lesion** usually causes a **purely vertical** or **purely torsional nystagmus**. Pure vertical nystagmus can only be induced by simultaneous stimulation of the same vertical canal on both sides. For example, a central lesion that affects the posterior canal projections from both sides leads to a static imbalance such that the combined action of anterior canal projections from both sides becomes unopposed. This results in a tonic bias for the eyes to rotate upward and hence a downbeat nystagmus. Pure torsional nystagmus, in contrast, can only be produced by stimulation of both the anterior and posterior canals on one side. For example, a central lesion that affects the anterior and posterior canals on the left side leads to a static imbalance such that the combined action of the anterior and posterior canals on the right side becomes unopposed. This results in a tonic bias for the eyes to rotate counterclockwise (from the patient's viewpoint) and hence a torsional nystagmus that beats clockwise.

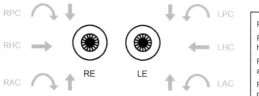

Direction of arrows = direction of slow phase of *both* eyes

| RE, LE = right, left eye |
| RHC, LHC = right, left horizontal canal |
| RAC, LAC = right, left anterior canal |
| RPC, LPC = right, left posterior canal |

Redrawn from Leigh RJ, Zee DS. The Neurology of Eye Movements. 3rd ed. New York: Oxford University Press; 1999. With permission of Oxford University Press.

Examples

1. Stimulate right horizontal canal (RHC): both eyes turn left (right medial rectus and left lateral rectus)

2. Stimulate left horizontal canal (LHC): both eyes turn right (right lateral rectus and left medial rectus)

3. Stimulate right anterior canal (RAC): both eyes rotate up and counterclockwise (from patient's point of view; i.e., right eye incyclotorts [right superior rectus] and left eye excyclotorts [left inferior oblique])

4. Stimulate left anterior canal (LAC): both eyes rotate up and clockwise (i.e., right eye excyclotorts [right inferior oblique] and left eye incyclotorts [left superior rectus])

5. Stimulate right posterior canal (RPC): both eyes rotate down and counterclockwise (i.e., right eye incyclotorts [right superior oblique] and left eye excyclotorts [left inferior rectus])

6. Stimulate left posterior canal (LPC): both eyes rotate down and clockwise (i.e., right eye excyclotorts [right inferior oblique] and left eye incyclotorts [left superior oblique])

Clinical Points

Peripheral vestibular lesion

- Lesion of LHC+LAC+LPC=Unopposed action of RHC+RAC+RPC= ↻ → (i.e., mixed horizontal and torsional nystagmus with slow phase to the left and counterclockwise from patient's point of view)

- Therefore, a peripheral vestibular lesion usually causes **mixed horizontal and torsional nystagmus**.

Central vestibular lesion

- Lesion of RPC+LPC=Unopposed RAC+LAC=↑ (downbeat nystagmus with upward slow phase)

- Lesion of LAC+LPC=Unopposed RAC+RPC=↻ (torsional nystagmus with counterclockwise slow phase from patient's point of view)

- Therefore, a central vestibular lesion causes **purely vertical** or **purely torsional nystagmus**.

The otolith–ocular reflex originates in the maculae of the otolith organs, the utricle and saccule, which act as linear accelerometers. Hair cells on the maculae have a wide range of polarization vectors. The cells in the **utricular macula** are oriented roughly in the horizontal plane, and, thus, the utricle is responsible for detecting horizontal translation and static head tilt. The cells in the **saccular macula**, in contrast, are oriented roughly in the vertical plane, parallel to the mid-sagittal plane. Thus, the saccule is responsible for detecting vertical translation, as well as static head tilt. The directions of the polarization vectors are reversed across a central zone in each macula called the **striola**. Thus, the otoliths have a more complex structure than the semicircular canals, both in spatial organization and in the distribution of polarization vectors.

The otolith organs suffer from a fundamental problem: they are unable to distinguish between tilt and translation. During **head tilt**, because the specific gravity of the otoconia is greater than that of the endolymph, the otoconia are displaced in the direction of gravity, causing the hair cells to bend toward the same direction as the head tilt. However, during linear **head translation**, the inertia of the otoconia and the endolymph causes the underlying hair cells to bend away from the direction of linear acceleration. Thus, for example, the same set of otolith hair cells that is activated by a head tilt toward the right ear is also activated equivalently by a translational acceleration toward the left ear. Because the required ocular response to a tilt is a combination of torsional and vertical eye movements, whereas that required for interaural translation is a horizontal eye movement, additional inputs or mechanisms are necessary for the brain to distinguish between tilt and translation.

Physiologic evidence suggests that the brain can distinguish between tilt and translation based on the frequency content of the linear acceleration input. Low-frequency linear acceleration is interpreted as tilt, and high-frequency stimuli is interpreted as translation. In addition, the "velocity storage integrator" network may also contribute by integrating angular head velocity signals detected by the canals to compute an internal estimate of gravity. Vestibular cells subsequently subtract this internal estimate of gravity from the net gravitoinertial acceleration signal detected by the otoliths to make an internal estimate of translation (see section 3.13).

Otolith Hair Cell Polarization

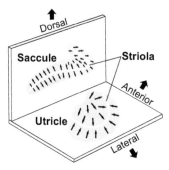

Redrawn from MacKay WA. Neuro 101: Neurophysiology Without Tears. 3rd ed. Toronto: Sefalotek; 1999. With permission of W. A. MacKay.

Polarization of otolith hair cells

- Hair cells on the macula of the otolith organs have a wide range of polarization vectors, with the directions of the vectors reversed across the striola.

- **Utricular macula**: oriented roughly in the horizontal plane; thus it detects horizontal translation and static head tilt

- **Saccular macula**: oriented roughly in the vertical plane, parallel to the midsagittal plane; thus it detects vertical translation and static head tilt

Static head tilt toward the right shoulder

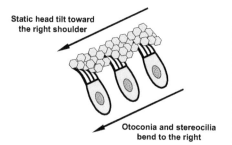

Otoconia and stereocilia bend to the right

During head tilt

Because the specific gravity of the otoconia is greater than that of the endolymph, the otoconia are displaced in the direction of gravity, causing the hair cells to bend toward the same direction as the head tilt.

Head translation (acceleration) to the left

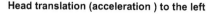
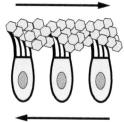

Otoconia and stereocilia bend to the right

During head translation

- The inertia of the otoconia and the endolymph causes the underlying hair cells to bend away from the direction of linear acceleration.

- The otoliths cannot by themselves distinguish between tilt and translation.

- To distinguish between tilt and translation, additional information is required, including:

  1. Frequency content of the stimulus (i.e., tilt [low frequency] vs. translation [high frequency])

  2. Extraotolith signals from the canals. The "velocity storage integrator" network computes an internal estimate of gravity by integrating angular head velocity signals detected by the canals.

Unlike the angular VOR pathway, which has been extensively elucidated, little is known about the precise anatomy of the translational VOR (otolith–ocular) pathway by which signals from the utricle and saccule reach the ocular motoneurons.

The utricle–ocular pathway has usually been assumed to be **disynaptic** through the vestibular nuclei, which are analogous to the canal–ocular pathway. For example, because of the inertia of the otoconia and endolymph, **head translation to the left** causes the stereocilia of the hair cells to bend toward the right, which leads to excitation of the hair cells that lie medial to the striola in the right utricle. Signals from the medial right utricle make excitatory connections to the ipsilateral vestibular nucleus, which then projects to ipsilateral abducens nucleus (this is in contrast to the canal pathway, where the medial vestibular nucleus projects to the contralateral abducens nucleus). The ipsilateral abducens nucleus in turn excites the ipsilateral abducens motoneurons and contralateral medial rectus motoneurons, via the abducens internuclear neurons, to generate compensatory eye movements to the right.

There is growing evidence that this disynaptic pathway is weak and that **polysynaptic** pathways play a more important role. The polysynaptic pathways originate from the lateral side of the striola in the utricle ipsilateral to the direction of head translation (i.e., the left utricle in this example). Signals from the lateral side of the left utricle then make connections to the ipsilateral vestibular nucleus, possibly via an extensive network of projections within the cerebellum, including the nodulus and ventral uvula, as well as the fastigial nucleus, the anterior vermis, and the flocculus/ventral paraflocculus. The ipsilateral vestibular nucleus then projects to the contralateral abducens nucleus to generate compensatory eye movements to the right.

Polysynaptic pathways are also responsible for generating compensatory torsional eye movements during static head tilt. For example, because the specific gravity of the otoconia is greater than that of the endolymph, **static head tilt** toward the right shoulder causes the otoconia and the stereocilia of the underlying hair cells to bend toward the right, which leads to excitation of the hair cells that lie medial to the striola in the right utricle. Signals from the medial right utricle make excitatory connections to the ipsilateral vestibular nucleus, which then makes polysynaptic excitatory connections to the contralateral trochlear nucleus (and thence to the ipsilateral or right superior oblique) and polysynaptic inhibitory connections to the ipsilateral inferior oblique subnucleus to inhibit the ipsilateral (right) inferior oblique.

At present, there is much less evidence for the involvement of the saccule, as opposed to the utricle, in evoking reflexive eye movements.

Connections from the utricle to extraocular muscles

To horizontal rectus muscles	To oblique muscles

Head Translation to the Left

Static Head Tilt to the Right Shoulder

Left panel (To horizontal rectus muscles):

RE — LR, MR
LE — MR, LR

III, IV, VI

Disynaptic pathway — weak contribution

Polysynaptic pathway (possibly via cerebellum) — strong contribution

Right utricle — VN — Scarpa's ganglion — Left utricle

Otoconia movement

Hair cells in lateral utricle inhibited / Hair cells in medial utricle activated

Hair cells in medial utricle inhibited / Hair cells in lateral utricle activated

Right panel (To oblique muscles):

RE — SO, IO
LE — SO, IO

III, IV, VI

Right utricle — VN — Scarpa's ganglion — Left utricle

Otoconia movement

Hair cells in lateral utricle inhibited / Hair cells in medial utricle activated

Hair cells in medial utricle inhibited / Hair cells in lateral utricle activated

Modified from Angelaki DE. Eyes on target: what neurons must do for the vestibuloocular reflex during linear motion. J Neurophysiol. 2004; 92:20–35. With permission of the American Physiological Society.

Modified from Uchino Y, Sasaki M, Sato H, Imagawa M, Suwa H, Isu N. Utriculoocular reflex arc of the cat. J Neurophysiol. 1996; 76:1896–903. With permission of the American Physiological Society.

LVN = lateral vestibular nucleus
VN = vestibular nucleus
MLF = medial longitudinal fasciculus
ATD = ascending tract of Dieters
III, IV, VI = third, fourth, sixth nerve nucleus
MR, LR, SR, IR = medial, lateral, superior, inferior rectus
SO, IO = superior, inferior oblique
——— = disynaptic excitatory connections
——— = polysynaptic excitatory (or disinhibitory) connections
·········· = polysynaptic inhibitory (or disfacilitatory) connections

Electrical stimulation of the left utricular nerve leads to a large incyclotorsion in the ipsilateral (left) eye and excyclotorsion in the contralateral (right) eye; an intermediate amount of elevation in the ipsilateral eye and depression in the contralateral eye; and a small adduction in the ipsilateral eye and abduction in the contralateral eye. Muscle tension also exhibits corresponding changes during stimulation: a large increase in the ipsilateral superior oblique and contralateral inferior oblique, a moderate increase in the ipsilateral superior rectus and contralateral inferior rectus, and a small increase in the ipsilateral medial rectus and contralateral lateral rectus. In addition, stimulation of the left utricular nerve results in a left (ipsilateral) head tilt via activation of the ipsilateral neck flexors and contralateral neck extensors.

Skew deviation is a vertical strabismus caused by a supranuclear lesion in the brainstem or cerebellum (see section 9.5.2). It has been attributed to an asymmetric disruption of the otolith–ocular pathway. Abnormal ocular torsion, pathologic head tilt, and abnormal tilt of the subjective visual vertical may be associated with skew deviation, constituting the **ocular tilt reaction** (OTR). Acute peripheral vestibulopathy can cause skew deviation and the complete OTR due to imbalanced inputs from the utricle. For example, a lesion of the right utricle or utricular nerve leads to a static imbalance so that the action of the left utricle or utricular nerve becomes unopposed. This tonic bias results in an ocular tilt reaction: hypotropia of ipsilesional (right) eye (i.e., skew deviation), excyclotorsion of ipsilesional (right) eye, and ipsilesional (right) head tilt.

After the utricular nerve projects to the vestibular nuclei, the otolith–ocular pathway crosses the midline and ascends to the midbrain via the MLF to contact the oculomotor and trochlear nuclei, as well as the interstitial nucleus of Cajal. Thus, a lesion in the MLF or midbrain causes a contralesional OTR. For example, a right MLF lesion results in a left OTR with hypotropia of the left eye, excyclotorsion of the left eye, and left head tilt.

RE   LE

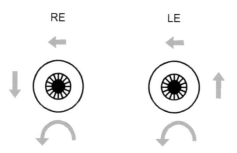

Redrawn from Suzuki JI, Tokumasu K, Goto K. Eye movements from single utricular nerve stimulation in the
cat. Acta Otolaryngol. 1969; 68:350–62.

Stimulating the left utricular nerve results in:

- Left eye (ipsilateral eye): incyclotorsion (superior oblique) > elevation (superior rectus) > adduction (medial rectus)

- Right eye (contralateral eye): excyclotorsion (inferior oblique) > depression (inferior rectus) > abduction (lateral rectus)

- Left (ipsilateral) head tilt: activation of ipsilateral neck flexors and contralateral neck extensors

Clinical Points

A lesion of the right utricular nerve leads to unopposed action of the left utricular nerve, and results in a right **ocular tilt reaction,** which is characterized by:
1. Skew deviation with hypotropia of the right eye (ipsilesional)
2. Excyclotorsion of right eye (and incyclotorsion of the left eye)
3. Right head tilt.

After the utricular nerve projects to the vestibular nuclei, the otolith–ocular pathway crosses the midline and ascends to the midbrain via the MLF to contact the oculomotor and trochlear nuclei, as well as the interstitial nucleus of Cajal. Therefore, a lesion in the MLF or midbrain causes a contralesional OTR (e.g., a right MLF lesion results in a left OTR with hypotropia of the left eye, excyclotorsion of the left eye, and left head tilt).

In addition to generating compensatory eye movements during head motion, the otolith organs, together with the semicircular canals, control posture and register the orientation of the eyes and body in three-dimensional space. This is achieved by orienting the eyes, head, and body to the **gravitoinertial acceleration vector** (GIA), which is the vector sum of gravitational acceleration (A_g) and inertial (or linear translational) acceleration (A_i).

In normal and pathological states, the torsional eye position is such that the eyes' vertical meridian is aligned with the GIA:

1. When the head is upright and stationary, the head's vertical axis and the eyes' vertical meridian are aligned with the GIA, which in turn is aligned with the gravitational acceleration vector A_g.

2. When the head is tilted counterclockwise statically (from the subject's viewpoint), the GIA remains vertical. The eyes compensate for the head tilt by rotating clockwise, so that the eyes' vertical meridian is realigned with the GIA. At the same time, the right eye depresses and the left eye elevates, so that the eyes' horizontal meridian is realigned with earth-horizontal.

3. When the head is translating to the right, the sum of A_g and A_i causes the GIA to tilt to the right, so that the GIA is no longer vertical. The eyes compensate by rotating clockwise, so that the eyes' vertical meridian is realigned with the new GIA. At the same time, both eyes rotate to the left to maintain fixation and compensate for the rightward head translation.

4. A lesion of the right otolith tilts the GIA to the right so that the patient's internal estimate of absolute vertical (gravity) is abnormally tilted to the right. In other words, the brain erroneously registers that the patient's head is tilted to the left. This results in a right OTR, which consists of a triad of abnormal head tilt to the right to realign the head's vertical axis with the new but abnormal GIA; clockwise rotation of the eyes to realign the eyes' vertical meridian with the new but abnormal GIA; and skew deviation (i.e., the right eye depresses and the left eye elevates) to realign the eyes' horizontal meridian with the new but abnormal internal estimate of the earth-horizontal.

Thus, in all four instances, the otolith–ocular reflex rolls the eyes toward the GIA. This mechanism is paralleled by the **vestibulo-collic reflex**, which orients the head to correspond to alterations in the GIA in space, as well as the **vestibulo-spinal reflex**, which readjusts the positions of the limbs to counter the alterations in the GIA and maintain postural stability.

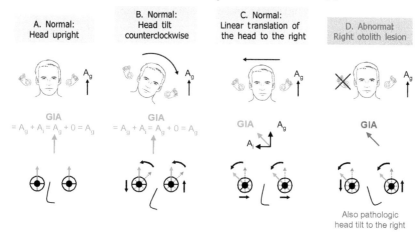

Gravitoinertial Acceleration (GIA)
= Gravitational Acceleration (A$_g$) + Inertial Acceleration (A$_i$)

In normal and pathological states, the torsional eye position is such that the eyes' vertical meridian is aligned with the GIA, which is the vector sum of gravitational acceleration (A_g) and inertial (or linear translational) acceleration (A_i).

A. When the head is *upright and stationary*, the head's vertical axis and the eyes' vertical meridian are aligned with the GIA, which, in turn, is aligned with the A_g vector.

B. When the head is *tilted counterclockwise* statically (from the subject's viewpoint), the GIA remains vertical. The eyes compensate for the head tilt by rotating clockwise, so that the eyes' vertical meridian is realigned with the GIA. At the same time, the right eye depresses and the left eye elevates, so that the eyes' horizontal meridian is realigned with earth-horizontal.

C. When the head is *translating to the right*, the sum of the A_g and A_i vectors cause the GIA to tilt to the right. The eyes compensate by rotating clockwise, so that the eyes' vertical meridian is realigned with new GIA. At the same time, both eyes rotate to the left to maintain fixation.

D. A *lesion of the right otolith* tilts the GIA to the right, meaning that the patient's internal estimate of absolute vertical (gravity) is abnormally tilted to the right (i.e., the brain erroneously registers that the patient's head is tilted to the left). This leads to a right **OTR**:

- Abnormal head tilt to the right to realign the head's vertical axis with the new but abnormal GIA
- Clockwise rotation of the eyes to realign the eyes' vertical meridian with the new but abnormal GIA
- Skew deviation (i.e., the right eye depresses and the left eye elevates) to realign the eyes' horizontal meridian with the new but abnormal internal estimate of the earth-horizontal

The VOR is a phylogenetically old brainstem reflex. It can nevertheless change to meet prevailing environmental circumstances. These changes may occur immediately or after several days to weeks and are classified as habituation and adaptation.

Although vision is the stimulus for many adaptive changes of VOR performance, the VOR may also show **habituation**, a reduction of response after repetitive stimulation in complete darkness. Habituation is most evident after repeated constant-velocity or low-frequency continuous oscillations. The functional significance of habituation is uncertain, although it may contribute to eliminating the spontaneous nystagmus that occurs after a unilateral labyrinthine lesion. Removal of the nodulus and uvula in monkeys prevents habituation and reverses habituation once it has occurred.

The VOR is an open-loop control system, meaning that the labyrinthine receptors, which provide the input of the reflex, receive no information about eye movements, the output of the reflex. In the absence of rapid feedback, the VOR must be continuously calibrated by short- and long-term adaptations to correct for any errors induced by visual or vestibular changes. These errors are sensed by vision, which recalibrates the VOR by a process called **motor learning** or **VOR adaptation**.

Adaptive changes in the VOR occur in response to certain visual stimuli. For example, due to rotational magnification, wearing magnifying glasses causes the angular VOR gain and the translational VOR sensitivity to increase, because the retinal image slip caused by magnifying glasses increases the amplitude of the eye movement relative to that of the head. Thus, a farsighted (hyperopic) person who habitually wears plus lenses has a higher VOR gain than an emmetropic person. Conversely, a nearsighted (myopic) person who habitually wears minus lenses has a lower gain. Individuals who wear contact lenses have no changes in gain because there is no rotational magnification or change in retinal image displacement.

More dramatic changes in VOR occur when subjects wear reversing prisms that laterally invert the world such that a head turn causes the environment to appear to move in the same direction as the head turn. After a short adaptation period, the eyes rotate in the same direction as the head (rather than in the opposite direction) to stabilize retinal image. Cross-axis adaptation also occurs in the VOR. When the head is rotated horizontally (about the yaw axis) while a visual display is synchronously rotated vertically (about the pitch axis), after a short training period, horizontal head rotations in darkness elicit vertical eye movements.

The sites of motor learning or VOR adaptation must be at points of convergence of visual and vestibular inputs, where visual–vestibular mismatch, in the form of retinal image slip, can recalibrate the VOR. This convergence occurs in the **flocculus** and **ventral paraflocculus**, and in the **vestibular nucleus**. The flocculus and ventral paraflocculus receive vestibular input from the vestibular nuclei via mossy fibers and visual input from the inferior olivary nucleus via climbing fibers, whereas the flocculus target neurons in the medial vestibular nucleus receive input from the flocculus and paraflocculus. Thus, a lesion of the flocculus and paraflocculus impairs VOR adaptation (see section 10.1.1). The y-group in the medulla may also contribute to vertical VOR adaptation (see section 9.2.3).

The vestibulocerebellum

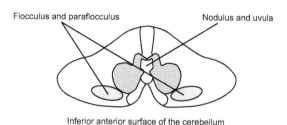

Flocculus and paraflocculus   Nodulus and uvula

Inferior anterior surface of the cerebellum

Effects of visual stimuli

1. Magnifying and minifying glasses

   - Due to rotational magnification, a farsighted (hyperopic) person who habitually wears plus lenses has a higher VOR gain than an emmetropic person.
   - A nearsighted (myopic) person who habitually wears minus lenses has a lower VOR gain.
   - Individuals who habitually wear contact lenses have no changes in gain because there is no rotational magnification.

2. Reversing prisms

   - Laterally invert the world such that a head turn causes the environment to appear to move in the same direction as the head turn
   - After a short period of adaptation, the eyes rotate in the same direction as the head.

3. Cross-axis adaptation

   - Coupling of horizontal head rotation (about the yaw axis) with a visual display that synchronously rotates vertically (about the pitch axis)
   - After a short training period, horizontal head rotation in darkness elicits vertical eye movements.

Two sites of VOR adaptation

1. **Flocculus and ventral paraflocculus** receive vestibular input from the vestibular nuclei via mossy fibers and visual input from the inferior olivary nucleus via climbing fibers.
2. **Flocculus target neurons** in the medial vestibular nucleus receive input from the flocculus and paraflocculus.

Clinical Point

Lesion of the flocculus and ventral paraflocculus impairs VOR adaptation (see section 10.1.1).

During sustained constant-velocity rotation (>10 sec), the hair cells are initially deflected, but they soon return to their resting position. The return of the hair cells to the resting position and the decline in activity of the vestibular nerve has a **time constant**, defined as the time required for a response to decline to 37% of its initial value, of about 5 sec. However, the VOR response (i.e., activity of vestibular neurons and compensatory eye movements) decays with a time constant of about 15 sec. Therefore, a central vestibular mechanism, called **velocity storage**, must have stored the activity from the hair cells to prolong VOR duration threefold.

The velocity storage mechanism is located in the **superior** and **medial vestibular nuclei**, and in the **vestibular commissure**, which contains fibers that connect the medial vestibular nuclei on both sides. The velocity storage mechanism enhances VOR response to low-frequency head movements (<0.03 Hz). It is also responsible for generating post-rotatory nystagmus, as well as optokinetic after-nystagmus (see section 3.14). The velocity storage mechanism may also provide extraotolith signals to distinguish between tilt and translation by computing an internal estimate of gravity (see section 3.8).

Velocity storage operates only during horizontal head rotation. During vertical or torsional head rotations, the VOR response declines with a time constant of about 7 sec, which is about the same as that of the vestibular afferents.

Purkinje cells in the nodulus of the cerebellum send inhibitory projections to the vestibular nucleus. A **lesion of the nodulus** removes this inhibition, resulting in an unstable velocity storage integrator. Thus, a lesion of the nodulus typically causes **periodic alternating nystagmus** in the dark. Periodic alternating nystagmus occurs in light and dark if the **flocculus and ventral paraflocculus** are also lesioned, by impairing visual fixation (see sections 7.5.5 and 10.1.2).

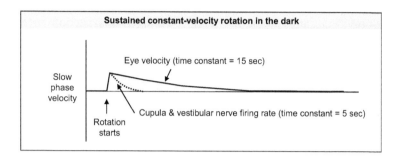

The velocity storage mechanism

- During sustained constant-velocity rotation, the hair cells are initially deflected, but they soon return to their resting position.
- The return of the hair cells to the resting position and the decline in activity of the vestibular nerve has a **time constant** of about 5 sec (time constant is defined as the time required for a response to decline to 37% of its initial value).
- The VOR response (i.e., activity of vestibular neurons and compensatory eye movements) decays with a time constant of about 15 sec.
- A central vestibular mechanism, called **velocity storage**, must have stored the activity from the hair cells to prolong VOR duration threefold.

Location of velocity storage

1. Superior and medial vestibular nuclei
2. Vestibular commissure, which contains fibers that connect the medial vestibular nuclei on both sides

Functions of velocity storage

1. Enhances VOR response to low-frequency head movements (<0.03 Hz)
2. Responsible for post-rotatory nystagmus, as well as optokinetic after-nystagmus (see section 3.14)
3. May provide extraotolith signals to distinguish between tilt and translation by computing an internal estimate of gravity (see section 3.8)

Clinical Points

Purkinje cells in the nodulus of the cerebellum send inhibitory projections to the vestibular nucleus. A **lesion of the nodulus** removes this inhibition, resulting in an unstable velocity storage integrator. Thus, a lesion of the nodulus typically causes **periodic alternating nystagmus** in the dark. If the flocculus and ventral paraflocculus are lesioned so that visual fixation is impaired, periodic alternating nystagmus occurs in light and dark (see sections 7.5.5 and 10.1.2).

Optokinetic nystagmus is induced reflexively by motion of a large visual scene, which causes an illusionary sensation of self-rotation (**circularvection**) in the opposite direction.

The function of the optokinetic system is to supplement the angular VOR. Whereas the angular VOR responds best to brief, high-frequency head rotation, the optokinetic system maintains retinal image stability during sustained, low-frequency rotation.

In the laboratory, during sustained head rotation in the dark, vestibular nystagmus (VN) subsides over about 60 sec as the cupula returns to its original position. If the rotation is suddenly stopped, **post-rotatory vestibular nystagmus** (PVN) begins with slow phases in the opposite direction. In another rather artificial situation when a normal subject sits with the head still inside a large, patterned, revolving drum (i.e., rotation of surroundings in light with the head stationary), **optokinetic nystagmus** develops. If the lights are suddenly turned off, the nystagmus does not stop immediately but gradually fades away as **optokinetic after-nystagmus** (OKAN). **Velocity storage**, discussed in section 3.13, is responsible for both post-rotatory nystagmus and OKAN. During the more natural situation when the head rotates in light, such that the environment sweeps across the retina in the opposite direction to head rotation, the nystagmus is the sum of VN and OKN. Thus, the optokinetic system sustains retinal image stability after the vestibular responses have ceased. If the rotation is suddenly stopped, PVN is balanced by OKAN, and no nystagmus occurs. Visual fixation also helps eliminate the post-rotatory nystagmus by shortening the time constant of velocity storage, a process called **visual dumping.**

Smooth pursuit and optokinetic responses are often activated simultaneously in naturally occurring situations, but the two systems are distinct. Whereas smooth pursuit is elicited voluntarily or induced by small objects whose images are guided to the foveal or parafoveal retina, OKN is induced reflexively by motion of a large visual scene that stimulates a large area of the retina. The smooth pursuit and optokinetic systems share similar neural pathways. Small, handheld drums or tapes used in the clinic do not elicit circularvection or OKAN. Both the smooth pursuit and optokinetic systems contribute to the optokinetic nystagmus evoked by such smaller field stimulation.

Just as the optokinetic smooth eye movements supplement the angular VOR during head rotation, an optokinetic subsystem, called **ocular following response** (OFR), supplements the linear VOR during head translation. The OFR has a very short latency and responds best to movement of large objects subtending about 40° of the visual field. It is enhanced when the background visual scene moves in the opposite direction.

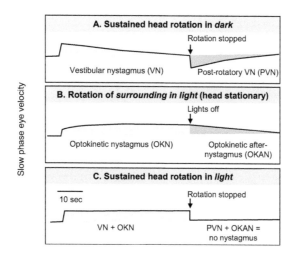

Redrawn from Cohen B, Raphan T. The physiology of the vestibuloocular reflex. In Highstein SM, Fay RR, Popper AN, eds. The Vestibular System. New York: Springer-Verlag; 2003:235-85. With permission of Springer Science and Business Media.

- Optokinetic nystagmus is induced reflexively by motion of a large visual scene, which causes an illusionary sensation of self-rotation (**circularvection**) in the opposite direction.
- Whereas the angular VOR responds best to brief, high-frequency head rotation, the optokinetic system maintains retinal image stability during sustained, low-frequency rotation:
  A. During sustained head rotation in the dark, vestibular nystagmus subsides over about 60 sec as the cupula returns to its original position. If the rotation is suddenly stopped, PVN begins, with slow phases in the opposite direction.
  B. During rotation of surroundings in light with the head stationary, OKN develops. If the lights are suddenly turned off, the nystagmus gradually fades away as OKAN.
  C. During sustained head rotation in light, the nystagmus is the sum of VN and OKN. Thus, the optokinetic system supplements the VOR after it ceases. If the rotation is suddenly stopped, PVN is balanced by OKAN, and no nystagmus occurs (visual fixation also contributes).
- Velocity storage is responsible for post-rotatory nystagmus, as well as OKAN (see section 3.13).
- The smooth pursuit and optokinetic systems share similar neural pathways.

Clinical Points

1. Small, handheld drums or tapes used in the clinic do not elicit circularvection or OKAN.
2. The optokinetic nystagmus evoked by this smaller field stimulation is elicited by both the smooth pursuit and optokinetic systems.

Several clinical tests are particularly useful to assess vestibular function without the need for sophisticated instruments.

1. To test for *static imbalance*, first inspect the eyes for **primary position nystagmus** while the patient fixes a distant target with the head stationary. In patients with **peripheral vestibular disorders**, the nystagmus usually has a mixed horizontal-torsional waveform (see section 3.7). Because peripheral vestibular nystagmus is often suppressed by visual fixation, the nystagmus may only be seen after fixation has been removed. Fixation can be removed in two ways. The first method is to have the patient wear a pair of Frenzel goggles. These goggles contain plus lenses that magnify the eyes, thus facilitating examination and effectively preventing the patients from fixing on anything in the environment. However, Frenzel goggles may not be readily available in the clinic, and they are expensive. The second way to remove fixation is by using the ophthalmoscope. While the examiner views the optic nerve head in one eye with the ophthalmoscope, occluding the fellow eye provides a sensitive method to detect nystagmus without fixation. Note that because the optic nerve head is behind the center of rotation of the eye, the direction of movement of the optic nerve head is opposite the direction of the nystagmus (which we observe by inspecting a landmark on the eye in front of the center of rotation). In contrast to peripheral vestibular nystagmus, the nystagmus in patients with **central vestibular disorders** usually has a purely vertical or purely torsional waveform (see section 3.7). Because central vestibular nystagmus is not suppressed by visual fixation, the nystagmus is present with or without fixation.

2. To test for *dynamic imbalance*, the **head thrust/impulse test** is performed. This test is particularly useful for identifying malfunction of a single canal in patients with peripheral vestibular disorder. The patient is asked to fix upon a distant target. To test the horizontal canals, the examiner briskly rotates the patient's head either to the right or to the left. Normally, the subject will be able to maintain fixation during head impulses in any direction. If the VOR is defective, the patient will not be able to maintain fixation and will need to make one or two refixating saccades. For example, if, in response to a leftward head impulse, the patient makes a rightward saccade to maintain fixation, this indicates that the left horizontal canal is not functioning properly. To test the vertical canals, the examiner briskly rotates the patient's head in the right anterior canal–left posterior canal or left anterior canal–right posterior canal planes (i.e., 45° from the mid-sagittal plane; see section 3.4) either forward or backward. For example, if, in response to a backward head impulse along left anterior canal–right posterior canal plane, the patient makes a downward saccade, this indicates that the right posterior canal is not functioning properly.

3. To test for **abnormalities in VOR gain**, the **head-shaking visual acuity** is assessed. The patient is asked to read the Snellen chart while the examiner rotates the head at about 2 Hz horizontally and then vertically. In a normal subject, the visual acuity will decrease by one or two lines. If the VOR gain is abnormal, visual acuity will decrease by several lines.

Tests	Peripheral vestibular disorder	Central vestibular disorder
Inspection for primary position nystagmus (static imbalance)	Mixed horizontal–torsional nystagmus	Purely vertical or purely torsional nystagmus
Head thrust/impulse test (dynamic imbalance)	Abnormal, refixation saccades when the head is rotated toward the lesioned canal	NA
Head-shaking visual acuity (abnormal VOR gain)	Decreased	Increased or decreased

Inspection for primary position nystagmus (test for static imbalance)

Observe any nystagmus when the patient fixes a distant target with the head stationary, first without and then with Frenzel goggles, which remove fixation.

- Peripheral vestibular disorders: mixed horizontal-torsional nystagmus; may only be seen after fixation has been removed by Frenzel goggles or by ophthalmoscope
- Central vestibular disorders: purely vertical or purely torsional nystagmus; present with or without fixation

Head thrust/impulse test (test for dynamic imbalance)

The patient is asked to fix upon a distant target. To test the horizontal canals, the examiner briskly rotates the patient's head either to the right or left.

- Normally, the subject will be able to maintain fixation during head impulses in any direction.
- If the VOR is defective, the patient will not be able to maintain fixation and will need to make one or two refixating saccades.
- Example: if during leftward head impulse, the patient makes a rightward saccade to maintain fixation, this indicates that the left horizontal canal is not functioning properly.

To test the vertical canals, the examiner briskly rotates the patient's head in the right anterior canal–left posterior canal or left anterior canal–right posterior canal planes (i.e., 45° from the mid-sagittal plane; see section 3.4) either forward or backward.

- Example: if during a backward head impulse along left anterior canal–right posterior canal plane, the patient makes a downward saccade, this indicates that the right posterior canal is not functioning properly.

Head-shaking visual acuity (test for abnormal VOR gain)

The patient is asked to read the Snellen chart while the examiner rotates the head at about 2 Hz horizontally and then vertically.

- Normally the visual acuity will decrease by one or two lines.
- If VOR gain is abnormal, visual acuity will decrease by several lines.

Chapter 4   *The Saccadic System*

Saccades are fast conjugate eye movements that move both eyes quickly in the same direction, so that the image of an object of interest is brought on the foveae. Saccades can be made not only toward visual targets, but also toward auditory and tactile stimuli, as well as toward memorized targets. Saccades can be generated reflexively, and they are responsible for resetting the eyes back to the mid-orbital position during vestibulo-ocular or optokinetic stimulation. Saccades need to be fast to get the eyes on the target as soon as possible. They also need to be fast because our eyes act like cameras with slow shutters—vision is so blurred during saccades that the eyes have to move quickly to minimize the time during which no clear image is captured on the foveae. Indeed, saccades are the fastest type of eye movements, and they are among the fastest movements that the body can make. Saccade speed is not under voluntary control but depends on the size of the movement, with larger saccades attaining higher peak velocities. It has been estimated that we make more than 100,000 saccades per day.

The burst neuron circuits in the brainstem provide the necessary motor signals to the extraocular muscles for the generation of saccades. There is a division of labor between the pons and the midbrain, with the pons primarily involved in generating horizontal saccades and the midbrain primarily involved in generating vertical and torsional saccades. However, because eye movements are a component of cognitive and purposeful behaviors in higher mammals, the process of deciding when and where to make a saccade occurs in the cerebral cortex. Not only does the cortex exert control over saccades through direct projections to the burst neuron circuits, it also acts via the superior colliculus. The superior colliculus is located in the midbrain and consists of seven layers: three superficial layers and four intermediate/deep layers. The three superficial layers receive direct inputs from both the retina and striate cortex, and they contain a retinotopic representation of the contralateral visual hemifield. The four intermediate and deep layers are primarily related to eye movements, but they also contain representations of the body surface and location of sound in space. In addition to receiving inputs from the frontal cortex, the superior colliculus receives powerful inhibitory inputs from the substantia nigra pars reticulata of the basal ganglia. These inhibitory inputs must be suppressed before the superior colliculus can drive a saccade. The cerebellum is important for maintaining saccade accuracy and for adaptation.

Because the brainstem provides the immediate premotor signals for saccades, damage to the burst neuron circuits affects both reflexive and volitional saccades. Because the cerebral cortex is primarily involved in higher-order, "executive" control of saccades, damage in cortical areas usually results in abnormal volitional saccades. Damage in the cerebellum causes saccades to over- or undershoot the target; this is the eye movement equivalent to limb dysmetria in cerebellar diseases.

In this chapter, the functions and characteristics of saccades are described. The anatomy and physiology of the burst neuron circuits in the brainstem that are responsible for generating horizontal, vertical, and torsional saccades are then described. The role of the cerebrum and cerebellum in the control of saccadic eye movements is also discussed. Finally, some tests of the saccadic system that could be performed at bedside are described.

4.1 Functions and Characteristics of Saccades

Saccades are fast eye movements that bring the image of an object of interest onto the fovea. They consist of a hierarchy of rapid eye movements, from the most rudimentary form, quick phases of vestibular and optokinetic nystagmus, to reflexive saccades made in response to the sudden appearance of a novel visual stimulus, to higher-level volitional saccades. Saccades have several characteristics:

1. **Saccadic velocity**. In normal subjects, the peak velocity of saccades varies from 30 to 700°/sec for amplitude ranging from 0.5 to 40°. The larger the saccades, the higher the peak velocity. This relationship between saccade amplitude and peak velocity has been called the **main sequence**. It can be used to determine whether a particular eye movement is a saccade or whether a patient's saccades are abnormally fast or slow.

2. **Saccadic duration**. The duration of saccades is approximately linearly related to the amplitude. It varies from 30 to 100 msec for amplitude ranging from 0.5 to 40°.

3. **Saccadic accuracy**. Small degrees of conjugate and disconjugate saccadic dysmetria are normal. A small overshooting (hypermetria) tends to occur with small-amplitude saccades, and a small undershooting (hypometria) occurs with larger amplitude saccades. The degree of dysmetria is normally about 10% of the amplitude of the initial saccade, but it is more prominent with increasing age, fatigue, or inattention.

4. **Saccadic latency (initiation time)**. The interval between the appearance of a target of interest and the onset of a saccade is normally about 150–250 msec. The introduction of a brief temporal gap of several hundred msec between the disappearance of an initial fixation target and the appearance of a peripheral target (i.e., the *gap paradigm*) leads to a reduction in saccadic latency to about 100 msec; these short-latency saccades are called **express saccades**. Conversely, if the initial fixation target remains while a saccade is made to a new target (i.e., the *overlap paradigm*), saccade onset is delayed to 200–250 msec. The gap and overlap paradigms illustrate the effects of fixation and attention on initiation of saccades. That is, disengagement of active fixation and attention allows faster onset of saccades.

In the clinical setting, each saccadic characteristic should be evaluated carefully because different disorders may affect one characteristic more than the others. For example, slow saccades are typically found in spinocerebellar ataxia type 2, whereas dysmetric saccades with normal velocity are typically exhibited in spinocerebellar ataxia type 6. Patients with ocular motor apraxia are unable to initiate voluntary saccades, leading to extremely prolonged latency, but their reflexive saccades are unaffected. Saccade hypermetria is often observed in patients with cerebellar lesions.

Function

Saccades bring the image of an object of interest onto the fovea.

Characteristics

1. Velocity
   - Normal range: 30–700°/sec for amplitude ranging from 0.5 to 40°
   - **Main sequence relationship**: Peak velocity increases with amplitude, and it saturates for large amplitude saccades.

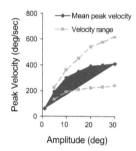

2. Duration: 30–100 msec for amplitude ranging from 0.5 to 40°
3. Accuracy: In normal subjects, a small overshooting (hypermetria) tends to occur with small-amplitude saccades, and a small undershooting (hypometria) occurs with larger amplitude saccades.
4. Latency (initiation time)
   a. Normal interval between appearance of a target and onset of saccades is 150–250 msec.
   b. Express saccades
      - Express saccades are elicited when a brief temporal gap of several hundred milliseconds is introduced between disappearance of an initial fixation target and appearance of a peripheral target (i.e., the gap paradigm).
      - Conversely, if the initial fixation target remains while a saccade is made to a new target (i.e., the overlap paradigm), saccade onset is delayed to 200–250 msec.
      - The gap and overlap paradigms illustrate the effects of fixation and attention on saccades initiation.

Clinical Points

The main sequence relationship can be used to determine whether a particular eye movement is a saccade or whether a patient's saccades are abnormally fast or slow.

Different disorders may affect one characteristic of saccades more than the others.

Abnormal velocity (e.g., saccades are too slow in spinocerebellar ataxia type 2)

Increased latency (e.g., ocular motor apraxia)

Inaccuracy (dysmetria; e.g., cerebellar lesions usually cause hypermetria)

Inappropriate saccades (e.g., saccadic intrusions and oscillations)

4.2 Pulse-Step of Innervation for Saccadic Eye Movement

The innervational changes during saccades consist of two components: a pulse and a step. A **pulse** of innervation consists of a high-frequency burst of phasic activity in agonist motoneurons. Phasic contraction of the agonist muscle overcomes viscous drag in the orbit and is responsible for the rapid eye movement. Once the eye has been brought to a new position, agonist motoneurons assume a new level of tonic innervation, higher than the resting level, constituting saccadic **step** of innervation, which holds the eye in its new position against orbital elastic recoiling forces.

The saccadic step, an eye position command, is created from the pulse (an eye velocity command) by a neural network that integrates, in the mathematical sense, conjugate eye-velocity commands into the appropriate position-coded information for the ocular motoneurons. This neural network is called the velocity-to-position **neural integrator**. For horizontal movements, the neural integrator consists of the **medial vestibular nucleus** and adjacent **nucleus prepositus hypoglossi** in the medulla. For vertical and torsional movements, the neural integrator is in the **interstitial nucleus of Cajal** in the midbrain. The neural integrator thus contributes to the gaze-holding mechanism, failure of which leads to gaze-evoked nystagmus. The cell groups of the paramedian tracts (PMT) may also contribute to gaze holding by relaying eye movement signals to the vestibulocerebellum. One component of the PMT cell groups is the medullary nucleus pararaphales, which receives eye position signals from the interstitial nucleus of Cajal. Thus, medullary lesions that damage this cell group may cause upbeat nystagmus (see section 9.2.3).

The pulse-step of innervation applies to all types of eye movements. When the discharge occurs for low-velocity eye movements (i.e., smooth pursuit, vestibular or optokinetic slow phases, and vergence), the phasic increase is usually smaller than that required for saccades.

From a pathophysiological standpoint, saccadic disorders can be the result of an abnormal pulse, an abnormal step, or a mismatch between the pulse and step of innervation. For example, a decrease in the height of the saccadic pulse, which reflects the firing rate of the motoneurons, causes *slow saccades*. A decrease in the amplitude of the saccadic pulse (i.e., height [firing rate] times width [duration of firing]), leads to *hypometric saccades*; conversely, an increase in pulse amplitude results in *hypermetric saccades*. ▸▸ If the saccadic step cannot be sustained despite a normal pulse, for example, due to a defective or leaky neural integrator, the eye drifts toward the central position at the end of each eccentric saccade, resulting in **gaze-evoked nystagmus** with corrective quick phases beating away from central position.

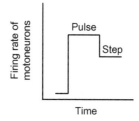

Pulse-step of innervation

Pulse. During a saccade, motoneurons and the agonist extraocular muscles exhibit a burst of high-frequency phasic activity, moving the eye quickly from one position to another against viscous drag of the orbit.

Step. After a saccade, motoneurons and the agonist extraocular muscles assume a new, higher level of tonic activity, holding the eye in its new position against the orbital elastic force, which tends to rotate the globe back to the mid-orbital position.

The step (an eye position command) is derived from the pulse (an eye velocity command). This is performed by the velocity-to-position **neural integrator**, which mathematically integrates a velocity command to yield a position command (**gaze-holding mechanism**).

- For horizontal movements, the neural integrator consists of the **medial vestibular nucleus** and **nucleus prepositus hypoglossi** in the medulla.
- For vertical and torsional movements, the neural integrator is the **interstitial nucleus of Cajal** in the midbrain.

The pulse-step of innervation applies to all types of eye movements, including saccades, pursuit, nystagmus slow phase, and vergence.

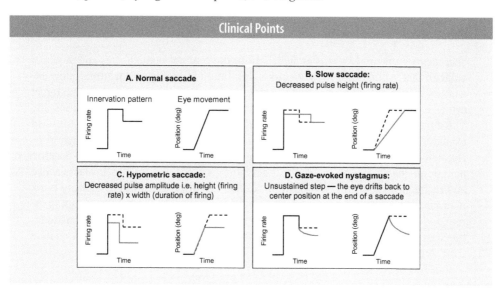

Redrawn from Leigh RJ, Zee DS. The Neurology of Eye Movements. 3rd ed. New York: Oxford University Press; 1999. With permission of Oxford University Press.

4.3 Brainstem Saccade Generation

Two classes of neurons in the brainstem are critical for the generation of saccades: burst neurons and omnipause neurons. Burst neurons are divided into excitatory and inhibitory types. **Excitatory burst neurons** (EBN) are further divided into medium-lead burst neurons and long-lead burst neurons. **Medium-lead** (also called short-lead) **burst neurons** generate the immediate premotor command for the saccadic pulse by activating motoneurons that innervate the agonist muscles. They discharge at a high frequency to motoneurons, 8–15 msec before and during saccades, but they are silent during fixation, pursuit, and vestibular and optokinetic eye movements. They reside within the nucleus reticularis pontis caudalis in the pontine paramedian reticular formation (PPRF) for horizontal saccades, and in the rostral interstitial nucleus of the medial longitudinal fasciculus (riMLF) for vertical and torsional saccades.

Long-lead burst neurons activate medium-lead EBN and inhibit omnipause neurons to release their tonic inhibition on EBN. They discharge irregularly for up to 100 msec before saccade onset. They are located predominantly in the rostral PPRF and the mesencephalic reticular formation. **Inhibitory burst neurons** (IBN) inhibit the motoneurons to antagonist muscles and discharge just before and during saccades. They reside within the nucleus paragigantocellularis dorsalis in the PPRF for horizontal saccades. For vertical and torsional saccades, IBN reside in the interstitial nucleus of Cajal and possibly within the riMLF.

Omnipause (pause) **neurons** tonically inhibit medium-lead burst neurons during fixation and smooth eye movements. They stop discharging 10–12 msec before and during saccades. When a saccade is called for, the omnipause cells are inhibited, (possibly by long-lead burst neurons) so that their inhibitory effects are removed from medium-lead burst neurons to allow saccade generation. Omnipause neurons lie within the nucleus raphe interpositus in the PPRF.

Model of Saccade Generation

Saccades are initiated by trigger signals from the cerebral hemispheres and superior colliculi that inhibit omnipause neurons. Inhibition of omnipause neurons allow excitatory burst neurons to discharge. A desired eye position signal (e.g., retinal target error), independent of the trigger signal, determines how long the burst neurons fire. The duration of their firing determines the amplitude of saccades. The medium-lead excitatory burst neurons generate an eye velocity command (the pulse), which is integrated to create a new eye position command (the step) by the velocity-to-position neural integrator. The pulse-step of innervation is sent to the motoneurons to move and maintain the eye in a new position. Collaterals of medium-lead excitatory burst neurons also activate inhibitory burst neurons, which inhibit antagonist motoneurons and omnipause neurons during the saccade. Once the actual eye position matches the desired eye position, the burst neurons cease firing, the omnipause cells resume their tonic activity, and the saccade stops.

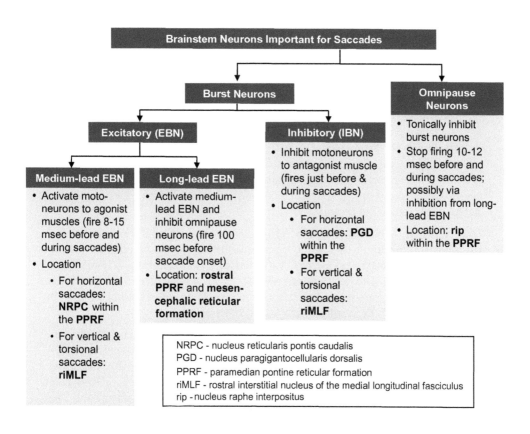

Brainstem Neurons Important for Saccades

Burst Neurons

Omnipause Neurons
- Tonically inhibit burst neurons
- Stop firing 10-12 msec before and during saccades; possibly via inhibition from long-lead EBN
- Location: **rip** within the **PPRF**

Excitatory (EBN)

Inhibitory (IBN)
- Inhibit motoneurons to antagonist muscle (fires just before & during saccades)
- Location
  - For horizontal saccades: **PGD** within the **PPRF**
  - For vertical & torsional saccades: **riMLF**

Medium-lead EBN
- Activate moto-neurons to agonist muscles (fire 8-15 msec before and during saccades)
- Location
  - For horizontal saccades: **NRPC** within the **PPRF**
  - For vertical & torsional saccades: **riMLF**

Long-lead EBN
- Activate medium-lead EBN and inhibit omnipause neurons (fire 100 msec before saccade onset)
- Location: **rostral PPRF** and **mesencephalic reticular formation**

NRPC - nucleus reticularis pontis caudalis
PGD - nucleus paragigantocellularis dorsalis
PPRF - paramedian pontine reticular formation
riMLF - rostral interstitial nucleus of the medial longitudinal fasciculus
rip - nucleus raphe interpositus

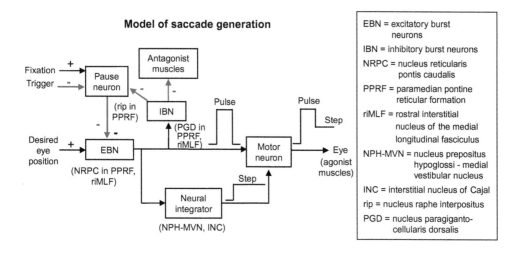

Model of saccade generation

EBN = excitatory burst neurons
IBN = inhibitory burst neurons
NRPC = nucleus reticularis pontis caudalis
PPRF = paramedian pontine reticular formation
riMLF = rostral interstitial nucleus of the medial longitudinal fasciculus
NPH-MVN = nucleus prepositus hypoglossi - medial vestibular nucleus
INC = interstitial nucleus of Cajal
rip = nucleus raphe interpositus
PGD = nucleus paragiganto-cellularis dorsalis

The paramedian pontine reticular formation (PPRF) receives bilateral projections from the **frontal eye field** (FEF) and contralateral projections from the **superior colliculus**, both of which carry trigger signals for the initiation of saccades. The medium-lead excitatory burst neurons (EBN) in the PPRF generate an eye velocity command (the pulse) and project to the abducens nucleus. Two populations of neurons reside within the abducens nucleus: the **abducens motoneurons**, which innervate the ipsilateral lateral rectus, and the **abducens internuclear neurons**, the axons of which cross the midline and ascend within the medial longitudinal fasciculus (MLF) to innervate the medial rectus motoneurons in the oculomotor nucleus on the opposite side. This internuclear pathway also transmits vestibulo-ocular reflex (VOR) and pursuit eye movement signals to the medial rectus. The abducens and medial rectus motoneurons activate the agonist muscles to move both eyes conjugately to the desired eye position.

The eye velocity command generated by the excitatory burst neurons in the PPRF is also sent to the velocity-to-position neural integrator, located within the **nucleus prepositus hypoglossi and medial vestibular nucleus complex** (NPH-MVN) for horizontal saccades. The neural integrator mathematically integrates the eye velocity command to create an eye position command (the step), which holds the eyes in their new position (i.e., gaze holding).

Because the PPRF excites both populations of neurons in the abducens nucleus (abducens motoneurons and internuclear neurons) and because it only carries saccadic signals, a discrete lesion of the PPRF causes a **conjugate horizontal saccadic palsy** to the same side (see section 9.3.2). For example, a right PPRF lesion causes a conjugate saccadic palsy to the right. In contrast, because the MLF carries not only saccadic signals, but also VOR and pursuit signals to the medial rectus, and because axons of the internuclear neurons cross the midline almost immediately after leaving the abducens nucleus, a lesion of the MLF causes an **ipsilesional adduction palsy**, which is the cardinal manifestation of **internuclear ophthalmoplegia** (see section 9.3.3). For example, a right MLF lesion (right internuclear ophthalmoplegia) results in adduction palsy, affecting adducting saccades, VOR, and pursuit of the right eye. A lesion of the NPH-MVN complex (also called a "leaky" neural integrator) results in failure of gaze holding, that is, an inability to sustain the saccadic step despite a normal saccadic pulse. The eyes thus drift toward the central position at the end of each eccentric saccade, which is followed by a corrective saccade toward the eccentric position, resulting in **gaze-evoked nystagmus**.

Excitatory burst neurons in the PPRF (and the riMLF for vertical and torsional saccades) are tonically inhibited by omnipause neurons in the nucleus raphe interpositus. Empirical evidence shows that a lesion of nucleus raphe interpositus causes **slow saccades** (rather than involuntary saccades).

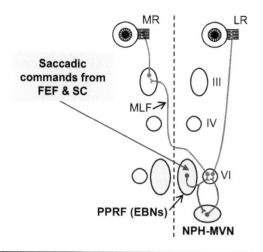

FEF = frontal eye field

SC = superior colliculus

EBNs = medium-lead excitatory burst neurons

PPRF = paramedian pontine reticular formation

NPH-MVN = nucleus prepositus hypoglossi - medial vestibular nucleus

III, IV, VI = third, fourth, sixth nerve nucleus

MLF = medial longitudinal fasciculus

MR, LR = medial rectus, lateral rectus

For horizontal saccades, excitatory burst neurons (EBNs) in **PPRF** send signals to:

1. **Abducens motoneurons** in the abducens nucleus, which generate a saccadic pulse to move the ipsilateral eye rapidly to a new position (ipsilateral lateral rectus).
2. **Abducens internuclear neurons** in the abducens nucleus, which send axons to the contralateral medial rectus subnucleus via the MLF. The medial rectus motoneurons then generate a saccadic pulse to move the fellow eye rapidly to a new position (the internuclear pathway also transmits VOR and pursuit eye movement signals to the medial rectus).
3. The **neural integrator (nucleus prepositus hypoglossi–medial vestibular nucleus [NPH-MVN])**, which generates a saccadic step to hold the eyes in new position (gaze holding).
4. **Omnipause neurons in nucleus raphe interpositus** tonically inhibit EBN in PPRF and in riMLF.

<table>
<tr><td>Clinical Points</td></tr>
</table>

A discrete lesion of the PPRF causes a *conjugate, horizontal saccadic palsy* to the same side (e.g., a right PPRF lesion causes a conjugate saccadic palsy to the right; see section 9.3.2).

Lesion of the MLF causes *ipsilesional adduction palsy,* the cardinal manifestation of *internuclear ophthalmoplegia* (INO) (e.g., a right MLF lesion [right INO] results in adduction palsy, affecting adducting saccades, VOR, and pursuit of the right eye; see section 9.3.3).

Lesion of NPH-MVN ("leaky integrator") causes *horizontal gazed-evoked nystagmus* because of failure of gaze holding.

Lesion of the nucleus raphe interpositus causes *slowing of saccades.*

The rostral interstitial nucleus of the medial longitudinal fasciculus (riMLF) receives ipsilateral projections from the frontal eye field. Medium-lead EBNs that generate upward and downward saccades are intermingled in the riMLF. Medium-lead EBNs responsible for upward saccades generate an eye velocity command (the pulse) and project via the MLF to the ipsilateral superior rectus and inferior oblique subnuclei of the oculomotor nucleus, with axon collaterals crossing within the oculomotor nucleus to innervate the contralateral superior rectus and inferior oblique subnuclei. Each riMLF, therefore, innervates all four elevator muscles in both eyes (i.e., both superior recti and inferior obliques). Medium-lead EBNs also send collateral axons to the interstitial nucleus of Cajal (INC) bilaterally, which integrates the pulse into a step command and transmits it to motoneurons.

Medium-lead EBNs responsible for downward saccades project via the MLF to the inferior rectus subnucleus of the oculomotor nucleus and to the trochlear nucleus on the same side. Inferior rectus motoneurons innervate the muscle of the ipsilateral eye, and superior oblique motoneurons innervate the muscle of the contralateral eye. Each riMLF, therefore, innervates two depressor muscles, one in each eye. Medium-lead EBNs also send collateral axons to the ipsilateral INC, which integrates the pulse into a step command and transmits it to motoneurons.

Although the riMLF contains burst neurons for both upward and downward saccades, each riMLF contains burst neurons that discharge for torsional saccades in one direction only: the right riMLF generates conjugate clockwise saccades, and the left riMLF generates conjugate counterclockwise saccades only (from the subject's point of view).

The omnipause neurons located in the nucleus raphe interpositus cease firing during vertical and torsional saccades as well as during horizontal saccades. Inhibitory burst neurons for vertical and torsional saccades reside within the INC and possibly the riMLF; they inhibit omnipause neurons and the antagonist muscles during saccades.

Because excitatory burst neurons responsible for upward saccades project bilaterally to the oculomotor nucleus, whereas EBNs responsible for downward saccades project ipsilaterally to motoneurons of the oculomotor and trochlear nuclei, isolated lesions of the riMLF are more likely to selectively impair downward saccades. A unilateral lesion of the riMLF thus causes slowing of downward saccades and loss of ipsitorsional saccades (e.g., clockwise saccades are lost with a right riMLF lesion; see section 9.4.1). In contrast, a bilateral lesion of the riMLF causes a vertical and torsional saccadic palsy in all directions. Empirical evidence shows that a unilateral lesion of the INC ("leaky integrator") causes torsional nystagmus with ipsilesional quick phase such that the upper poles of both eyes beat toward the side of lesion.

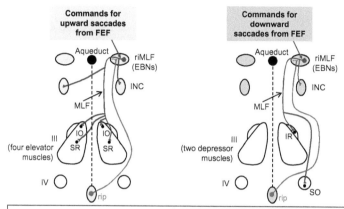

FEF = frontal eye field; riMLF = rostral interstitial nucleus of the medial longitudinal fasciculus
EBNs = excitatory burst neurons; INC = interstitial nucleus of Cajal; rip = nucleus raphe interpositus
MLF = medial longitudinal fasciculus; III, IV, VI = third, fourth, sixth nerve nucleus
SR, IR = superior and inferior rectus; IO, SO = inferior and superior oblique

For **upward saccades:**

- EBNs generate a saccadic pulse and project via the MLF to the ipsilateral superior rectus and inferior oblique subnuclei of the oculomotor nucleus, with axon collaterals crossing within the oculomotor nucleus to innervate the contralateral superior rectus and inferior oblique subnuclei.
- EBNs also send collaterals to INC bilaterally, which integrates the pulse into a step command.

For **downward saccades:**

- EBNs project via the MLF to the ipsilateral inferior rectus subnucleus of the oculomotor nucleus and to the ipsilateral trochlear nucleus, the axons of which decussate to innervate the superior oblique of the opposite eye.
- EBNs also send collaterals to ipsilateral INC, which integrates the pulse into a step command.

For **torsional saccades,** each riMLF contains EBNs that discharge for torsional saccades in one direction only. The right riMLF generates conjugate clockwise saccades, and the left riMLF generates conjugate counterclockwise saccades only (from the subject's point of view).

Clinical Points

Unilateral lesion of riMLF causes slowing of downward saccades and loss of ipsitorsional saccades (e.g., clockwise saccades are lost with right riMLF lesion; see section 9.4.1).
Bilateral lesion of riMLF causes vertical and torsional saccadic palsy in all directions.
Unilateral lesion of INC ("leaky integrator") causes torsional nystagmus with ipsilesional quick phase (i.e., upper poles of both eyes beat toward the side of lesion).

Cerebral Control of Saccades

The saccade subregion of the frontal eye field (FEFsac), the supplementary eye field, and the dorsolateral prefrontal cortex, as well as the parietal eye field (PEF) and area 7a in the parietal cortex, participate in the control of saccades. These areas initiate saccades by sending trigger signals to the omnipause neurons in the pons, and they encode saccade amplitude and direction. The PEF initiates visually guided (reflexive) saccades and projects to the ipsilateral superior colliculus and to the FEF.

The FEFsac initiates volitional and visually guided (reflexive) saccades and projects to the superior colliculus (SC) directly and via the PEF. The FEFsac also projects to the caudate nucleus, which sends inhibitory projections to the nucleus substantia nigra pars reticulata (SNpr) in the basal ganglia. The SNpr, in turn, sends inhibitory projections to the superior colliculus. The SNpr tonically discharges during fixation, and when it pauses, it disinhibits the SC, which discharges before and during voluntary and visually evoked saccades. Thus, the FEFsac has a powerful two-pronged effect on the SC: one direct and the other through the basal ganglia (i.e., the caudate and SNpr). The FEFsac and SC project directly to the PPRF and riMLF in the brainstem. Each FEFsac and SC generates contralateral horizontal saccades, whereas vertical and torsional saccades are generated by simultaneous activation of both frontal eye fields or both superior colliculi.

Together, the FEFsac and SC form an obligatory route for saccadic commands originating in the cerebrum. A lesion of both the FEFsac and SC, but not either alone, causes defective saccade generation. A lesion of either the FEFsac or the SC alone causes subtle abnormalities: mildly hypometric and delayed (increased latency) saccades.

Cerebellar Control of Saccades

The cerebellum regulates the size of saccades (dorsal oculomotor vermis and the fastigial nucleus) and participates in the repair of saccade inaccuracy (flocculus and paraflocculus). The **dorsal "oculomotor" vermis** (lobules VI and VII) receives saccadic input from, among other structures, the nucleus reticularis tegmenti pontis and discharges before saccades. The nucleus reticularis tegmenti pontis in turn sends inhibitory projections to an ellipsoidal region in the caudal fastigial nucleus, the fastigial oculomotor region, which is important in the control of saccade accuracy and consistency. Projections of the fastigial nucleus decussate within the cerebellum to reach the brainstem, where they terminate onto burst neurons, omnipause neurons, and the rostral pole of the superior colliculus. The flocculus and paraflocculus are important for the adaptation of the pulse and pulse-step mismatch for saccades.

A lesion of the **dorsal vermis** results in dysmetric and slow saccades (i.e., hypometric ipsilesional saccades and mild hypermetric contralesional saccades). A lesion of the **fastigial nucleus** also leads to dysmetric and slow saccades, but saccades are hypermetric toward the side of the lesion (i.e., ipsipulsion; hypermetric ipsilesional and hypometric contralesional saccades) because projections of the fastigial nucleus decussate within the cerebellum to reach the brainstem. A lesion of the flocculus and paraflocculus results in postsaccadic drift because adaptation to pulse-step mismatch of saccades is lost.

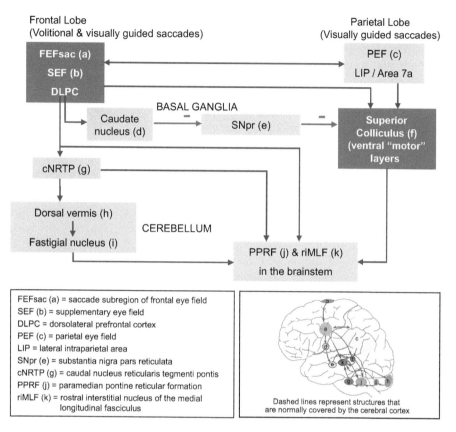

Frontal Lobe
(Volitional & visually guided saccades)

Parietal Lobe
(Visually guided saccades)

FEFsac (a)
SEF (b)
DLPC

PEF (c)
LIP / Area 7a

BASAL GANGLIA

Caudate
nucleus (d)

SNpr (e)

Superior
Colliculus (f)
(ventral "motor"
layers

cNRTP (g)

Dorsal vermis (h)

CEREBELLUM

Fastigial nucleus (i)

PPRF (j) & riMLF (k)
in the brainstem

FEFsac (a) = saccade subregion of frontal eye field
SEF (b) = supplementary eye field
DLPC = dorsolateral prefrontal cortex
PEF (c) = parietal eye field
LIP = lateral intraparietal area
SNpr (e) = substantia nigra pars reticulata
cNRTP (g) = caudal nucleus reticularis tegmenti pontis
PPRF (j) = paramedian pontine reticular formation
riMLF (k) = rostral interstitial nucleus of the medial
            longitudinal fasciculus

Dashed lines represent structures that
are normally covered by the cerebral cortex

Redrawn from Leigh RJ, Zee DS. The Neurology of Eye Movements. 3rd ed. New York: Oxford University Press; 1999.
With permission of Oxford University Press.

- Activation of the frontal eye field (FEFsac) and superior colliculus (SC) on one side generates contralateral horizontal saccades.

- Simultaneous activation of FEFsac on both sides or SC on both sides generates vertical and torsional saccades.

Clinical Points

Lesion both FEFsac and SC: defective saccade generation

Lesion either FEFsac or SC: mildly hypometric and delayed (increased latency) saccades

Lesion of the dorsal vermis: dysmetric and slow saccades (hypometric ipsilesional saccades and mild hypermetric contralesional saccades)

Lesion of the fastigial nucleus: dysmetric and slow saccades (ipsipulsion; i.e., hypermetric ipsilesional and hypometric contralesional saccades)

Saccades consist of a hierarchy of rapid eye movements, from the most rudimentary form, **quick phases** of vestibular and optokinetic nystagmus, or automatic resetting movements in response to spontaneous drift of the eyes, to **visually guided (reflexive) saccades** that are generated in response to the sudden appearance of a novel visual stimulus, to higher-level **volitional (voluntary) saccades**. Volitional saccades can be further divided into four categories: (1) saccades **to command**—saccades generated on cue; (2) **predictive, anticipatory saccades**—saccades generated in anticipation of or in search of the appearance of a target at a particular location; (3) **memory-guided saccades**—saccades generated to a location in which a target was previously present; and (4) **antisaccades**—saccades generated in the opposite direction to a suddenly appearing target. Attention and volitional effort are especially demanded when making antisaccades because reflexive saccades to the visual target must be suppressed.

Saccades are best examined clinically by having a patient look alternately at two targets held apart horizontally or vertically, such as the examiner's finger and nose. The velocity, latency, accuracy, trajectory, and conjugacy should be noted. If a saccade abnormality is identified, one should localize the disturbance within the hierarchical organization of saccades by assessing first whether the most rudimentary quick phases are affected. This can be done by spinning the patient in a swivel chair to elicit vestibular nystagmus or by using an optokinetic drum to elicit optokinetic nystagmus. Loss of quick phases is usually due to a **lesion of premotor burst neurons** in the brainstem.

Next, determine if the patient can generate visually guided (reflexive) saccades by presenting the patient with a suddenly appearing visual target. Then examine the ability of the patient to make voluntary saccades in response to command by asking the patient to make saccades rapidly between two stationary targets. Loss of voluntary saccades with preservation of quick phases and visually guided (reflexive) saccades is characteristic of **acquired ocular motor apraxia**.

Other voluntary saccades can also be tested. To test predictive, anticipatory saccades, the examiner holds both hands up and asks the patient to make a saccade when one of the examiner's fingers moves. With predictable timing, the examiner moves first a finger on one hand and then a finger on the other and repeats this cycle several times. By occasionally not moving one finger, one can determine if the patient makes a predictive saccade without a visual stimulus. Defects of predictive saccadic control are common in **Parkinson's disease**. Antisaccades can be assessed by the examiner holding both hands up and moving a finger on one hand suddenly. The patient is required to look away from the moving finger (i.e., to look to the finger that does not move). Errors on antisaccade tasks are common in **lesions of the prefrontal cortex**.

1. Test saccades by having a patient look alternately at two targets held apart horizontally or vertically, such as the examiner's finger and nose.
2. Note velocity, latency, accuracy, trajectory, and conjugacy.
3. Localize any saccade abnormality within the hierarchy of saccades by assessing (in order):

Quick phases

- Spin the patient in a swivel chair to elicit VOR or use an optokinetic drum to elicit OKN.
- Loss of quick phases is usually due to **lesion of premotor burst neurons** in the brainstem.

Visually guided (reflexive) saccades
- Present the patient with a suddenly appearing visual or auditory target.

Voluntary saccades to command
- Ask the patient to make saccades rapidly between two stationary targets.
- Loss of voluntary saccades with preservation of quick phases and visually guided (reflexive) saccades is characteristic of **acquired ocular motor apraxia**.

Predictive, anticipatory saccades
- Hold both hands up and ask the patient to make a saccade when one of your fingers moves. With predictable timing, move first a finger on one hand and then a finger on the other, and repeat this cycle several times, occasionally not moving one finger to determine if the patient makes a predictive saccade.
- Defects of predictive saccadic control are common in **Parkinson's disease**.

Antisaccades
- Hold both hands up and move a finger on one hand suddenly. Ask the patient to look away from the moving finger (i.e., look to the finger that does not move).
- Errors on antisaccade task are common in **lesions of the prefrontal cortex**.

Hierarchy (lowest to highest)	Definition
Quick phases	Quick phases of VOR or OKN, or automatic resetting movements in response to spontaneous drift of the eyes
Visually guided (reflexive) saccades	Saccades generated in response to the sudden appearance of a novel visual stimulus (also to auditory or tactile stimuli)
Volitional (voluntary) saccades	Elective saccades made as part of purposeful behavior
1. To command	• Saccades generated on cue
2. Predictive, anticipatory	• Saccades generated in anticipation of or in search of the appearance of a target at a particular location
3. Memory guided	• Saccades generated to a location in which a target has been previously present
4. Antisaccades	• Saccades generated in the opposite direction to a sudden-appearing target (need to suppress reflexive saccades)

VOR, vestibulo-ocular reflex; OKN, optokinetic nystagmus.

Chapter 5

The Smooth Pursuit System

Smooth pursuit consists of conjugate eye movements that allow both eyes to smoothly track a slowly moving object so that its image is kept on the foveae. For example, smooth pursuit eye movements are used when you track a child on a swing. Only animals with foveae make smooth pursuit eye movements. Rabbits, for instance, do not have foveae, and their eyes cannot track a small moving target. However, if a rabbit is placed inside a rotating drum painted on the inside with stripes so that the rabbit sees the entire visual field rotating en bloc, it will track the stripes optokinetically. Humans have both smooth pursuit and optokinetic eye movements, but pursuit predominates. When you track a small, moving object against a detailed stationary background, such as a bird flying against a background of leaves, the optokinetic system will try to hold your gaze on the stationary background, but it is overridden by pursuit.

Pursuit works well at speeds up to about 70°/sec, but top athletes may generate pursuit as fast as 130°/sec. Pursuit responds slowly to unexpected changes—it takes about 100 msec to track a target that starts to move suddenly, and this is why we need the faster acting vestibulo-ocular reflex (VOR) to stabilize our eyes when our heads move. However, pursuit can detect patterns of motion and respond to predictable target motion in much less than 100 msec.

Pursuit cannot be generated voluntarily without a suitable target. If you try to pursue an imaginary target moving across your visual field, you will make a series of saccades instead of pursuit. However, the target that evokes pursuit does not have to be visual; it may be auditory (e.g., a moving, beeping pager), proprioceptive (e.g., tracking your outstretched finger in the dark), tactile (e.g., an ant crawling on your arm in the dark), or cognitive (e.g., tracking a stroboscopic motion in which a series of light flashes in sequence, even though no actual motion occurs).

The neural pathway that controls pursuit eye movements is not completely understood. Visual information is relayed from the striate cortex to the extrastriate areas, where neurons are specialized for motion, with large receptive fields, strong direction selectivity, and activity that encodes both target and eye motions. These extrastriate areas have projections directly to the brainstem, as well as to other cortical areas. The cerebellum receives input from the brainstem and is critical in generating smooth pursuit. Recent evidence suggests that the pursuit system has a functional architecture similar to that of the saccadic system. Rather than being controlled primarily by areas in extrastriate cortex specialized for processing visual motion, pursuit involves an extended network of cortical areas (e.g., frontal eye field) and other subcortical structures (e.g., superior colliculus and basal ganglia) that are also important for saccadic eye movements. Thus, although the traditional view is that pursuit and saccades are two distinct systems, it may be more accurate to consider the two movements as different outcomes from a shared cascade of sensorimotor functions.

Clinically, when pursuit fails to track a target, a series of catch-up saccades are exhibited. Because the smooth pursuit system involves many brain structures, pursuit deficits do not usually have any localizing value; other neurological and eye movement abnormalities are needed to pinpoint the location of a lesion.

In this chapter, the functions and characteristics of smooth pursuit are discussed. The putative neural pathway that controls pursuit eye movements is then discussed. Finally, some tests of the pursuit system that could be performed at bedside are described.

5.1 Functions and Characteristics of Smooth Pursuit

Functions

1. Stabilizes the image of a small moving target on the fovea

2. Cancels the VOR during combined eye–head tracking (i.e., VOR cancellation). During smooth tracking of a target that moves in the same direction as the head, smooth pursuit cancels VOR; otherwise, the VOR would move the eyes opposite the direction of intended gaze.

3. Cancels optokinetic nystagmus during tracking of a small, moving target against a detailed stationary background. For example, during smooth tracking of a bird flying against a background of leaves, the optokinetic system will try to hold the gaze on the stationary background, but it is overridden by pursuit.

Characteristics

1. **Velocity**: 0.1–70°/sec (top athletes may show pursuit as high as 130°/sec)

2. **Latency (initiation time)**: 100–130 msec (i.e., much longer than VOR [about 15 msec], but shorter than saccades [about 200 msec])

3. **Gain**: eye velocity/target velocity = 1.0 (ideal)

4. **Two phases of smooth pursuit**:

   Open loop phase (pursuit initiation): during the latency period
   - Guided by target motion (i.e., retinal slip velocity)
   - Initial acceleration (first 20–40 msec) is very stereotypic and does not depend on initial target velocity.
   - After this, there is a variable component in which pursuit acceleration depends on the initial target velocity.

   Closed loop phase (pursuit maintenance or **steady state)**: after the latency period
   - During open loop phase, retinal slip is reduced to a fraction of target speed.
   - To maintain pursuit, the brain adds an extraretinal feedback of eye velocity (i.e., an **efference copy**) to retinal slip velocity to compute the target velocity.

5. **Predictive character of smooth pursuit**
   - If target motion is unpredictable, pursuit shows a phase lag behind the target (about one latency period), as when tracking a flying insect.
   - If target motion is predictable, pursuit will track with no phase lag such that the object is perfectly centered on the fovea, as when tracking a child on a swing.

6. **Stimuli for smooth pursuit**
   - Target velocity (i.e., retinal slip velocity; a velocity error) is the primary stimulus
   - Position of target (a position error)
   - Motor command to the eye (efference copy)
   - Proprioception (afferent input) e.g., tracking one's outstretched finger in the dark; also uses knowledge of motor command to the limb
   - Perception of motion (requires high-level integration of many motion cues; e.g., stroboscopic motion in which one infers motion of an object from a series of flashes, even though no actual motion occurs)

Smooth pursuit can be examined clinically by asking the patient to track a small target with the head still, such as a pencil tip held at 1 meter away. When the gain is low, **catchup saccades** are seen, giving the appearance of saccadic pursuit. Conversely, when the gain is high, **backup saccades** are observed.

A useful clinical tool to test smooth pursuit is the handheld optokinetic drum. Although it does not adequately elicit optokinetic nystagmus, the optokinetic drum can be used to assess smooth pursuit by rotating the drum in front of the patient in both horizontal and vertical directions. The direction and nature of slow phases are then analyzed. **Pursuit asymmetry** is commonly seen in cerebral hemispheric disease. For example, a patient with a left posterior cerebral lesion may show fewer corrective quick phases when the drum is rotated to his or her left, due to low pursuit gain to the left. **Pursuit reversal**, which is corrective quick phases that beat toward the same direction as that of drum rotation, can be seen in some patients with infantile nystagmus syndrome.

Because smooth pursuit cancels the VOR, smooth pursuit function can be inferred by testing VOR cancellation. This can be done by spinning the patient in a swivel chair while the patient fixates on his or her outstretched thumb. Normally, the eyes should be able to maintain steady fixation. With inadequate VOR cancellation, the eyes are taken off target by VOR slow phases, which lead to corrective saccades. For example, deficient VOR cancellation on rotation to the left corresponds to low pursuit gain to the left.

A lesion in MT and MST causes two types of pursuit defects: retinotopic and directional (see section 11.3.3). A unilateral lesion in V1 or MT causes retinotopic pursuit defects (**scotoma of motion**), which consist of lower smooth pursuit speed and inaccurate saccades in all directions in the contralateral hemifield. In contrast, a unilateral lesion in MST causes **directional pursuit defects**, which consist of lowered smooth pursuit speed toward the side of the lesion, regardless of the hemifield where the target lies; saccades are not affected. Lesions in the smooth pursuit subregion of the frontal eye field (FEFsem), the DLPN, or the NOT cause deficits in ipsiversive horizontal pursuit. A lesion in the rostral nucleus reticularis tegmenti pontis (rostral NRTP) causes deficits in upward pursuit.

Lesions in different areas of the cerebellum have different effects on smooth pursuit. Bilateral lesions of the flocculus have no effects on pursuit. Unilateral lesions of the ventral paraflocculus (VPF) cause mild deficits in horizontal and vertical pursuit (both directions) and VOR cancellation, whereas bilateral lesions of the flocculus and VPF cause severe deficits in horizontal and vertical pursuit (both directions) and VOR cancellation. Therefore, VPF is the primary structure involved in pursuit and VOR cancellation. Lesions of the vermis result in deficits in ipsiversive horizontal pursuit, whereas lesions in the fastigial nucleus lead to deficits in contraversive horizontal pursuit. Lesions involving the rest of the pursuit pathway (i.e., starting from the level of medial vestibular nucleus) will also affect the VOR because pursuit and the VOR share similar pathways from this point forward.

1. Ask the patient to track a small target with the head still (e.g., a pencil tip held at 1 meter away).

   ▪ **Catch-up saccades** (saccadic pursuit) are seen when the gain is low.

   ▪ **Backup saccades** are observed when the gain is high.

2. Rotate a handheld optokinetic drum in both horizontal and vertical directions, and analyze the direction and nature of slow phases.

   ▪ **Pursuit asymmetry** is common in cerebral hemispheric disease.

   ▪ **Pursuit reversal** is seen in infantile nystagmus syndrome (i.e., quick phases toward the same direction as that of drum rotation).

3. To test VOR cancellation, spin the patient in a swivel chair while the patient fixes on his or her outstretched thumb.

   ▪ Normally, the eyes should be able to maintain steady fixation.

   ▪ With inadequate VOR cancellation, the eyes are taken off target by VOR slow phases, which results in corrective saccades (e.g., deficient VOR cancellation on rotation to the left corresponds to low pursuit gain to the left).

Clinical Points

Lesion in V1 or MT causes *scotoma of motion* (i.e., impaired horizontal pursuit [both directions] in the affected contralateral hemifield). See section 11.3.3.

Lesion in MST causes *directional pursuit deficit* (i.e., impaired horizontal pursuit toward the side of lesion, regardless of the hemifield where the target lies). See section 11.3.3.

Lesion in the FEFsem, DLPN, or NOT causes deficits in *ipsiversive horizontal pursuit*.

Lesion in the rostral NRTP causes deficits in *upward pursuit*.

Lesion in the cerebellum:

▪ **Flocculus and VPF**

   a. Bilateral lesions of the flocculus: no effect on pursuit

   b. Unilateral lesion of the VPF: mild deficit in horizontal and vertical pursuit (both directions) and VOR cancellation

   c. Bilateral lesion of the flocculus and VPF: severe deficit in horizontal and vertical pursuit (both directions) and VOR cancellation. Therefore, VPF is the primary structure involved in pursuit and VOR cancellation.

▪ **Lesion in the vermis:** deficit in ipsiversive horizontal pursuit

▪ **Lesion in the fastigial nucleus:** deficit in contraversive horizontal pursuit

Lesions involving the rest of the pursuit pathway (i.e., starting from the level of medial vestibular nucleus) will also affect the VOR because pursuit and the VOR share similar pathways from this point forward.

Chapter 6 | *The Vergence System*

Vergence eye movements shift the gaze point between near and far, such that the image of a target is maintained simultaneously on both foveae. Unlike other eye movement systems, vergence movements are disjunctive, meaning that the eyes move in opposite directions. To move from a far to a near target, the eyes converge (i.e., rotate toward the nose) so that the lines of sight of the two eyes intersect at the target. To aim at a target farther away, the eyes diverge (i.e., rotate toward the temples). When the target is located at optical infinity, the lines of sight are parallel. During deep sleep, deep anesthesia, and coma, the eyes diverge beyond parallel, indicating that eye alignment is normally actively maintained by the brain because the orbits, in which the eyeballs are located, are divergent.

The vergence system is believed to be relatively new evolutionarily. Just as a new version of computer software tends to have bugs, perhaps it is for this reason that vergence is the last of the eye movement systems to reach full development in children, that it is often the first system to be affected by fatigue, alcohol, and other drugs, and that defective vergence is a common cause of strabismus and diplopia.

Vergence eye movements are very slow, lasting 1 sec or longer. One reason for this may be that vergence, unlike saccades, is driven by visual feedback, which normally takes at least 80 msec. Another reason may be that the speed of vergence movements is limited by how fast the lenses change shape (accommodation) and how fast the pupils constrict. There may simply be no advantage for vergence to take place quickly and then wait for the lenses and pupils to catch up. The triad of convergence, accommodation, and pupillary constriction constitutes the near triad.

The two most important stimuli for vergence are retinal image blur and retinal disparity. If the retinal image of an object is blurred, the target is either too near or too far away. This results in a change in accommodation, which is accompanied by a change in pupillary size, as well as a change in vergence. Similarly, if a single object casts its image on noncorresponding points on the two retinas, vergence eye movements are elicited to realign the lines of sight to achieve single binocular vision.

Whereas other eye movements can be directed along any meridian, vergence is most robust along the horizontal meridian. This is because the eyes are separated horizontally in the head, and so horizontal vergence is functionally most useful. Although vertical and torsional vergence can be elicited by vertical and torsional disparities, their amplitudes are much smaller than that of horizontal vergence. This explains why a vertical or torsional strabismus is often poorly tolerated.

The neural pathway that controls vergence eye movements is not completely understood. Binocularly driven neurons are present in the visual cortex and other brain areas, and no motor neurons are devoted exclusively to drive vergence. One can speculate that these binocularly driven neurons must project to the oculomotor nuclear complex, so that both medial rectus muscles are activated simultaneously to generate vergence eye movements.

Malfunction of vergence accounts for a number of common disorders. Convergence insufficiency causes diplopia at near distances and is commonly seen in young adults who complain of eyestrain, periocular headache, and blurred vision after brief periods of reading. Convergence insufficiency is also often found in patients with Parkinson's disease or progressive supranuclear palsy. An abnormal synkinetic relationship between vergence and accommodation is a common cause of childhood strabismus.

In this chapter, the functions and characteristics of vergence eye movements are discussed. The putative neural pathway that controls vergence is then discussed. Finally, some tests of the vergence system that could be performed at bedside are described.

6.1 Functions and Characteristics of Vergence Eye Movements

Vergence eye movements are disjunctive movements that move the eyes in opposite direction (i.e., convergence or divergence). They hold the images of a single object simultaneously on both foveae. Vergence eye movements have several characteristics:

1. **Velocity.** Vergence movements show two types of responses: (a) Fast vergence is observed in response to a large and abrupt change in disparity—for example, when one abruptly changes focus from near to far. (b) Slow vergence is seen in response to a small and slow change in disparity—for example, tracking a target that moves slowly in depth. Similar to saccades, peak velocity of vergence increases with its amplitude (i.e., follows main sequence [see section 4.1]). Convergence speed is usually greater than divergence speed.

2. **Latency.** The latency of a vergence movement is about 200 msec for retinal blur stimuli and about 80–160 msec for retinal disparity stimuli.

3. **Waveform/trajectory.** For convergence, the trajectory is one of increasing (exponential) velocity waveform, whereas for divergence, it is of decreasing (exponential) velocity waveform. The time constant is about 150–200 msec, reflecting the viscosity and elasticity of the eye muscles and connective tissues, and implies a step or tonic change in innervation. However, motoneurons actually show pulse-step discharge during vergence.

4. Vergence consists of two phases: (a) In the **initiation (transient/open loop) phase**, fast vergence is triggered in response to large retinal disparity with dissimilar features (shape, contrast, spatial frequency). This phase may be responsible for coarse stereopsis. (b) In the **completion (sustained/closed loop) phase**, slow eye movements complete the vergence response via negative visual feedback. This phase responds well to small disparity with similar features and may be responsible for fine stereopsis. The horizontal fusional vergence system maintains correspondence of retinal images in both eyes with precision but is not perfect. The remaining disparity is called **fixation disparity**, which is a small residual disparity that acts as a steady-state vergence error to provide a negative feedback signal for sustained vergence. This small disparity is also responsible for stereopsis.

5. **Vergence and saccade interaction.** Most vergence eye movements are accompanied by disconjugate saccades, and saccades speed up vergence (several times faster). During horizontal saccades, the eyes transiently diverge and then converge, aligning 30–100 msec after completion of saccades. During upward saccades, there is often an initial divergence, and during downward saccades, there is an initial convergence.

6. **Stimuli for vergence.** Vergence can be elicited by two primary stimuli: (a) **retinal blur**, due to loss of image sharpness, eliciting **accommodative vergence**; and (b) **retinal disparity**, due to separation of images of a single object such that they fall on noncorresponding parts of the retina, eliciting **fusional/disparity vergence**. Other stimuli, such as (c) **proximity of targets** (i.e., proximal vergence; based on cues such as perspective); (d) **change in size**, or **looming**; and (e) **monocular cues derived from motion**, may also evoke vergence. There is also a resting level of vergence tone, called **tonic vergence**, about which changes in vergence induced by new sensory cues take place. Vergence can also be generated voluntarily.

Vergence eye movements are **disjunctive movements** that move the eyes in opposite direction (i.e., convergence or divergence). Their function is to hold the images of a single object simultaneously on both foveae.

Characteristics

1. **Velocity**
   - Fast vergence is a response to a large and abrupt change in disparity (e.g., changing focus abruptly from near to far).
   - Slow vergence is a response to a small and slow change in disparity (e.g., tracking a target that moves slowly in depth).
   - Peak velocity increases with amplitude of vergence (i.e., follows main sequence).
   - Convergence speed is usually greater than divergence speed.

2. **Latency**
   - Retinal blur stimuli: 200 msec
   - Retinal disparity stimuli: 80–160 msec

3. **Waveform** or **trajectory**
   - Convergence: increasing velocity waveform
   - Divergence: decreasing velocity waveform
   - Time constant: 150–200 msec (this reflects the viscosity and elasticity of the eye muscles and connective tissue and implies a step or tonic change in innervation, but motoneurons actually show pulse-step discharge during vergence)

4. **Two phases of vergence eye movements**
   a. **Initiation/transient**
      - Fast, open-loop response that completes within a few hundred msec
      - Responds to large disparity with dissimilar features (shape, contrast, spatial frequency) and may be responsible for coarse stereopsis

   b. **Completion/sustained**
      - Slow response that completes vergence via negative visual feedback
      - Responds to small disparity with similar features and may be responsible for fine stereopsis
      - Fixation disparity: a small residual disparity for stereopsis and acts as steady-state vergence error to provide negative feedback signal for sustained vergence

5. **Vergence and saccade interaction**: Most vergence eye movements are accompanied by disconjugate saccades, and saccades speed up vergence (several times faster).

6. **Stimuli**
   - Retinal blur (loss of image sharpness) elicits **accommodative vergence**.
   - Retinal disparity (separation of images of a single object such that they fall on noncorresponding parts of the retina) elicits **fusional/disparity vergence.**
   - Proximity of targets (i.e., **proximal vergence**; based on cues such as perspective)
   - Change in size (looming)
   - Monocular cues derived from motion
   - **Tonic vergence** (resting level of vergence tone)
   - **Voluntary vergence**

Cerebral Control of Vergence

Information about the role of cortical areas in vergence is relatively sparse. In the striate/primary visual cortex (area V1), three types of disparity neurons are present. (1) **Tuned-zero/near-zero neurons** respond to binocular stimuli over a narrow range about the fixation point. They may be responsible for fine stereopsis, and they provide input for ultra-short latency vergence response (60–85 msec) to small disparities in a large field, which may help stabilize the visual scene during self-motion. (2) **Tuned-far neurons** respond to binocular stimuli that are farther from fixation. They may be responsible for coarse stereopsis, and they provide input for vergence response to large disparities. (3) **Tuned-near neurons** respond to binocular stimuli that are nearer than fixation. Like tuned-far neurons, they may be responsible for coarse stereopsis, and they provide input for vergence response to large disparities. Other cerebral areas that participate in vergence include the frontal cortex immediately anterior to the saccade subregion of the frontal eye field, the frontal cortex within the pursuit subregion of the frontal eye field, the lateral intraparietal area in the parietal cortex, the middle temporal (MT), and medial superior temporal (MST) areas.

Brainstem Premotor and Motor Commands for Vergence

Neurons in the supra-oculomotor area within the **mesencephalic reticular formation** (MRF), 1–2 mm dorsal to the oculomotor nucleus, are involved in the control of vergence, and they presumably send premotor commands to ocular motor neurons. Three main types of neurons are present in the MRF: (1) **vergence tonic cells**, which discharge in relation to vergence angle; (2) **vergence burst cells**, which discharge in relation to vergence velocity; and (3) **vergence burst-tonic cells**, which discharge in relation to both vergence velocity and angle.

Some motoneurons in the abducens and oculomotor nuclei play a more important role in vergence. The medial rectus is innervated by three separate subgroups of motor neurons. The cells in the dorsomedial part of the oculomotor nucleus (subgroup C) have the smallest cell bodies and innervate the tonic fibers in the outer orbital layer of the medial rectus. These cells are believed to be principally concerned with vergence movements.

Cerebellar Control of Vergence

The medial part of **nucleus reticularis tegmenti pontis** (NRTP) in the basal pons contains neurons that discharge during vergence. The NRTP receives input from the frontal eye field and projects to the **dorsal vermis** and the **nucleus interpositus** in the cerebellum of monkeys (which corresponds to the **emboliform and globose nuclei** in humans). The dorsal vermis and the posterior nucleus interpositus contain neurons that discharge during far response. The dorsal vermis projects to the fastigial nucleus, which contains neurons that are active during near response. The **flocculus** contains neurons that discharge in relation to the angle of vergence eye position.

Lesions of the NRTP lead to impaired holding of vergence angle. Lesions of the dorsal vermis result in esodeviation (excess convergence); whereas lesions of the fastigial oculomotor region lead to exodeviation (excess divergence).

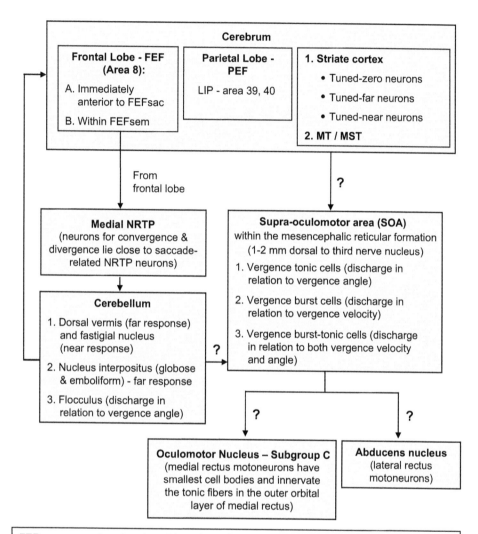

FEFsac = saccade subregion of frontal eye field; FEFsem = pursuit subregion of frontal eye field; PEF = parietal eye field; LIP = lateral intraparietal area; MT = middle temporal visual area; MST = medial superior temporal visual area; NRTP = nucleus reticularis tegmenti pontis

Clinical Points

Lesion of NRTP leads to impaired convergence.

Lesion of dorsal vermis leads to esodeviation (excess convergence).

Lesion of fastigial oculomotor region leads to exodeviation (excess divergence).

Both fusional and accommodative vergence can be assessed simultaneously by measuring the **near point of convergence** (NPC). Ask the patient to fixate on a small target as it is brought toward the nose. The NPC is the point at which fusion can no longer be maintained and divergent movement occurs. **Convergence insufficiency**, with abnormally high NPC, is commonly seen in Parkinson's disease and progressive supranuclear palsy.

To test fusional vergence only, ask the patient to fixate on a distant target. Put a horizontal prism in front of one eye to induce a fusional vergence movement, which is often accompanied by a saccade. By progressively increasing the amplitude of the prism until diplopia occurs (the breaking point of fusion), one can measure the range of fusional amplitude for both convergence and divergence.

The **near triad** consists of convergence, accommodation, and pupillary constriction. The **AC/A ratio** is the synkinetic relationship between accommodative-linked convergence and accommodation, and it normally ranges from 3 to 5. Accommodative vergence is often measured by the AC/A ratio. To calculate the AC/A ratio, first perform the cover–uncover test and use one of the following three methods:

1. **Clinical method**

$$\text{AC/A} = (D_n - D_d)/\text{accommodation}$$

where D_n and D_d are deviation at near and at distance, respectively, and accommodation (in diopters) = (1/distance at near) – (1/distance at far).

2. **Lens gradient method**

$$\text{AC/A} = (D_{cc} - D_{sc})/\text{power of lens}$$

where D_{cc} and D_{sc} is deviation with and without lens, respectively.

3. **Heterophoria method**

$$\text{AC/A} = \text{PD} + (D_n - D_d)/\text{accommodation}$$

where PD is pupillary distance in centimeters, and accommodation (in diopters) = (1/distance at near) – (1/distance at far).

The **CA/C ratio** is the synkinetic relationship between convergence-linked accommodation and convergence, and it normally ranges from 0.1 to 0.15. High AC/A ratio is usually associated with low CA/C ratio and vice versa.

To test both fusional and accommodative vergence simultaneously, measure the **near point of convergence**.

- Ask the patient to fixate on a small target as it is brought toward the nose. The NPC is the point at which fusion can no longer be maintained and divergent movement occurs.
- **Convergence insufficiency,** with abnormally high NPC, is common in Parkinson's disease and progressive supranuclear palsy.

To test fusional vergence only

- Ask the patient to fixate on a distant target. Put a horizontal prism in front of one eye to induce a fusional vergence movement, which is often accompanied by a saccade.
- By progressively increasing the amplitude of the prism until diplopia occurs (the breaking point of fusion), one can measure the range of fusional amplitude for both convergence and divergence.

To test accommodative vergence only

- The **near triad** consists of convergence, accommodation and pupillary constriction.
- The **AC/A ratio** is the synkinetic relationship between accommodative-linked convergence and accomodation (normal AC/A ratio is 3 to 5).
- Perform cover–uncover test and calculate AC/A ratio (three methods):

1. **Clinical method:**

$$AC/A = (D_n - D_d)/\text{accommodation (in diopters)},$$

where D_n and D_d are deviation at near and at distance, respectively, and accommodation $= (1/\text{distance at near}) - (1/\text{distance at far})$.

2. **Lens gradient method:**

$$AC/A = (D_{cc} - D_{sc})/\text{power of lens},$$

where D_{cc} and D_{sc} is deviation with an without lens, respectively.

3. **Heterophoria method:**

$$AC/A = PD \text{ (in cm)} + (D_n - D_d)/\text{accommodation},$$

where PD is pupillary disctance, and accomodation $= (1/\text{distance at near}) - (1/\text{distance at far})$.

- The **CA/C ratio** is the synkinetic relationship between convergence-linked accommodation and convergence (normal CA/C ratio is 0.1–0.15). High AC/A ratio is usually associated with low CA/C ratio and vice versa.

Part II

Nystagmus, Saccadic Dyskinesia, Other Involuntary Eye Movements, and Gaze Deviations

The word *nystagmus* comes from a Greek word for drowsiness or nodding, as in "nodding off to sleep." The idea is that a drowsy person's head shows the same alternating slow-quick pattern as ocular nystagmus; the head of a drowsy person drifts downward slowly and then snaps up in an attempt to regain wakefulness, before again resuming a downward drift.

By definition, nystagmus consists of involuntary oscillations of the eyes that are initiated by slow eye movements. If both phases are slow eye movements, it is called pendular nystagmus. If one phase is a saccade (quick phase), which alternates with a slow phase, it is called jerk nystagmus. Although the fundamental defect in nystagmus is an imbalance of slow eye movements that drives the eyes off their target, the direction of nystagmus is conventionally named in the direction of the corrective quick phases that return the eyes toward their target. The slow-eye-movement imbalance may due to defects in the vestibulo-ocular, smooth pursuit, optokinetic, or gaze-holding systems, or rarely in the vergence system.

Saccadic dyskinesia includes saccadic intrusions and oscillations. These are abnormal fast eye movements that drive the eyes away from their target and disrupt visual fixation. Involuntary fast eye movements that intermittently take the fovea off a target are called saccadic intrusions, whereas sustained abnormal fast eye movements are called saccadic oscillations. Some saccadic intrusions and oscillations have an interval between sequential saccades (e.g., square wave jerks, macro-square wave jerks, square wave oscillations, macrosaccadic oscillations), whereas others do not. The presence of an **intersaccadic interval** signifies the integrity of both pause cells that stop saccades and the neural integrator that sustains eye position between saccades. Saccadic dyskinesia usually occurs with lesions of the cerebellum or brainstem.

Both nystagmus and saccadic dyskinesia move the fovea off target, which results in a decrease in vision. They also cause oscillopsia, an illusion of motion in the stationary environment. When examining a patient with oscillopsia, it is crucial to ask him or her whether the oscillopsia is present only during head movements or whether it is present with or without head movements. Oscillopsia that is present during head movements usually occurs in patients with bilateral peripheral lesions of the vestibular end-organs or nerves, or in patients with central vestibular dysfunction as a result of lesions in the brainstem or cerebellum. Oscillopsia that is present independent of whether the head is stationary or moving is commonly seen in nystagmus and saccadic dyskinesia. This condition may also be seen in patients with extraocular muscle paresis because of abnormal gain of the vestibuloocular reflex, and rarely it is present with seizure or occipital lobe infarct (see section 7.2 for differential diagnosis of oscillopsia).

In this part, nystagmus is classified and discussed based on a pathophysiological approach (chapter 7). In chapter 8, saccadic dyskinesia, as well as other involuntary eye movements and gaze deviations, are discussed.

Nystagmus is involuntary eye oscillations initiated by slow eye movements that drive the eye away from the target. In contrast, saccadic dyskinesia consists of involuntary, fast eye movements that take the fovea off target. Nystagmus usually arises from lesions in the

1. Vestibulo-ocular system (VOR)
2. Gaze-holding system
3. Smooth pursuit and optokinetic system.

Characteristics of Nystagmus

1. Pendular versus jerk
   - Pendular (see A in the figure below): both phases are slow eye movements.
   - Jerk (see B, C, and D in the figure below): one phase consists of fast eye movements (quick phase), and the other consists of slow eye movements. By convention, the direction of nystagmus is named after the direction of quick phases that return the eye to the target.
2. Plane: horizontal, vertical, torsional, or combined form (e.g., rotary, elliptical)
3. Conjugacy
   - Conjugate: Both eyes move in the same direction with similar amplitude and frequency.
   - Disconjugate: Both eyes move in the same direction with different amplitude and frequency (e.g., internuclear ophthalmoplegia).
   - Disjunctive: The eyes move in opposite directions (e.g., oculomasticatory myorhythmia seen in Whipple's disease).
4. Amplitude
5. Frequency
6. Slow-phase waveform: decreasing, increasing, or constant velocity (see B, C, and D in the figure below)

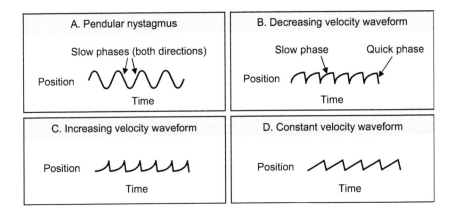

7.2 Differential Diagnosis of Oscillopsia

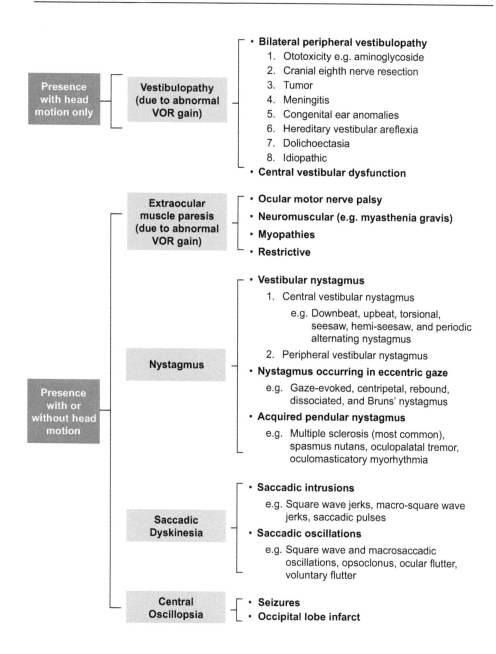

Presence with head motion only

Vestibulopathy (due to abnormal VOR gain)
- Bilateral peripheral vestibulopathy
  1. Ototoxicity e.g. aminoglycoside
  2. Cranial eighth nerve resection
  3. Tumor
  4. Meningitis
  5. Congenital ear anomalies
  6. Hereditary vestibular areflexia
  7. Dolichoectasia
  8. Idiopathic
- Central vestibular dysfunction

Extraocular muscle paresis (due to abnormal VOR gain)
- Ocular motor nerve palsy
- Neuromuscular (e.g. myasthenia gravis)
- Myopathies
- Restrictive

Presence with or without head motion

Nystagmus
- Vestibular nystagmus
  1. Central vestibular nystagmus
     e.g. Downbeat, upbeat, torsional, seesaw, hemi-seesaw, and periodic alternating nystagmus
  2. Peripheral vestibular nystagmus
- Nystagmus occurring in eccentric gaze
  e.g. Gaze-evoked, centripetal, rebound, dissociated, and Bruns' nystagmus
- Acquired pendular nystagmus
  e.g. Multiple sclerosis (most common), spasmus nutans, oculopalatal tremor, oculomasticatory myorhythmia

Saccadic Dyskinesia
- Saccadic intrusions
  e.g. Square wave jerks, macro-square wave jerks, saccadic pulses
- Saccadic oscillations
  e.g. Square wave and macrosaccadic oscillations, opsoclonus, ocular flutter, voluntary flutter

Central Oscillopsia
- Seizures
- Occipital lobe infarct

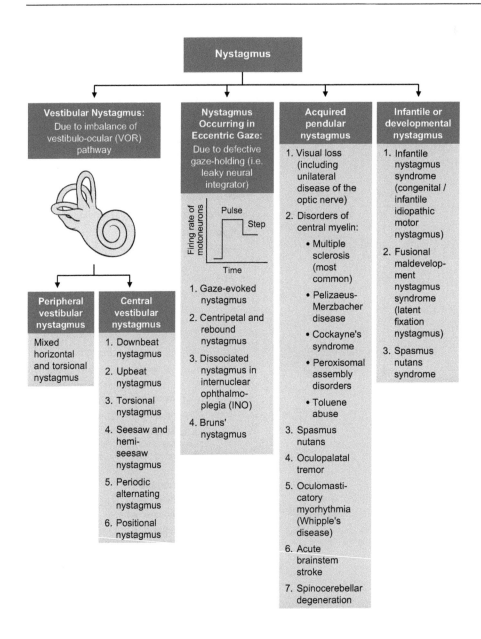

7.4 Peripheral Versus Central Vestibular Nystagmus

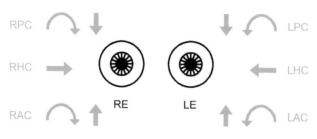

RE, LE = right, left eye

RHC, LHC = right, left horizontal canal

RAC, LAC = right, left anterior canal

RPC, LPC = right, left posterior canal

Direction of arrows = direction of slow phase of *both* eyes

Redrawn from Leigh RJ, Zee DS. The Neurology of Eye Movements. 3rd ed. New York: Oxford University Press; 1999. With permission of Oxford University Press.

Peripheral Vestibular Nystagmus

Caused by unilateral diseases of the vestibular organ and nerve (bilateral symmetric peripheral vestibulopathy does not cause nystagmus; instead, it causes oscillopsia from abnormal VOR gain).

1. Waveform
   - Mixed horizontal–torsional (e.g., $RHC + RAC + RPC = \curvearrowright \rightarrow$)
   - Linear (constant) velocity waveform
   - Jerk nystagmus
2. Unidirectional: follows **Alexander's law**, which states that nystagmus intensity increases during gaze in the direction of the quick phases
3. Suppressed by vision and smooth pursuit
4. Adaptation: nystagmus subsides in days
5. Other vestibular symptoms: vertigo, hearing loss, tinnitus
6. No other neurological signs

Central Vestibular Nystagmus

Caused by diseases of the brainstem and its connection with the vestibulocerebellum (i.e., flocculus, paraflocculus, and nodulus).

1. Waveform
   - Purely vertical, torsional, horizontal, or mixed (e.g., $RAC + LAC = \uparrow$ or $RAC + RPC = \curvearrowright$)
   - Linear, increasing, or deacreasing velocity waveforms
   - Jerk nystagmus
2. Reverse direction with gaze or unidirectional
3. Not suppressed by vision or smooth pursuit
4. No adaptation: nystagmus often persists
5. No other vestibular symptoms
6. Other brainstem or cerebellar signs present

- Peripheral vestibular diseases often cause a **positioning nystagmus**, which is caused by the actual head movement (this is in contrast to *positional* nystagmus, which is caused by a specific head position secondary to a central lesion).

- Positioning nystagmus is paroxysmal, and can be found in disorders such as benign paroxysmal positioning vertigo (BPPV), Ménière's disease, perilymph fistula, vestibular atelectasis, physiological "head extension vertigo" or "bending over vertigo."

7.5 Central Vestibular Nystagmus

7.5.1 Downbeat Nystagmus ▸▸

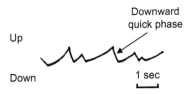

Characteristics

- Occurs in primary position
- Nystagmus intensity increases on lateral gaze (highly characteristic)
- Most are conjugate

Causes

1. Arnold-Chiari malformation (23%)
2. Cerebellar degeneration (23%)
3. Vertebrobasilar infarction (12%)
4. Multiple sclerosis (8%)
5. Drugs (e.g., phenytoin, carbamazepine, or lithium intoxication) (6%)
6. Idiopathic (21%)

Location of Lesion

1. Pontomedullary junction
2. Flocculus of the cerebellum

Pathogenesis

Disruption of posterior canal projections to brainstem tegmentum, leading to an upward bias (i.e., upward slow phase; see section 3.6).

Treatment

Suboccipital craniotomy for Arnold-Chiari malformation (see section 7.9).

7.5.2 Upbeat Nystagmus ▸▸

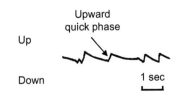

Characteristics

- Occurs in primary position
- Nystagmus intensity increases on upgaze (i.e., follows Alexander's law)
- Most are conjugate

Causes

1. Cerebellar degeneration (20%)
2. Brainstem and cerebellar infarct (20%)
3. Multiple sclerosis (13%)
4. Tumors (12%)
5. Others: vascular, infection, inflammation, metabolic, toxic, trauma

Location of Lesion

1. Superior cerebellar peduncle (i.e., brachium conjunctivum)
2. Bilateral midline lesions in pontomesencephalic or pontomedullary junction (damage in the nucleus prepositus hypoglossi, or the perihypoglossal nuclei, especially the nucleus intercalatus, or the cell groups of the paramedian tract; see section 9.2.3)

Pathogenesis

Disruption of anterior canal projections to the brainstem (via the brachium conjunctivum and ventral brainstem tegmentum), leading to a downward bias (i.e., downward slow phase).

Treatment

See section 7.9 for treatment details.

7.5.3 Torsional Nystagmus ▸▸

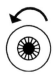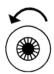

7.5.4 Seesaw and Hemi-Seesaw Nystagmus ▸▸

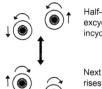

Half-cycle: RE falls & excyclotorts, LE rises & incyclotorts

Next half-cycle: RE rises & incyclotorts, LE falls & excyclotorts

Characteristics

- Upper pole of the eye beats away from the side of the lesion
- Most are conjugate

Causes

1. Infarction (37%)
2. Multiple sclerosis (20%)
3. Venous angioma (10%)
4. Arnold-Chiari malformation (7%)
5. Tumor (5%)
6. Encephalitis (5%)
7. Trauma (5%)
8. Seizure (5%)
9. Idiopathic (5%)

Location of lesion

1. Pontomedullary junction
2. Cerebellar or midbrain lesions are less common.

Pathogenesis

Disruption of anterior and posterior canal projections on the same side (see section 3.7).

Treatment

There is no definitive treatment.

Characteristics

- One half-cycle consists of depression and excyclotorsion of one eye and synchronous elevation and incyclotorsion of the fellow eye; during the next half-cycle, the movements reverse in each eye.
- If the waveform is pendular, it is called seesaw nystagmus; if it is jerk (i.e., one half-cycle being a quick phase), then it is called hemi-seesaw nystagmus.

Causes

1. Parasellar tumor (e.g., pituitary adenoma, craniopharyngioma; 13%)
2. Infarct or hemorrhage (9%)
3. Trauma (7%)
4. Congenital (7%)
5. Visual loss (5%)

Location of lesion

1. Pendular: diencephalic-midbrain lesion (often with bitemporal hemianopia)
2. Jerk (hemi-seesaw): unilateral midbrain or lateral medullary lesion

Pathogenesis

1. Abnormal central otolith projection to the interstitial nucleus of Cajal
2. Optic chiasmal lesion leads to damage of subcortical pathway to the inferior olivary nucleus and flocculus.

Treatment

See section 7.9 for treatment details.

7.5.5 Periodic Alternating Nystagmus ▸▸

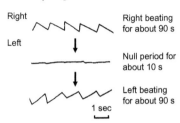

Right — Right beating for about 90 s

Left — Null period for about 10 s

Left beating for about 90 s

1 sec

Characteristics

- Right beating for about 90 sec (crescendo–decrescendo), stops for 5–20 sec (null period), then left beating for about 90 sec (crescendo–decrescendo)
- Follows Alexander's law: Nystagmus intensity increases on gaze in the direction of the quick phase
- May have periodic alternating head-turn to minimize nystagmus (i.e., head turn toward the direction of quick phases)

Causes

1. Congenital (may occur in albinism)
2. Arnold-Chiari malformation
3. Cerebellar degeneration
4. Multiple sclerosis
5. Infections
6. Tumors
7. Visual loss

Location of lesion

Lesions are located in the nodulus and uvula.

Pathogenesis

1. Increased gain of the central velocity storage mechanism of the VOR (see section 3.13) results in PAN in dark
2. Together with lack of visual input to the VOR from lesions in the flocculus, results in PAN in light

Treatment

See section 7.9 for treatment details.

7.5.6 Positional Nystagmus

Characteristics

- A new head position (detected by the otolith) causes the nystagmus, which continues as long as the head remains in the precipitating position.
- Due to lesions of the vestibulocerebellum or dorsolateral to the fourth ventricle

Types

1. Positional downbeat nystagmus
   - Due to lesions of the nodulus
   - A frequent and often the only clinical sign in neurologic patients
   - May spontaneously resolve or persist
2. Central positional nystagmus without vertigo
   - May beat diagonally or toward the undermost or uppermost ear (i.e., may change direction with head position)
   - Indicative of posterior fossa disease
3. Central positional nystagmus and vertigo (central BPPV or pseudo-BPPV; Note: BPPV is a peripheral vestibular disorder)
   - Lesions of the posterior cerebellar vermis
   - Purely torsional or purely vertical waveform
   - Often has other ocular motor signs (e.g., saccadic pursuit and gaze-evoked nystagmus)
4. Basilar insufficiency: nystagmus, vertigo, and postural imbalance induced with head maximally rotated or extended while standing; terminated abruptly by returning the head to a neutral, upright position

7.6.1 Physiological End-Point Nystagmus

Physiological end-point nystagmus is a normal phenomenon during extreme gaze. There are three types:

1. Unsustained end-point nystagmus—occurs for a few beats
2. Sustained end-point nystagmus—normal if present in both horizontal directions and low in amplitude ($<4°$)
3. Fatigue-induced end-point nystagmus—occurs after eccentric fixation for >30 sec

7.6.2 Gaze-Evoked Nystagmus ▶▶

The most common form of nystagmus, gaze-evoked nystagmus occurs during lateral or upward gaze (seldom on downward gaze) with quick phases beating away from primary position (i.e., centrifugal quick phases with centripetal slow drift).

Gaze-evoked nystagmus (GEN)

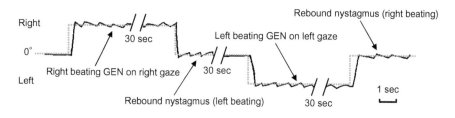

Pathogenesis

Pathogenesis involves defective gaze holding:

- Normal pulse but unsustained step, so that the eye drifts back to primary position after it moves to an eccentric position (see section 4.2)
- Due to "leaky" integrator: medial vestibular nucleus-nucleus prepositus hypoglossi (MVH-NPH) for horizontal gaze and intersitial nucleus of Cajal for vertical gaze

Causes

1. Drugs (e.g., alcohol, anticonvulsants [phenytoin, carbamazepine], sedatives [phenobarbiturates], and antidepressants [lithium])
2. Lesions in the cerebellum (especially the flocculus) and its projection to the brainstem (e.g., spinocerebellar degeneration, episodic ataxia type 2, multiple sclerosis, cerebellar or brainstem ischemia, and posterior fossa tumors)

7.6.3 Centripetal and Rebound Nystagmus

- Seen in some patients with gaze-evoked nystagmus

- On sustained eccentric gaze (>30 sec), gaze-evoked nystagmus decreases in amplitude, or it may even reverse direction, so that the eyes begin to drift centrifugally (away from primary position), resulting in a **centripetal nystagmus** (beating toward primary position).

- When the eyes return to primary position, **rebound nystagmus** occurs with quick phases beating in opposite direction to the gaze-evoked nystagmus when the eyes are in eccentric gaze, lasting for a few seconds (see figure on previous page).

- Rebound nystagmus typically occurs in patients with cerebellar disease and with experimental lesions of the MVH-NPH.

- Both centripetal and rebound nystagmus beat in the same direction and may represent an attempt by the brainstem or cerebellum to correct for the centripetal drift of the gaze-evoked nystagmus.

- Gaze-evoked, centripetal, and rebound nystagmus are seldom visually disabling unless severe because the eye drifts are minor when the eyes are close to central position.

7.6.4 Dissociated Nystagmus in Internuclear Ophthalmoplegia ▸▸

Dissociated nystagmus occurs during gaze away from the side of the lesion: The abducting eye exhibits an abducting centrifugal nystagmus (i.e., beating away from primary position), while the adducting eye on the same side of the MLF lesion exhibits a small or no nystagmus (see section 9.3.3). There are three possible explanations:

1. The abducting nystagmus may represent an attempt by the brain to adaptively correct for hypometric saccades due to the weak medial rectus. By adaptively increasing the innervation to the weak adducting eye, Hering's law dictates a conjugate increase of innervation to the abducting eye. This results in overshooting saccades and post-saccadic drift in the abducting eye. Because saccades initiate the oscillations, abducting "nystagmus" is not a true nystagmus, but rather a series of saccadic pulses.

2. The abducting nystagmus is a dissociated gaze-evoked nystagmus caused by interruption of the paramedian tracts, which are important for gaze holding. The nystagmus appears more prominent in the abducting eye because of adduction weakness in the adducting ipsilesional eye.

3. The abducting nystagmus is a result of an increased convergence tone, which leads to centripetal drift of contralesional eye with correcting saccades.

7.6.5 Bruns' Nystagmus

Brun's nystagmus is caused by cerebellopontine angle tumors (e.g., schwannoma of the eighth cranial nerve). This condition consists of

- Low frequency, large-amplitude horizontal nystagmus when the patient looks toward the side of lesion, due to defective gaze holding

- High frequency, small-amplitude nystagmus when the patient looks away from the side of lesion, due to vestibular imbalance

Characteristics

- **Acquired pendular nystagmus** is one of the more common types of nystagmus and is often associated with constant oscillopsia. It usually has horizontal, vertical, and torsional components with the same frequency, and one component may predominate. In contrast, congenital pendular nystagmus is predominantly horizontal, with a small torsional and negligible vertical component. (See table on next page)

- The nystagmus trajectory depends on the phase relationship between the different components. If the horizontal and vertical components are in phase, the trajectory is oblique. If the horizontal and vertical components are 180° out of phase, the trajectory is elliptical. If the horizontal and vertical components are 90° out of phase and have the same amplitude, the trajectory is circular.

- The nystagmus may be conjugate, disconjugate (sometimes appearing monocular), or disjunctive (convergent-divergent), but the frequency is usually the same in both eyes.

Etiology of Acquired Pendular Nystagmus
Visual loss (including unilateral disease of the optic nerve)
Disorders of central myelin
• Multiple sclerosis (most common)
• Pelizaeus-Merzbacher disease (see section 11.3.5)
• Cockayne's syndrome
• Peroxisomal assembly disorders
• Toluene abuse
Spasmus nutans (see section 7.8.3)
Oculopalatal tremor (see section 9.2.2)
Oculomasticatory myorhythmia (Whipple's disease; see section 9.4.4)
Acute brainstem stroke
Spinocerebellar degeneration

Pathogenesis

Acquired pendular nystagmus most likely results from an abnormality in the internal feedback circuits between brainstem nuclei and the cerebellum (e.g., the gaze-holding network), which are important for long-term recalibration using visual input.

Treatment

See section 7.9 for treatment.

Acquired pendular nystagmus with visual loss

- Most commonly caused by optic nerve disease; may resolve when vision is restored
- In unilateral optic nerve disease, the nystagmus mainly affects the abnormal eye (monocular nystagmus), with a prominent vertical, low-frequency, pendular waveform, and a less prominent horizontal jerk waveform.
- In bilateral optic nerve disease, the amplitude of the nystagmus is usually greater in the eye with poorer vision (i.e., the Heimann-Bielschowsky phenomenon). The **Heimann-Bielschowsky phenomenon** is also present with severe amblyopia, dense cataract, and high myopia.

	Acquired Pendular Nystagmus	Congenital pendular nystagmus
Waveform	Usually sinusoidal	Variable
Dissociation between eyes	Frequent (i.e., disconjugate or disjunctive)	Rare (i.e., usually conjugate)
Direction	Horizontal, vertical, or torsional	Horizontal and uniplanar (rarely vertical or torsional)
OKN reversal or inverted pursuit	No	Yes
Oscillopsia	Frequent	Rare

OKN, optokinetic nystagmus.

7.8 Infantile or Developmental Nystagmus

7.8.1 Infantile Nystagmus Syndrome (Congenital/Infantile Idiopathic Motor Nystagmus) ▸▸

Congenital jerk nystagmus

Right

Increasing velocity waveform

0°

Left

1 sec

Congenital pendular nystagmus

Right

Foveation periods

0°

Left

Characteristics

1. Usually horizontal (may be vertical or elliptical)

2. Most common waveform is jerk (with increasing velocity slow phase) or pendular

3. Conjugate

4. Uniplanar (i.e., the plane of nystagmus remains unchanged in all position of gaze). Uniplanar nystagmus is seen in only three conditions: congenital nystagmus, peripheral vestibular nystagmus, and periodic alternating nystagmus.

5. Intensity increases with fixation; decreases in darkness and with convergence (nystagmus blockage syndrome)

6. May be associated with head oscillation or latent nystagmus

7. No oscillopsia (i.e., oscillopsia is minimized by central suppression of image motion on the retina).

8. Foveation period (i.e., a brief [< 100 msec] period when the eye is closest to primary position). Visual acuity is related to the duration of the foveation periods.

9. Reversed optokinetic nystagmus (OKN) and inverted pursuit:

   - With an OKN drum, quick phases beat in the same direction as the drum rotation.

   - Velocity signals may be processed incorrectly with an inversion of sign, leading to wrongly directed smooth pursuit commands.

10. Null zone (i.e. an eye position in which nystagmus intensity is minimum and visual acuity is optimal). May adopt a head turn to keep the eyes in the null zone.

Management

- Cycloplegic refraction (astigmatism is frequently associated)

- Base-out prism stimulates convergence and may dampen nystagmus

- **Kestenbaum procedure** is a surgical procedure that places the null zone in primary position. For example, for left head turn, perform lateral rectus recession and medial rectus resection in the right eye, and medial rectus recession and lateral rectus resection in the left eye.

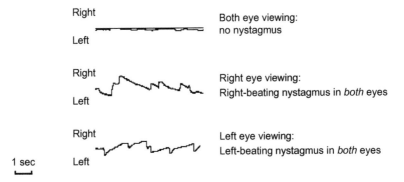

Characteristics

- Evoked or enhanced by covering one eye (i.e., during monocular viewing)
- Conjugate, horizontal nystagmus with quick phases of both eyes beating toward the fixating eye
- Direction of nystagmus reverses instantaneously when the fixating eye is switched to the fellow eye; a characteristic that differentiates it from acquired forms of nystagmus.
- Ophthalmoscopy of optic disc is a sensitive method to detect latent nystagmus. (Note that because the optic disc is behind the center of rotation of the globe, the direction of movement of the optic disc is opposite to the direction of the nystagmus.)

Associated ophthalmic and medical conditions

- Infantile esotropia (most common). Persists into adulthood despite surgical realignment.
- Any lesion that disrupts binocular development in the first six months of life, such as monocular cataract, glaucoma, corneal leukoma, marked anisometropia, constant infantile exotropia, or hypertropia.
- Down's syndrome

Associated eye movement abnormalities

Smooth pursuit and OKN asymmetry during monocular viewing

- Robust response when a target moves toward the nose, away from the temple
- Weak response when a target moves away from the nose, toward the temple

Dissociated vertical deviation ▸▸

- When the examiner covers one eye, the covered eye moves upward while the viewing eye maintains fixation.
- However, when the covered eye is now uncovered (i.e., both eyes viewing), the previously covered eye moves down to primary position, without any corresponding downward movement of the previously fixating eye, in violation of Herring's law.

7.8.3 Spasmus Nutans ▸▸

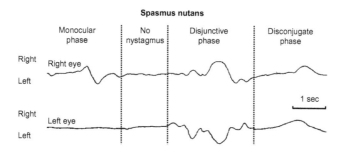

Spasmus nutans

Monocular phase | No nystagmus | Disjunctive phase | Disconjugate phase

Right eye
Right
Left

Left eye
Right
Left

1 sec

Spasmus nutans consists of a triad of nystagmus, head nodding, and abnormal head position.

Course

- Onset usually in first year of life
- No neurologic abnormalities
- Spontaneous remission usually within one to two years after onset; may persist more than eight years. Remission may reflect structural maturation of the central nervous system or "full calibration" of eye movements.

Characteristics of the Nystagmus

- Pendular: intermittent, small amplitude, and high frequency (3–11 Hz)
- Variable: conjugate, disconjugate, disjunctive, or monocular over the course of seconds to minutes
- Plane: predominantly horizontal, but may have a vertical or torsional component
- Intensity: greater intensity in the abducting eye and during convergence

Characteristics of Head Nodding

- Irregular with horizontal and vertical components (frequency ~3 Hz)
- Increases during attention
- In some patients, head nodding causes the nystagmus to cease.

Characteristics of Abnormal Head Posture

- Head tilt or head turn
- Present in about two-thirds of patients

Workup

1. MRI of the head to rule out tumor of the visual pathway, particularly optic chiasmal glioma
2. Differentiate spasmus nutans from infantile nystagmus. The nystagmus in spasmus nutans is intermittent, dissociated, and of higher frequency.

7.9 Treatment for Nystagmus

1. Treat underlying causes, such as drug intoxication, metabolic derangement, infection, and structural lesion.

2 Treat if patient is symptomatic (e.g., oscillopsia, decreased visual acuity, abnormal head posture).

3. There are only a few controlled treatment trials; thus, treatment is often based on a trial-and-error approach.

4. Listed in the table below are some medications reported to be effective. For nystagmus types that are not listed, there is little evidence for any drug benefit.

Nystagmus type	Treatment
Peripheral vestibular nystagmus	• Usually resolves spontaneously due to central compensation. Acute pharmacologic treatment should be used for up to 48 h to prevent delay in central compensation • Diphenhydramine (25–50 mg orally every 4–6 h) • Promethazine (12.5–25 mg orally every 4–6 h) • For **benign paroxysmal positional vertigo**, perform modified Epley procedure
Downbeat nystagmus	• 3,4-diaminopyridine (5–10 mg orally, 4–5 times per day, with maximum daily dose of 80 mg) • 4-aminopyridine (10 mg orally per day) • Clonazepam (1.5 mg orally per day in 3 divided doses; increase by 0.5–1.0 mg every 3 days to a maximum daily dose of 20 mg) • Baclofen (5 mg orally, 3 times per day; increase by 5 mg per week to a maximum daily dose of 80 mg) • Acetazolamide for nystagmus associated with **episodic ataxia type 2** (250 mg orally per day; increase by 250 mg every 3 days to a maximum daily dosage of 3 g) • Suboccipital craniotomy for **Arnold-Chiari malformation**
Upbeat nystagmus	• Baclofen (same dosage as for downbeat nystagmus)
Seesaw nystagmus	• Baclofen (same dosage as for downbeat nystagmus) • Clonazepam (same dosage as for downbeat nystagmus) • Gabapentin (100 mg orally, 3 times per day; increase by 100 mg every 3 days to a maximum dose of 1200 mg 3 times per day) • Alcohol

continued

Nystagmus type	Treatment
Periodic alternating nystagmus	• Baclofen (same dosage as for downbeat nystagmus)
Acquired pendular nystagmus	• Memantine (5 mg orally per day; increase by 5 mg per week to a maximum daily dose of 10 mg twice per day) • Gabapentin (same dosage as for seesaw nystagmus) • Clonazepam (same dosage as for downbeat nystagmus) • Valproate (10–60 mg/kg orally per day) • Scopolamine (1.5 mg transdermally every 3 days)

Chapter 8

*Saccadic Dyskinesia, Other Involuntary
Eye Movements, and Gaze Deviations*

8.1.1 Square Wave Jerks ▸▸

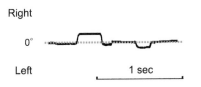

Right

0°

Left   1 sec

Characteristics

- A small saccade of 0.5–3° that takes the eye away from fixation, followed by a saccade that returns the eye back to fixation after about 200 msec (i.e., presence of intersaccadic interval during which visual feedback occurs)

- So named because of its appearance in eye movement tracings (see figure above)

- Normal subjects often have square wave jerks (SWJ), but the rate is only 4–6 per minute.

- Pathologic SWJ occurs at a rate of >15 per minute.

Etiology

- Cerebellar diseases (e.g., cerebellar degeneration, masses, multiple sclerosis)

- Basal ganglion diseases (e.g.. Parkinson's disease, progressive supranuclear palsy, multiple system atrophy)

- Cerebral cortical diseases

Pathogenesis

Square wave jerks result from damage of projections from the frontal eye field, rostral pole of the superior colliculus, and the central mesencephalic reticular formation to the omnipause cells in the pons.

Treatment

If symptomatic, SWJ may be treated with methylphenidate, diazepam, phenobarbital, or amphetamines.

8.1.2 Macro-Square Wave Jerks

Characteristics

Macro-square wave jerks are similar to SWJ but with amplitudes ranging from 4 to 50°, and they occur in burst.

Etiology

Macro-square wave jerks are associated with cerebellar or brainstem diseases affecting cerebellar outflow (e.g., spinocerebellar degeneration, masses, multiple sclerosis, Arnold-Chiari malformation, Friedreich's ataxia).

Pathogenesis

Macro-square wave jerks result from defective GABA (γ-aminobutyric acid) inhibition of the superior colliculus by substantia nigra pars reticulata.

Treatment

Diazepam or phenobarbital may be used to treat macro-square wave jerks.

Right

0°

Left

Characteristics

- Burst of saccades with defective steps of innervation (i.e., stepless saccades)
- Conjugate or monocular

Etiology

Saccadic pulses are associated with multiple sclerosis.

Pathogenesis

Saccadic pulses result from damage of omnipause cells or the neural integrator. A pulse of innervation drives the eye to a new position; however, there is no step to hold the eye in its new position, so the eye drifts back to its previous position (with decreasing velocity exponential waveform)

8.2 Saccadic Oscillations: Continuous Disruptions of Fixation (Salvos of Saccadic Intrusions)

8.2.1 Square Wave Oscillations

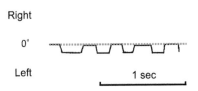

Right

0°

Left

1 sec

8.2.2 Macrosaccadic Oscillations ▸▸

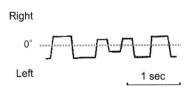

Right

0°

Left

1 sec

Characteristics

Square wave oscillations are similar to SWJ, but they occur continuously rather than sporadically.

Etiology

Square wave oscillations are associated with Parkinson's disease with alcoholic cerebellar degeneration and with progressive supranuclear palsy.

Characteristics

- A series of large saccades that straddle fixation (i.e., passing from one side to the other side of the target), overshooting it each time without foveation of the target.

- Intersaccadic intervals of 200 msec when the eye is stationary in the eccentric position

- Characteristic spindle shape on eye movement recordings: The amplitude of the saccades increases and then decreases within a burst.

- Triggered by saccades

- Vanish in darkness and are replaced by more irregular saccadic eye movements

Etiology

Macrosaccadic oscillations result from deep cerebellar lesions affecting the vermis and paramedian nuclei (e.g., hemorrhage, tumor, or multiple sclerosis, and paraneoplastic syndrome).

Pathogenesis

Macrosaccadic oscillations arise from abnormal calibration of saccadic size by the cerebellum with excessive gain, resulting in hypermetric primary and corrective saccades that oscillate around the desired eye position.

8.2.3 Opsoclonus and Ocular Flutter ▶▶

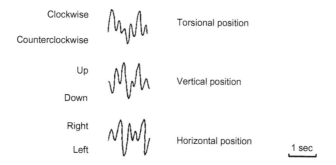

Clockwise / Counterclockwise — Torsional position

Up / Down — Vertical position

Right / Left — Horizontal position

1 sec

Characteristics

- Consist of saccadic oscillations with no intersaccadic interval

  Ocular flutter is confined to one plane, usually horizontal.

  Opsoclonus involves all three planes (horizontal, vertical, and torsional). Other terms for opsoclonus include saccadomania, "dancing eyes," and ocular myoclonus.

- High-frequency oscillations (10–15 Hz) with large and variable amplitude
- Present during fixation, pursuit, convergence, sleep, and eyelid closure

Etiology of Opsoclonus and Ocular Flutter

In Children

Encephalopathic or parainfectious (e.g., rubella, mumps, coxsackie B virus).
Paraneoplastic (neuroblastoma is responsible for the majority of paraneoplastic opsoclonus).

- Other signs: myoclonus, ataxia (i.e., opsoclonus–myoclonus syndrome)
- 2% of neuroblastoma patients present initially with opsoclonus–myoclonus.
- 59% of patients with opsoclonus–myoclonus have occult neuroblastoma
- Peak incidence: 18 months

Neonatal (e.g., intrauterine anoxia, intracranial hemorrhage)
Idiopathic
Others: hydrocephalus, thallium intoxication, *Haemophilus influenza,* poliomyelitis vaccination, or infection

In Adults

Encephalopathic (usually occurs in patients < 40 years old; e.g., viral)
Paraneoplastic (usually occurs in patients > 40 years old; e.g., lung or breast carcinoma)
Toxic-metabolic: medications (lithium, amitriptyline), toxins (strychnine, cocaine, thallium, organophosphates), metabolic (hyperosmolar coma)
Idiopathic (50%)
Others: vascular, head trauma, multiple sclerosis, tumor

Pathogenesis

- Disinhibition of the **fastigial nucleus** in the cerebellum due to malfunctioning of Purkinje cells in the dorsal vermis that normally inhibit the fastigial nucleus
- Damage to omnipause cells in the pons
- Changes in synaptic organization of excitatory and inhibitory saccadic burst neurons in the brainstem may cause saccadic oscillations whenever omnipause cells are inhibited.

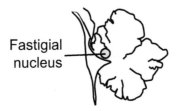

Fastigial nucleus

Mid-sagittal section of the cerebellum

Workup

1. Neuroimaging results are usually normal.
2. Lumbar puncture results are usually normal; they may show mild pleocytosis or protein elevation.
3. Antineuronal antibodies tests (e.g., Ri, Yo, Hu, Ma1, Ma2, amphiphysin, CV2, CRMP-5, neurofilaments).
   - The majority of patients do not have specific antineuronal antibodies; therefore, the presence of antibodies confirm the diagnosis, but their absence does not exclude the diagnosis.
   - The tumor and the central nervous system share a common epitope, which elicits an immune response against both the tumor and normal neural tissue.
   - Children with paraneoplastic opsoclonus have a better oncologic prognosis, regardless of disease stage, due to a single copy of N-*myc* oncogene.
4. Systemic workup in children
   - Computed tomography or MRI of chest and abdomen
   - Urinary catecholamines (vanillyl mandelic acid, homovanillic acid)
   - If negative, consider total-body scintigraphy with metaiodobenzylguanidine, which has a sensitivity of 95% and specificity of 100% for neuroblastoma
   - If all of the above tests are negative, repeat evaluation after several months.
5. Systemic workup in adults
   - Computed tomography or MRI of chest and abdomen
   - Gynecological exam and mammography for women
   - If negative, consider [^{18}F]fluorodeoxyglucose-positron emission tomography whole-body scan

Treatment

For idiopathic or parainfectious/encephalopathic opsoclonus, treatment consists of corticosteroids, propranolol, verapamil, clonazepam, and thiamine. For paraneoplastic opsoclonus, treat the underlying cause.

Children

1. Corticosteroids or adrenocorticotropic hormone (ACTH)
2. May try intravenous immunoglobulin (IVIG)

Adults

1. Corticosteroids or ACTH (results not consistent)
2. May try plasmapheresis, IVIG, immunoadsorption, and biotin

Course and prognosis

Children with paraneoplastic or idiopathic conditions

- Multiple relapses require prolonged treatment.
- Significant developmental sequelae occur even with treatment (motor, cognitive, language, and psychological deficits).

Adults

- Idiopathic/parainfectious conditions are monophasic with good recovery. In older patients, relapses and residual gait ataxia may occur.
- Paraneoplastic conditions present a more severe course despite treatment. Without treatment of the underlying tumor, mortality rate is high. With treatment of the underlying tumor, most have complete or partial neurological recovery.

8.2.4 Voluntary Flutter (Voluntary Nystagmus) ▸▸

Voluntary nystagmus is present in about 8% of normal population and may occur as a familial trait.

Characteristics

- Horizontal, conjugate, saccadic oscillations that can be initiated at will, with frequency and amplitude similar to those seen in opsoclonus and ocular flutter
- Can only be maintained briefly (at most, about 30 sec)
- Often initiated by convergence
- Often accompanied by fluttering of the eyelids (which is not in synchrony with the eye oscillations), pupillary constriction, and contraction of other facial muscles in an expression of effort
- Oscillopsia and decreased vision during the oscillations

Workup

1. Usually completely normal neurologically
2. Look for signs that indicate a pathologic process (e.g., ocular dysmetria, cerebellar ataxia, and shivering myoclonus)

8.3.1 Ocular Bobbing

Typical bobbing (initial phase: fast and down)

- Rhythmic, downward jerks, followed by slow return to mid-position
- Associated with *bilateral horizontal gaze palsy* (including horizontal vestibulo-ocular response [VOR]; i.e., no response to caloric testing)

Causes

1. Intrinsic pontine lesion (e.g., infarct or hemorrhage)
2. Cerebellar hemorrhage compressing the pons
3. Subarachnoid hemorrhage from aneurysms of the posterior circulation

Atypical bobbing (initial phase: fast and down)

Atypical bobbing is similar to typical bobbing, but with some *residual horizontal gaze* (i.e., can have full horizontal eye movements, or internuclear ophthalmoplegia, or unilateral or bilateral abducens palsy).

Causes

1. Pontine hemorrhage
2. Central pontine myelinolysis (see section 9.3.1)
3. Metabolic, hepatic, or hypoxic encephalopathy
4. Obstructive hydrocephalus
5. Cerebellar hematoma

Pretectal V-pattern pseudo-bobbing (initial phase: fast and down)

- Downward and convergent jerks, slow return to mid-position
- Associated with other pretectal signs (see section 9.4.3)

Cause

Acute obstructive hydrocephalus including shunt malfunction.

Reverse bobbing (initial phase: fast and up)

Reverse bobbing is characterized by upward jerks, followed by slow return to mid-position.

Causes

Metabolic encephalopathy, phenothiazine and benzodiazepine intoxication.

Ocular dipping or inverse bobbing (initial phase: slow and down)

Ocular dipping is characterized by slow, downward movements over 2 sec, which remain tonically depressed for 2–10 sec, followed by rapid return to mid-position.

Causes

Anoxic coma, carbon monoxide poisoning, status epilepticus, or head trauma.

Converse bobbing (initial phase: slow and up)

- Also referred to as "inverse/reverse ocular bobbing"
- Slow, upward movements over 1–5 sec, which remain tonically elevated for 1–10 sec, followed by rapid return to mid-position

Causes

Pontine infarction, AIDS-related cryptococcal meningitis, or lithium and carbamazepine toxicity.

8.3.2 Gaze Deviations

Horizontal Gaze Deviations

Sustained

1. Ipsilesional deviation: acute cerebral hemispheric infarcts, especially with right-sided large and posterior lesion
2. Contralesional "wrong-way" deviation: thalamic lesions; pontine lesions (below the oculomotor decussation at the pontomesencephalic junction); other supratentorial diseases such as frontoparietal hemorrhages (rare)

Intermittent

1. Epileptic seizures
2. Periodic alternating gaze deviation
   - Conjugate horizontal gaze deviation that changes direction every 1–2 min
   - Causes: Arnold-Chiari malformation, medulloblastoma, Creutzfeldt-Jacob disease, or hepatic encephalopathy
   - Pathogenesis: related to periodic alternating nystagmus; likely due to the same VOR disinhibition from dysfunction of the nodulus and uvula in the cerebellum
3. Ping-pong gaze
   - Slow, conjugate horizontal gaze deviation that changes direction every few seconds
   - Causes: bilateral cerebral infarction or posterior fossa hemorrhage

Upward Gaze Deviations

Sustained

1. Hypoxic-ischemic insult
2. Oculogyric crisis and other drug effects (see section 11.2.2)
3. Lesion in the periaqueductal gray matter

Intermittent: paroxysmal tonic upgaze of childhood with ataxia

1. Age of onset: 2–20 months
2. Characteristics
   - Consists of tonic or intermittent upward deviation lasting seconds to minutes, frequently recurring over minutes to hours, with or without brief downbeating jerks
   - Tendency to adopt a chin-down head posture during prolonged episodes
   - Truncal and gait ataxia
   - Self limiting, but may last months to a few years
3. Treatment: levadopa, 100–150 mg daily, may be effective

Downward Gaze Deviations

Sustained

1. Compressive lesions on the dorsal midbrain (e.g., tumor, hemorrhage, and hydrocephalus)
2. Thalamic hemorrhage
3. Healthy neonates
   - Full range of eye movements
   - Normal imaging
   - Resolves by six months
4. Premature infants with intraventricular hemorrhage and hydrocephalus
   - Accompanied by upgaze paresis and large-angle esotropia (due to damage of pretectal structures; see section 9.4.3)
   - The combination of downward gaze deviation and lid retraction is known as the "setting sun" sign

Intermittent

Paroxysmal downward gaze deviation is seen in periventricular leukomalacia (e.g., premature infants with cerebral palsy, retardation, and visual impairment).

Part III

Supranuclear and Internuclear Ocular Motor Disorders

Supranuclear and internuclear ocular motor disorders are caused by damage in different parts of the brain before eye movement signals reach the ocular motor nuclei. This damage may include lesions in the brainstem (medulla, pons, and midbrain), cerebellum, and cerebrum (thalamus, basal ganglia, and cerebral hemispheres). In this part of the book, clinical–pathological correlations for supranuclear and internuclear ocular motor disorders are discussed using an anatomic approach.

A number of structures in the medulla are particularly important for eye movement control. They include the medial vestibular nucleus and the adjacent nucleus prepositus hypoglossi, which are critical for horizontal and vertical gaze-holding, as well as the inferior olivary nucleus and its projections, via the inferior cerebellar peduncle, to the cerebellum. Lateral medullary syndrome and oculopalatal tremor are the most recognized syndromes that feature prominent ocular motor abnormalities in lesions involving the medulla.

Structures in the pons that are important for horizontal eye movements include the abducens nucleus, the paramedian pontine reticular formation, and the medial longitudinal fasciculus (MLF). In the midbrain, structures that are critical for vertical eye movements include the rostral interstitial nucleus of the medial longitudinal fasciculus, the interstitial nucleus of Cajal, and the posterior commissure. Although lesions in the pons commonly cause abnormal horizontal eye movements, and lesions in the midbrain commonly cause disturbances in vertical eye movements, this is an oversimplification. For example, lesions in the pons that damage the MLF commonly cause internuclear ophthalmoplegia—a combination of adducting deficit in the ipsilesional eye and abducting nystagmus in the contralesional eye. However, because the MLF also carries fibers for vertical gaze-holding, smooth pursuit, and the vestibulo-ocular reflex (VOR), bilateral lesions of the MLF in the pons also cause disturbances of vertical eye movements. The specific ocular motor abnormalities seen in lesions in different parts of the brainstem are discussed in chapter 9. Inflammatory, infectious, toxic, and degenerative diseases, as well as vergence disorders, in which supranuclear and internuclear eye movement disorders are prominent are also discussed in chapter 9.

Lesions involving the cerebellum cause abnormal eye movements in two ways. First, cerebellar lesions are often associated with damages in the brainstem, which can produce cerebellar dysfunctions by virtue of its projections to cerebellar Purkinje cells via the climbing fiber. Second, cerebellar lesions alone can also cause specific eye movement abnormalities. Three principal syndromes are observed: the syndrome of the flocculus and ventral paraflocculus, the syndrome of the nodulus and uvula, and the syndrome of the dorsal vermis and its underlying fastigial nuclei. The main features of these syndromes are discussed in chapter 10.

The manifestations of abnormal eye movements in cerebral diseases are varied. Thalamic lesions cause disturbances of both horizontal and vertical gaze. A number of conditions that affect the basal ganglia, including Parkinson's disease and Huntington's disease, also cause abnormal eye movements. The ocular motor disturbances that result from lesions in the cerebral hemispheres depend on a number of factors, including the duration (acute vs. chronic), size (diffuse vs. focal), location, and the laterality (unilateral vs. bilateral) of the lesions. Chapter 11 presents the specific ocular motor abnormalities seen in lesions in different parts of the cerebrum.

Chapter 9

Ocular Motor Disorders Caused by Lesions in the Brainstem

9.1 Important Brainstem Structures for Ocular Motor Control

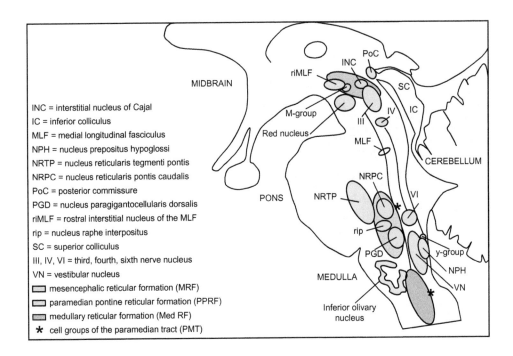

INC = interstitial nucleus of Cajal
IC = inferior colliculus
MLF = medial longitudinal fasciculus
NPH = nucleus prepositus hypoglossi
NRTP = nucleus reticularis tegmenti pontis
NRPC = nucleus reticularis pontis caudalis
PoC = posterior commissure
PGD = nucleus paragigantocellularis dorsalis
riMLF = rostral interstitial nucleus of the MLF
rip = nucleus raphe interpositus
SC = superior colliculus
III, IV, VI = third, fourth, sixth nerve nucleus
VN = vestibular nucleus
▭ mesencephalic reticular formation (MRF)
▭ paramedian pontine reticular formation (PPRF)
▭ medullary reticular formation (Med RF)
✱ cell groups of the paramedian tract (PMT)

Medulla	Pons	Midbrain

1. Perihypoglossal nucleus
  ▪ Nucleus prepositus hypoglossi (NPH)
  ▪ Nucleus interclatatus
  ▪ Nucleus of Roller
2. Vestibular nucleus
3. Medullary reticular formation
4. Inferior olivary nucleus
5. Inferior cerebellar peduncle (restiform body)
6. Cell groups of the paramedian tracts
7. y-group
	1. Abducens nucleus
	2. Paramedian pontine reticular formation
	  ▪ Nucleus reticularis pontis caudalis
	  ▪ Nucleus raphe interpositus
	  ▪ Nucleus paragiganto-cellularis dorsalis
	  ▪ Cell groups of the paramedian tract
	3. Medial longitudinal fasciculus
	4. Nucleus reticularis tegmenti pontis
	5. Dorsolateral pontine nuclei (not shown in figure above)
		1. Rostral interstitial nucleus of the MLF (riMLF)
		2. Interstitial nucleus of Cajal
		3. Posterior commissure
		4. Nucleus of the posterior commissure (not shown in the figure above)
		5. Medial longitudinal fasciculus
		6. Oculomotor (III) and trochlear (IV) nucleus
		7. Central mesencephalic reticular formation
		8. M-group

9.2 Ocular Motor Syndromes Caused by Lesions in the Medulla

9.2.1 Lesions in the Lateral Medulla: Lateral Medullary Syndrome (Wallenberg's Syndrome)

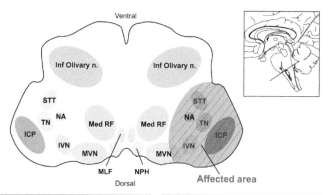

Affected structures:
- MVN = Medial vestibular nucleus
- IVN = Inferior vestibular nucleus
- ICP = Inferior cerebellar peduncle
- TN = Spinal nucleus of trigeminal nerve & tract
- STT = Spinothalamic tract
- NA = Nucleus ambiguus

NPH = Nucleus prepositus hypoglossi
Med RF = Medullary reticular formation
Inf olivary n. = Inferior olivary nucleus
MLF = Medial longitudinal fasciculus

Clinical Features of Lateral Medullary Syndrome

Ipsilesional

- Lateropulsion (i.e., a compelling sensation of being pulled toward the side of the lesion) results from involvement of the inferior cerebellar peduncle.
- Ipsilesional limb ataxia results from involvement of the inferior cerebellar peduncle.
- Ipsilesional impairment of pain and temperature sensation of the face results from involvement of the spinal nucleus of trigeminal nerve and its tract.
- Ipsilesional dysarthria, dysphagia, loss of gag reflex, and hoarseness results from involvement of the nucleus ambiguus.
- Ipsilesional Horner's syndrome results from involvement of descending sympathetic fibers from the hypothalamus.

Contralesional

Contralesional impairment of pain and temperature sensation of the trunk and limbs results from involvement of the spinothalamic tract.

Vertigo

Vertigo results from involvement of the vestibular nucleus.

Hiccups

The cause of hiccups is unknown; they may result from involvement of the medullary reticular formation.

Occlusion of ipsilateral vertebral artery (most common)

Occlusion of posterior inferior cerebellar artery

Dissection of vertebral artery (spontaneous or traumatic)

Demyelinating disease

Eye Movement Abnormalities in Lateral Medullary Syndrome

Ipsipulsion of saccades[1] ▶▶

- Ipsipulsion of horizontal saccades: hypermetric ipsilesional saccades, and hypometric contralesional saccades
- Ipsipulsion of vertical saccades: inappropriate horizontal component toward the side of the lesion, causing an oblique trajectory of vertical saccades
- Torsipulsion (i.e. inappropriate torsional "blips") which may occur during horizontal saccades

Deviation of the eyes toward the side of the lesion (lateropulsion)

Occurs behind closed lids, in darkness, or with a blink

Impaired contralesional smooth pursuit

Ocular tilt reaction[2] (OTR)

Ipsilesional hypotropia, ipsilesional head tilt, excyclotorsion of the ipsilesional eye, and tilt of subjective visual vertical toward the side of lesion (e.g. the whole room tilts on its side or even upside down, but is usually transient; see section 9.5.2)

Spontaneous nystagmus in central position

- Mixed horizontal–torsional waveform ▶▶
- Slow phases may be directed toward or away from the side of the lesion.
- Lid nystagmus presents as twitching of lids synkinetic with horizontal quick phases

Head nystagmus[3]

---

1. Lateropulsion and ipsipulsion of saccades results from involvement of inferior cerebellar peduncle (restiform body), which carries olivocerebellar projections from the inferior olivary nucleus. This results in an interruption of climbing fiber input from the inferior cerebellar peduncle to the dorsal vermis, thus releasing Purkinje cell inhibition on the fastigial nucleus, leading to findings similar to those found in lesions of the fastigial nucleus (see section 10.2.2).

2. OTR results from an imbalance of otolithic input.

3. Head nystagmus may reflect a lesion in vestibulospinal and reticulospinal projections to cervical motoneurons.

9.2.2 Lesions in the Inferior Olivary Nucleus: Oculopalatal Tremor ▸▸

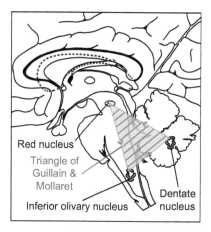

Red nucleus
Triangle of Guillain & Mollaret
Inferior olivary nucleus
Dentate nucleus

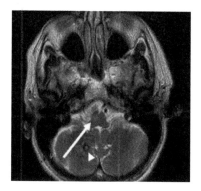

Axial MRI showing hypertrophic degeneration of the inferior olivary nucleus (arrow) in the medulla and a cavernoma with hemorrhage in the cerebellum (arrowhead).

Oculopalatal tremor usually occurs many months after an initial insult, due to neural deafferentation. It rarely resolves spontaneously. Treatment is with gabapentin, ceruletide, or anticolinergic agents.

Etiology of Oculopalatal Tremor
Infarct
Hemorrhage
Demyelination (rare)

Eye Movement Abnormalities in Inferior Olivary Nucleus Lesion: Oculopalatal Tremor
Vertical pendular nystagmus[1]
Synchronous rhythmic movements of the pharynx, face, tensor tympani, vocal cords, shoulders, and respiratory muscles[2]

---

1. Pathogenesis of vertical pendular nystagmus: results from involvement of the **Triangle of Guillain and Mollaret**, which consists of:

- Red nucleus in the midbrain (which projects to the inferior olivary nucleus via the central tegmental tract)
- Inferior olivary nucleus in the medulla (which projects to the contralateral dentate nucleus via the olivocerebellar tract in the inferior cerebellar peduncle)
- Contralateral dentate nucleus in the cerebellum (which projects to the red nucleus via the superior cerebellar peduncle)

Hypertrophic degeneration of inferior olivary nucleus (which contains increased acetylcholine-esterase reaction product) is necessary but not sufficient for the genesis of the nystagmus

2. Pathogenesis of palatal tremor: results from rostral cerebellar or brainstem damage that denervates the dorsal cap of inferior olivary nucleus.

9.2.3 Other Medullary Lesions

Paramedian medulla

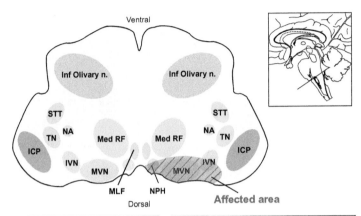

Affected structures:
- NPH = nucleus prepositus hypoglossi
- MVN = medial vestibular nucleus
- IVN = inferior vestibular nucleus
- Ventral tegmental tract
- Cell groups of the paramedian tracts i.e. the medullary nucleus pararaphales

Med RF = medullary reticular formation
Inf Olivary n. = inferior olivary nucleus
MLF = medial longitudinal fasciculus
ICP = inferior cerebellar peduncle

Eye Movement Abnormalities in Paramedian Medullary Lesion

Upbeat nystagmus (most common)[1]

Horizontal nystagmus with gaze-evoked component[2]

---

1. Upbeat nystagmus may be a result of:
- Lesion in the ventral tegmental pathway for upward VOR (which is mediated by anterior canals), leading to a downward vestibular bias, and thus, upbeat nystagmus (see section 7.5.2); or
- Lesion in one component of the cell groups of the paramedian tracts (PMT), the medullary nucleus pararaphales, which receives vertical eye position signals from the interstitial nucleus of Cajal (INC) for vertical gaze-holding

2. Horizontal nystagmus with gaze-evoked component may result from lesion in the medial vestibular nucleus and nucleus prepositus hypoglossi (MVN-NPH), which are important for horizontal gaze-holding.

The y-group

The y-group is a small group of cells that lies rostral to the inferior cerebellar peduncle.

It receives inputs from the saccule (part of the otolith) and from Purkinje cells of the flocculus, and it projects to the oculomotor and trochlear nuclei via the superior cerebellar peduncle and a crossing ventral tegmental tract.

Functions

1. Discharge during upward smooth pursuit, optokinetic, and combined eye-head tracking (VOR cancellation), but not during VOR in darkness (see sections 3.14 and 5.2)
2. Together with the flocculus and ventral paraflocculus, may contribute to vertical VOR adaptation (see section 3.12)

No known documented clinical correlate

Cell groups of the paramedian tracts

Collections of neurons scattered along the midline fiber tracts in the pons and medulla, including:

1. The **nucleus pararaphales** in the medulla, which receives vertical eye position signals from the INC, and projects to the flocculus and ventral paraflocculus
2. The **nucleus incertus** in the pons, which contains burst-tonic neurons that mainly discharge in relation to horizontal eye movements, and projects to the flocculus

   Function: may send an "efference copy" of eye movement commands to the flocculus for gaze holding or longer term adaptation

   No known documented clinical correlate

9.3.1 Lesions in the Abducens Nucleus

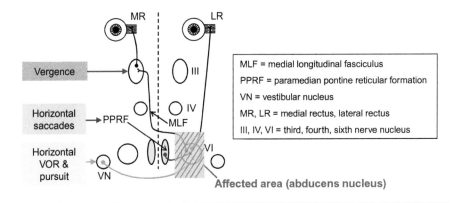

MLF = medial longitudinal fasciculus
PPRF = paramedian pontine reticular formation
VN = vestibular nucleus
MR, LR = medial rectus, lateral rectus
III, IV, VI = third, fourth, sixth nerve nucleus

Affected area (abducens nucleus)

The abducens nucleus contains:

1. Abducens motoneurons that innervate the ipsilateral lateral rectus
2. Abducens internuclear neurons, the axons of which cross the midline and ascend via the MLF to innervate the contralateral medial rectus motoneurons in the oculomotor nucleus.
3. Neurons that project to the cerebeller flocculus

The abducens nucleus is the final common motor pathway for horizontal conjugate eye movements, as it receives input for horizontal saccades, VOR, and smooth pursuit.

Eye Movement Abnormalities in Abducens Nucleus Lesion: Horizontal Conjugate Gaze Palsy

Ipsilesional horizontal gaze palsy
- loss of all conjugate movements (saccades, pursuit, VOR) toward the side of the lesion
- sparing of vertical movements and vergence[1]

Acutely, manifests as contralesional gaze deviation.

Horizontal gaze-evoked nystagmus occurs on looking contralesionally, with quick phases directed away from the side of the lesion.[2]

Ipsilesional facial palsy[3]

---

1. Vergence is spared because vergence commands are sent directly to medial rectus motoneurons in the oculomotor nucleus, without passing through the abducens nucleus or the MLF.

2. Horizontal gaze-evoked nystagmus may be a result of interruption of fibers of passage from the medial vestibular nucleus, or from the cell groups of the paramedian tracts (PMT), both of which are involved in gaze-holding.

3. Ipsilesional facial palsy results from involvement of the genu of the facial nerve which loops around the abducens nucleus (see section 12.4.1).

Congenital diseases

- Bilateral Duane's syndrome
- Möbius syndrome
- Horizontal gaze palsy and progressive scoliosis (HGPPS)
- Congenital horizontal gaze paralysis and ear dysplasia
- Familial congenital paralysis of horizontal gaze

Lesions in the brainstem

- Pontine lesions: glioma, hemorrhage, infarct, mass, or arteriovenous malformation
- Foville's syndrome (lesions in the abducens nucleus and/or fascicle)
- One-and-a-half syndrome (lesions in the abducens nucleus and adjacent MLF)
- Anterior inferior cerebellar artery syndrome (see section 10.5.3)
- Central pontine myelinosis[1]

Large cerebellar mass

Neurodegenerative diseases

- Wernicke's encephalopathy
- Gaucher's disease
- Leigh's syndrome

Typical bobbing

---

1. **Central pontine myelinosis** is a complication of severe and prolonged hyponatremia (particularly when corrected too rapidly) which results in concentrated, frequently symmetric, non-inflammatory demyelination within the central basis pontis. In 10% of patients, demyelination also occurs in extrapontine areas, including the midbrain, thalamus, basal nuclei, and cerebellum.

- Clinical features
  1. Delirium, spastic quadriplegia, pseudobulbar palsy (e.g. head and neck weakness, dysphagia, and dysarthria)
  2. Horizontal gaze paralysis, vertical gaze paralysis (caused by demyelination in the midbrain), atypical bobbing (see section 8.3.1)
- MRI brain reveals intense symmetric demyelination in the pons with or without extension to extrapontine areas
- Treatment
  1. Supportive
  2. Correct hyponatremia at a rate of 10 μmol/L every 24 h to avoid hypernatremia
  3. Vitamin supplementation for alcoholic patients
- Prognosis
  1. Death is common; maximum recovery may require several months.
  2. Chronic neurologic deficits: "locked-in" syndrome, spastic quadriparesis, as well as tremor and ataxia (from extrapontine lesions)

9.3.2 Lesions in the Paramedian Pontine Reticular Formation

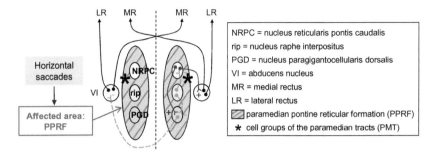

The paramedian pontine reticular formation (PPRF) contains:

1. **Excitatory burst neurons (EBN)** in the dorsomedial nucleus reticularis pontis caudalis (NRPC) that
   - Project to the ipsilateral abducens nucleus to generate ipsilateral, conjugate, horizontal saccades
   - Project to inhibitory burst neurons in the nucleus paragigantocellularis dorsalis (PGD) and receive inhibitory inputs from omnipause neurons in nucleus raphe interpositus (rip)
2. **Inhibitory burst neurons** in the PGD that
   - Project to the contralateral abducens nucleus to inhibit the antagonist muscles
   - Receive inhibitory inputs from omnipause neurons and excitatory inputs from ipsilateral excitatory burst neurons
3. **Omnipause neurons** in the nucleus raphe interpositus (rip) that
   - Project to excitatory and inhibitory burst neurons to inhibit horizontal and vertical saccades
   - Receive inputs from long-lead burst neurons in rostral PPRF, the rostral pole (fixation zone) of the superior colliculus, and the fastigial nucleus
4. **Cell groups of the PMT** send efference copy to the cerebellar flocculus for gaze holding and longer term adaptation.
5. **Fibers of passage that send horizontal VOR, pursuit, and gaze-holding signals** to the abducens nucleus

Eye Movement Abnormalities in PPRF Lesion: Horizontal Conjugate Saccadic Palsy

Unilateral lesion

- Ipsilesional horizontal saccadic palsy, with or without involvement of ipsilesional smooth pursuit and VOR (depends on whether fibers of passage for horizontal VOR, pursuit, and gaze-holding are involved)
- Acutely, manifests as contralesional gaze deviation
- Horizontal gaze-evoked nystagmus on looking contralesionally, with quick phases directed away from the side of the lesion

Bilateral lesion

Bilateral lesion results in total horizontal gaze palsy (involvement of fibers of passage for horizontal VOR, pursuit and gaze-holding) and slowing of vertical saccades (involvement of omnipause neurons).

9.3.3 Lesions in the Medial Longitudinal Fasciculus: Internuclear Ophthalmoplegia ▸▸

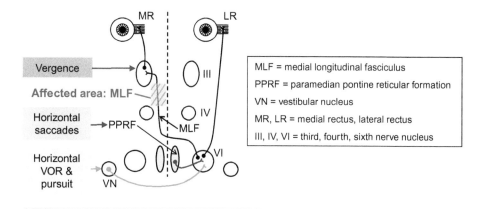

The MLF contains fibers important for both horizontal and vertical eye movements.

For horizontal gaze:

- The MLF contains axons from abducens internuclear neurons, which carry signals for horizontal saccades, VOR, and smooth pursuit
- Projects to medial rectus motoneurons in the contralateral oculomotor nucleus

For vertical gaze:

- The MLF contains axons from the riMLF, which carries vertical saccadic signals (see section 9.4.1)
- Contains axons from the vestibular nuclei, which carry signals for vertical VOR, smooth pursuit (see section 9.4.2), gaze holding, and otolith–ocular reflex
- Projects to the oculomotor and trochlear nuclei, as well as the INC

Etiology of Internuclear Ophthalmoplegia

Multiple sclerosis and other demyelinating diseases (commonly bilateral)

Brainstem infarction (commonly unilateral)

Brainstem and fourth ventricular tumor

Arnold-Chiari malformation

Hydrocephalus

Trauma

Infectious: bacterial, viral, spirochetal, AIDS

Metabolic: hepatic encephalopathy, maple syrup urine disease, Fabry's disease

Nutritional: Wernicke's encephalopathy, pernicious anemia

Drug intoxication: barbiturates, lithium, narcotics, phenothiazine, propanolol, tricyclic antidepressants

Carcinomatous infiltration or remote effect of cancer (i.e., paraneoplastic)

Progressive supranuclear palsy

Right INO

On left gaze:

Right eye: Left eye:
Adducting deficit   Abducting nystagmus

Eye Movement Abnormalities in MLF Lesion: Internuclear Ophthalmoplegia (INO)

Unilateral INO

- Ipsilesional adducting deficit (MR weakness) during conjugate horizontal eye movement
    1. Often manifests as slowing of adducting saccades, leading to "adduction lag"
    2. Adduction may be intact during convergence.[1]
- Abducting nystagmus of contralesional eye (i.e. a "dissociated nystagmus")[2]
- Skew deviation i.e., hypotropia in contralesional eye (due to interruption of the otolith-ocular pathway)
- Dissociated vertical nystagmus i.e., downbeat in the ipsilesional eye and torsional in the contralesional eye[3]

Bilateral INO

- Same as unilateral INO, plus abnormal vertical movements, including vertical gaze-evoked nystagmus, impaired vertical pursuit, VOR, OKN, and VOR cancellation
- Saccadic intrusions (result from brainstem involvement in addition to MLF)
- Walled-eyed bilateral INO (WEBINO) i.e., an exotropia which may result from a loss of convergence

---

1. Convergence may be intact or impaired. The former may imply a more caudal lesion (i.e. posterior INO of Cogan), whereas the latter may imply a more rostral lesion (i.e. anterior INO of Cogan).

2. Possible explanations

 a. The abducting nystagmus may represent an attempt by the brain to adaptively correct for hypometric saccades due to the weak medial rectus. By adaptively increasing the innervation to the weak adducting eye, Hering's law dictates a conjugate increase of innervation to the abducting eye. This results in overshooting saccades and postsaccadic drift in the abducting eye. Since saccades initiate the oscillations, abducting "nystagmus" is not a true nystagmus, but rather a series of saccadic pulses.

 b. The abducting nystagmus is a dissociated gaze-evoked nystagmus caused by interruption of the paramedian tracts which is important for gaze-holding. The nystagmus appears more prominent in the abducting eye because of adduction weakness in the ipsilesional eye.

 c. The abducting nystagmus is a result of an increased convergence tone which leads to centripetal drift of contralesional eye with correcting saccades.

3. Possible explanations

 a. Downbeat nystagmus may be due to an upward bias from intact anterior canal (AC) pathways that do not pass through the MLF (i.e. posterior canal pathways pass through the MLF, but some AC pathways do not).

 b. Torsional nystagmus may be due to interruption of pathways between the vestibular nucleus and the interstitial nucleus of Cajal (INC).

9.3.4 Combined Lesions in the Abducens Nucleus and MLF: One-and-a-half Syndrome

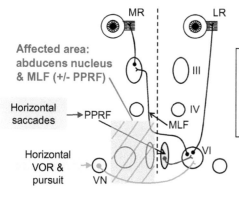

Affected area: abducens nucleus & MLF (+/- PPRF)

Horizontal saccades → PPRF

Horizontal VOR & pursuit

MLF = medial longitudinal fasciculus

PPRF = paramedian pontine reticular formation

VN = vestibular nucleus

MR, LR = medial rectus, lateral rectus

III, IV, VI = third, fourth, sixth nerve nucleus

Eye Movement Abnormalities in Combined Abducens Nucleus and MLF (with or without PPRF) Lesion: One-and-a-half Syndrome

Ipsilesional horizontal gaze palsy and INO, with abduction of the contralesional eye being the only preserved movement

Example: Right one-and-a-half syndrome

- On right gaze: horizontal conjugate gaze palsy (involvement of the right abducens nucleus)
- On left gaze: adducting deficit in right eye, abducting nystagmus in left eye (involvement of the right MLF)

Paralytic pontine exotropia: on looking straight ahead, the contralesional eye is deviated outward due to unopposed action of the lateral rectus, which is innervated by the intact contralesional abducens nucleus.

Vertical and vergence eye movements may be spared.

Etiology of One-and-a-Half Syndrome

Multiple sclerosis

Brainstem ischemia

Tumor

Hemorrhage

Trauma

9.3.5 Other Pontine Lesions

Nucleus reticularis tegmenti pontis

- The nucleus reticularis tegmenti pontis has three anatomical and functional subdivisions:
    1. Caudal NRTP encodes saccades in three dimensions (horizontal, vertical, and torsional)
    2. Medial NRTP encodes vergence
    3. Rostral NRTP encodes smooth pursuit (especially upward pursuit)
- The caudal NRTP receives input from the superior colliculus, whereas the medial NRTP receives input from the frontal and supplementary eye field.
- The NRTP projects to the dorsal vermis, fastigial nucleus, and interposed nucleus, as well as the flocculus and paraflocculus of the cerebellum.

Eye Movement Abnormalities in NRTP Lesion
Abnormal saccades with torsional errors, in violation of Listing's law
Impaired convergence
Lesion of the rostral NRTP causes deficit in upward pursuit
Ablation of the cerebellar vermis results in esodeviation

Dorsolateral pontine nucleus

The dorsolateral pontine nucleus encodes smooth pursuit. It receives input from the middle temporal visual area, the medial superior temporal visual area, the frontal eye field, and the nucleus of the optic tract and projects to the flocculus, paraflocculus, and dorsal vermis of the cerebellum. A lesion in the dorsolateral pontine nucleus results in impaired ipsilateral pursuit (see section 5.2).

9.4 Ocular Motor Syndromes Caused by Lesions in the Midbrain

9.4.1 Lesions in the Rostral Interstitial Nucleus of the Medial Longitudinal Fasciculus

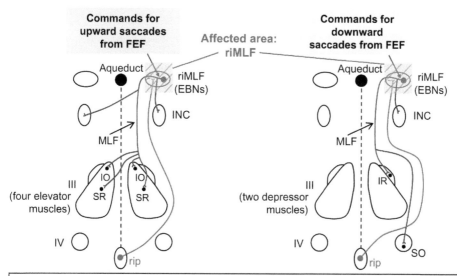

FEF = frontal eye field; riMLF = rostral interstitial nucleus of the medial longitudinal fasciculus
EBNs = excitatory burst neurons; INC = interstitial nucleus of Cajal; rip = nucleus raphe interpositus
MLF = medial longitudinal fasciculus; III, IV, VI = third, fourth, sixth nerve nucleus
SR, IR = superior and inferior rectus; IO, SO = inferior and superior oblique

The rostral interstitial nucleus of the medial longitudinal fasciculus (riMLF):

Contains burst neurons (medium-lead EBN) for vertical and torsional saccades

- Each riMLF projects bilaterally to motoneurons for the elevator muscles (superior rectus and inferior oblique), but ipsilaterally to motoneurons for the depressor muscles (inferior rectus and superior oblique).

- Although each riMLF contains burst neurons for upward or downward saccades, the right riMLF is responsible for conjugate clockwise saccades and the left riMLF is responsible for conjugate counterclockwise saccades (from patient's point of view).

Receives inputs from long-lead burst neurons in the midbrain and rostral PPRF, superior colliculus, cerebellar fastigial nucleus, nucleus of the posterior commissure, omnipause neurons in rip, and contralateral riMLF via the ventral commissure

Projects predominantly to the ipsilateral oculomotor and trochlear nuclei; it also projects to the ipsilateral INC, cell groups of the paramedian tracts, and the spinal cord (for head movements)

Most common etiology of riMLF lesions is infarcts in the distribution of the posterior thalamosubthalamic paramedian artery, which may by paired or single

Eye Movement Abnormalities in riMLF Lesion: Abnormal Vertical and Torsional Saccades

Unilateral lesion

- Mild slowing of downward saccades because projections to depressors are ipsilateral, whereas those to elevators are bilateral.
- Torsional nystagmus beating contralateral to the side of the lesion
- Loss of ipsitorsional quick phases (e.g., right riMLF lesion results in a loss of clockwise quick phases, from patient's point of view)
- Static, contralesional torsional deviation
- Vertical one-and-a-half syndrome, manifested as either
  1. An upgaze palsy in both eyes and monocular paresis of depression in the ipsilateral eye or
  2. A downgaze palsy in both eyes and monocular paresis of elevation in the ipsilateral eye

Bilateral lesion

- Common because both riMLFs are often supplied by a single posterior thalamosubthalamic paramedian artery
- Vertical and torsional saccades are abolished (may be more pronounced for downward than for upward saccades).
- Vertical pursuit, VOR, and gaze holding, as well as horizontal saccades, are spared.

9.4.2 Lesions in the Interstitial Nucleus of Cajal

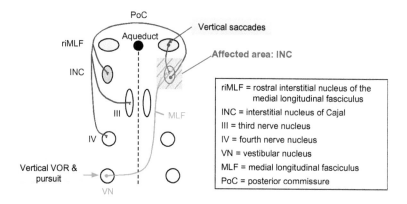

The interstitial nucleus of Cajal (INC):

Contains two populations of neurons that are responsible for

- Neural integration (i.e., gaze holding) during vertical and torsional movements
- Eye–head coordination in the roll plane

Receives inputs from burst neurons (medium-lead excitatory burst neurons) in the riMLF, the vestibular nuclei, and the y-group

Projects via the posterior commissure to the contralateral oculomotor and trochlear nucleus as well as to the contralateral INC. The INC also sends ascending projections to mesencephalic reticular formation, zona incerta, riMLF, and nuclei of the central thalamus and descending projections to nucleus gigantocellularis of pontine reticular formation (for head movements), vestibular nuclei, PMT cell groups in medulla, and cervical cord.

Eye Movement Abnormalities in INC Lesion

Unilateral lesion

- Impaired gaze holding in vertical and torsional planes
- Ocular tilt reaction: skew deviation (contralesional hypotropia), excyclotorsion of the contralesional eye (and incyclotorsion of the ipsilesional eye), and contralesional head tilt
- Torsional nystagmus that has ipsilesional quick phases (i.e., beats in opposite direction to that caused by a riMLF lesion), with or without a downbeat component

Bilateral lesion

- All vertical movements (saccades, pursuit, and VOR) are impaired (saccadic speed is normal).
- Impaired gaze holding in vertical and torsional planes
- Upbeat nystagmus
- Neck retroflexion

9.4.3 Lesions in the Posterior Commissure and the Nucleus of the Posterior Commissure: Vertical Gaze Palsy and Pretectal Syndrome ▸▸

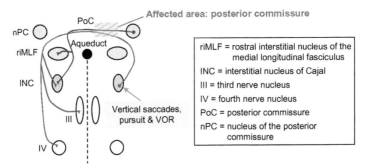

The posterior commissure

1. Contains axons from neurons in the INC that project to the contralateral oculomotor and trochlear nucleus, as well as to the contralateral INC

2. Contains axons from neurons in the nucleus of the posterior commissure that project to the contralateral riMLF and INC (may be important for upgaze) and the M-group (important for lid–eye coordination during vertical saccades).

Eye Movement Abnormalities in Posterior Commissure Lesion: Pretectal Syndrome

Vertical gaze palsy and loss of vertical gaze-holding (neural integrator) function
- Upward eye movements are predominantly affected: loss of upward saccades, pursuit, VOR, and Bell's phenomenon
- Downward saccades and smooth pursuit may be impaired, but VOR is relatively preserved.
- Downward gaze deviation, especially in premature infants with intraventricular hemorrhage (a combination of downgaze deviation and lid retraction is known as the "setting sun" sign).
- Downbeat nystagmus

Convergence-retraction nystagmus consists of asynchronous convergent saccades (i.e., not a true nystagmus) and is evoked by attempted upward saccades.

Light-near dissociation of the pupils (see below)

Pathologic lid retraction while looking straight ahead (Collier's sign)

Skew deviation

Disturbances of vergence eye movements:
- Paralysis or spasm of convergence
- Paralysis of divergence

Accommodation spasm or paresis

Others
- Square-wave jerks
- A- or V-pattern exotropia
- Pseudo-abducens palsy i.e., the abducting eye moves slower than the adducting eye
- Pretectal V-pattern pseudo-bobbing (see section 8.3.1)

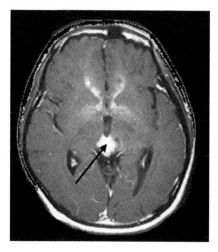

Axial MRI showing a pineal gland tumor (arrow) involving the pretectal area.

Differential Diagnosis of Vertical Gaze Palsy

Pretectal syndrome (the most common causes by age group)

Infant: Congenital aqueductal stenosis, leading to hydrocephalus, which stretches or compresses the posterior commissure

Age 10–20 years: Pineal gland tumor (e.g., germinoma), causing direct compression on the posterior commissure or obstructive hydrocephalus

Age 21–30 years: Head trauma, leading to subdural hematoma

Age 31–40 years: Vascular malformation (e.g., midbrain or thalamic hemorrhage)

Age 41–50 years: Multiple sclerosis

Age 51–60 years: Basilar artery stroke or infarction

Other causes

Metabolic: Niemann-Pick disease (type C), Gaucher's disease, Tay-Sachs disease, maple syrup urine disease, Wilson's disease, kernicterus

Drug-induced: barbiturates, carbamazepine, neuroleptic agents

Degenerative: progressive supranuclear palsy, Huntington's disease, Lytico-Bodig, corticobasal ganglionic degeneration, Lewy bodies disease

Infectious/inflammatory: Whipple's disease, encephalitis, syphilis, tuberculoma

Miscellaneous: hypoxia, benign transient vertical gaze palsy in childhood, mesencephalic clefts

Light-near dissociation of the pupils in pretectal syndrome

The Pupillary Light Reflex Pathway

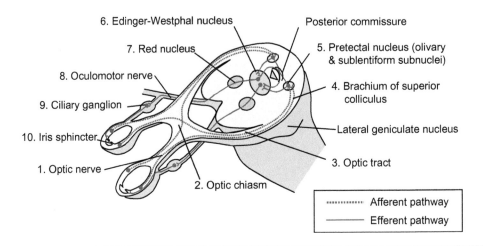

- The optic nerve carries monocular light information to the optic chiasm, where nasal retinal fibers (temporal field) decussate to the contralateral optic tract, and temporal retinal fibers (nasal field) remain uncrossed and continue in the ipsilateral optic tract.

Clinical Point

Lesion in optic tract causes a relative afferent pupillary defect in the contralateral eye because the temporal visual field is 60–70% larger than the nasal field (see also section 12.3.1).

- Before synapsing at the lateral geniculate nucleus, some retinal ganglion cell axons that carry light-related signals leave the optic tract, enter the brachium of superior colliculus at the level of the midbrain, and synapse at the pretectal nucleus (the pretectal nucleus also receives input from the superior colliculus, which carries descending accommodation-related signals from the retina and cortical areas, including the lateral suprasylvian area, to the pretectal nucleus).

- The pretectal nucleus projects to the Edinger-Westphal nucleus (EWN), a parasympathetic nucleus.

- The EWN then sends out parasympathetic fibers, which travel along the ipsilateral oculomotor nerve and synapse at the ciliary ganglion. There are two subtypes of parasympathetic fibers: (1) pupillomotor fibers (3%), whose cell bodies lie in the EWN caudally and innervate the iris sphincter, and (2) accommodative fibers (97%), whose cell bodies lie in the EWN more rostrally and innervate the ciliary muscle. These two types of fibers enter the eye via the short posterior ciliary nerves.

In **pretectal syndrome**, the lesion damages the pretectal (light) fibers that enter the EWN caudally, sparing fibers for near response (accommodative) that enter the EWN more rostrally. This results in light-near dissociation of the pupils.

9.4.4 Other Midbrain Lesions

Central mesencephalic reticular formation

The function of the central mesencephalic reticular formation (cMRF) is to program horizontal and vertical saccades via reciprocal connections with the superior colliculus, supplementary eye field, and PPRF.

Lesion in central mesencephalic reticular formation causes:

1. Ipsilesional gaze shift
2. Hypometria of ipsilesional and downward saccades and hypermetria of contralesional and upward saccades
3. Square-wave jerks

M-group

The M-group coordinates lid–eye movement during vertical saccades.

Paramedian Midbrain

Lesion in the paramedian midbrain causes midbrain paresis of horizontal gaze:

1. Impaired horizontal ipsilesional pursuit and contralesional saccades, with sparing of the horizontal VOR (**Roth-Bielschowsky phenomenon**)
2. Nuclear oculomotor nerve palsy (bilateral ptosis, elevation palsy, and dilated pupils; see section 12.2.1)

Periaqueductal Gray

Lesion in periaqueductal gray causes selective loss of downgaze with tonic upward gaze deviation

Double elevator palsy (monocular elevator palsy)

Characterisitics

1. Limited elevation of one eye (affects both elevators; i.e., the superior rectus and inferior oblique)
2. Orthotropic in primary position but limited elevation on upgaze, resulting in a vertical deviation
3. May be associated with limited depression of the contralateral eye

Etiology

Congenital

Midbrain infarct or tumor, ipsilateral or contralateral to the side of lesion

Possible mechanisms

- Lesions in the oculomotor fascicle that selectively affect the superior rectus and inferior oblique bundles (the most plausible mechanism)
- Prenuclear lesion, but the lesion has to be very close to the oculomotor complex because each riMLF projects bilaterally to the elevators

---

- Double elevator palsy cannot be caused by a nuclear lesion because the inferior oblique is supplied by the ipsilateral oculomotor nucleus, whereas the superior rectus is supplied by the contralateral oculomotor nucleus (see section 12.2.1)

Progressive supranuclear palsy (Steele-Richardson-Olszewski Syndrome)

A neurodegenerative disease that affects eye movements, cognition, and posture. Usually fatal within approximately six years of onset, commonly from aspiration pneumonia. It occurs sporadically although a few familial cases have been reported.

Clinical features

1. Supranuclear ophthalmoplegia
2. Cognitive changes
3. Pseudobulbar palsy (dysarthria, dysphagia), prominent neck dystonia, parkinsonism, and gait disturbances that cause imbalance and frequent falls

---

Eye Movement Abnormalities in Progressive Supranuclear Palsy

Impaired saccades:
1. Vertical saccades
   - Abnormal vertical saccades result from involvement of the riMLF, brainstem reticular formation, and omnipause cells in nucleus raphe interpositus (rip)
   - Early stage: slow saccades, especially downward, with normal range of movement (in contrast to Parkinson's disease, which causes hypometric upward saccades with normal velocity – see section 11.2.2)
   - Later stage: loss of vertical saccades and quick phases
   - Advanced disease: vertical gaze palsy
2. Horizontal saccades: slow and hypometric
3. Increased inaccuracy of antisaccades (results from involvement of substantia nigra pars reticulata via its projection to the superior colliculus)

Impaired horizontal and vertical smooth pursuit with catch-up saccades (results from involvement of the DLPN)

Normal eye-head tracking (especially vertical) and sparing of VOR

Square-wave jerks (result from involvement of the rostral pole of the superior colliculus and the cMRF)

Internuclear ophthalmoplegia

Loss of convergence

Eyelid disorders: apraxia of lid opening, lid lag, blepharospasm, inability to suppress a blink to a bright light (visual "glabellar" or Myerson's sign), absent Bell's phenomenon

---

Neuropathology

- Neurofibrillary tangles, neuronal loss, and gliosis in subcortical and brainstem areas (including the globus pallidus, substantia nigra pars compacta and reticulata, periaqueductal gray, brainstem reticular formation, and superior colliculi)

- Abnormality of the microtubule-binding protein τ, which is misfolded, tangled, and twisted to form neurofibrillary tangles

Treatment

Progressive supranuclear palsy may be treated with dopamine agonists, tricyclic antidepressants, and methysergide.

Whipple's disease

Whipple's disease is a rare, relapsing, infectious disease caused by the bacteria *Tropheryma whippelii.*

Clinical features

1. Fever of unknown origin

2. Polyarthralgia

3. Chronic diarrhea (involving the small intestine)

4. Lymphadenopathy

5. Involvement of the central nervous system can be the sole presentation of Whipple's disease, which may present as altered mentation, polydipsia, hyperphagia, or myoclonus

6. Ocular manifestations: chronic uveitis, keratitis, retinitis, vitritis, vitreous hemorrhage, or papilledema

---

Eye Movement Abnormalities in Whipple's Disease

Vertical gaze palsy (mimic progressive supranuclear palsy)

- Initially, slow vertical saccades and quick phases

- Eventually, all eye movements are impaired.

Oculomasticatory myorhythmia consisting of: ▸▸

1. Pendular, usually convergence–divergence (occasionally vertical) oscillations

   - Frequency of about 1 Hz

   - Pathognomonic for Whipple's disease

   - Persists during sleep

2. Concurrent regular, repetitive contractions (1–2 Hz) of the facial, masticatory, and pharyngeal muscles, with or without limb involvement

---

Diagnosis

- Small-intestine biopsy: foamy macrophages containing periodic acid-Schiff-positive, gram-positive bacilli in the lamina propria of the mucosa
- Polymerase chain reaction analysis

Treatment

Treatment of Whipple's disease is with antibiotics such as trimethoprim-sulfamethoxazole.

9.5 Ocular Motor Syndromes Caused by Lesions in Multiple Sites in the Brainstem, Cerebellum, or Cerebrum

9.5.1 Slow Saccades

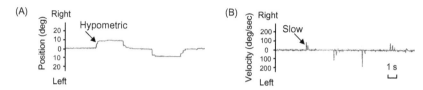

Eye movement recordings in a patient with right abducens nerve palsy showing slow and hypometric abducting saccades. (A) Eye position vs. time; (B) Eye velocity vs. time.

Differential Diagnosis of Slow Saccades[1,2]

Lesions in the pons

- Spinocerebellar ataxias, especially SCA2 which is associated with slow horizontal saccades
- Lesions of the PPRF: bilateral lesion causes slow vertical saccades and total horizontal gaze palsy
- Internuclear ophthalmoplegia: slow adducting saccades
- Paraneoplastic syndrome

Lesions in the midbrain

- Progressive supranuclear palsy (PSP): slowing of vertical saccades first, then horizontal saccades
- Whipple's disease: slowing of vertical saccades first, then horizontal saccades
- Amyotrophic lateral sclerosis: slow vertical saccades in some cases

Lesions in the basal ganglion

- Advanced Parkinson's (i.e., early stage is characterized by hypometric horizontal and vertical saccades, not slow saccades) and related diseases; Lytico-Bodig
- Huntington's disease: slow vertical saccades
- Creutzfeldt-Jakob disease: slow horizontal and vertical saccades

Others

- In dementia: Alzheimer's disease (stimulus-dependent), AIDS
- Drug intoxications: anticonvulsants, benzodiazepines
- Peripheral nerve palsy, diseases affecting neuromuscular junction and extraocular muscle, restrictive ophthalmopathy
- Miscellaneous: lipid storage diseases, Wilson's disease, tetanus

---

1. Pathologic mechanisms of slow saccades:
   - Lesions of excitatory burst neurons in NRPC of the PPRF, or riMLF, or both or
   - Lesions of the omnipause cells in rip of the PPRF or
   - Abnormal inputs to the PPRF from lesions of the frontal eye field or superior colliculus
2. Blinking of eyelids may speed up slow saccades. This is probably due to the effects of blinking on omnipause and burst neurons rather than the effects of momentary deprivation of vision.

9.5.2 Skew Deviation and the Ocular Tilt Reaction

Skew deviation is a vertical misalignment of the visual axes caused by a disturbance of prenuclear inputs, with or without abnormal torsion. The vertical misalignment may be comitant (nearly the same in all positions of gaze) or incomitant (vary with eye position). Rarely, it alternates with eye position (e.g., right hypertropia on right gaze and left hypertropia on left gaze). Skew deviation is associated with other central neurologic signs and may be part of the ocular tilt reaction (OTR).

Right Ocular Tilt Reaction (OTR)

1. Right hypotropia (skew)
2. Excyclotorsion of the right eye and incyclotorsion of the left eye

3. Right head tilt

Eye Movement Abnormalities in Ocular Tilt Reaction

Skew deviation (e.g., hypotropia of the right eye in right OTR)

Ocular torsion with upper poles of the eyes rotated toward the lower ear (e.g., in right OTR, excyclotorsion of the right eye and incyclotorsion of the left eye)

- This is in contrast to physiologic counterrolling, in which the upper poles of the eyes rotate toward the higher ear
- May be dissociated between the two eyes

Head tilt (e.g., right head tilt in right OTR)

Acutely, may have associated torsional nystagmus

Deviation of the subjective visual vertical (e.g., tilting of subjective visual vertical to the right in right OTR)

Pathogenesis of skew deviation and OTR

Disruption of the otolith–ocular pathway in the vestibular periphery, brainstem, or the cerebellum leads to an abnormal internal estimate of the gravitoinertial acceleration (see section 3.11).

Acute peripheral vestibulopathy

Lesions of the vestibular organ or its nerve cause an ipsilesional OTR (e.g., a right utricular nerve lesion results in hypotropia of the right eye, excyclotorsion of the right eye and incyclotorsion of the left eye, and right head tilt).

The **Tullio phenomenon** (an irritative/excitatory phenomenon) is

- Caused by a perilymph fistula or abnormalities of the ossicular chain or its connection with the membranous labyrinth
- Characterized by sound-induced vestibular symptoms; for example, stimulation of the left ear with a specific auditory tone causes hypotropia of the right eye, excyclotorsion of the right eye and incyclotorsion of the left eye, and right head tilt (i.e., similar effects as a lesion in the right ear).

Lesions in the vestibular nuclei

Lesions in the vestibular nuclei that occur as part of lateral meduallary syndrome, for example, lead to ipsilesional OTR with disconjugate torsion. The constellation of symptoms includes ipsilesional hypotropia, ipsilesional head tilt, and disconjugate torsion (i.e., excyclotorsion of the ipsilesional eye, but small or absent incyclotorsion of the contralesional eye).

Lesions in the cerebellum

Lesions in the cerebellum lead to sustained or alternating skew deviation.

Lesions in the medial longitudinal fasciculus

Lesions in the MLF, such as in INO, lead to contralesional OTR because otolithic projections from the vestibular nuclei cross the midline and ascend in the MLF. For example, a right MLF lesion results in a left OTR with hypotropia of the left eye, excyclotorsion of the left eye and incyclotorsion of the right eye, and left head tilt.

Lesions in the midbrain and interstitial nucleus of Cajal

May present as one of the following:

1. Sustained contralesional OTR
2. Paroxysmal skew deviation/OTR; an irritative phenomenon that causes an ipsilateral OTR (ipsilateral to the side of irritation)
3. Periodic alternating skew deviation that alternates between the eyes or varies in magnitude over the course of a few minutes (rare)

Raised intracranial pressure

Supratentorial tumors or pseudotumor cerebri may raise intracranial pressure, leading to skew deviation and OTR.

9.5.3 Multiple Sclerosis

Multiple sclerosis is an idiopathic, inflammatory, demyelinating disease of the central nervous system.

- Most common debilitating illness among young adults aged 20–40
- Incidence is 0.5–1 per 1000; with higher incidence in Caucasians and in temperate climates
- Affects females more often, with a female-to-male ratio of 2:1

Clinical Features of Multiple Sclerosis

Classic presentation

- Optic neuritis
- Transverse myelitis (e.g., bladder, bowel, and sexual dysfunction) (Devic syndrome is an acute transverse myelitis accompanied by bilateral optic neuritis.)
- Internuclear ophthalmoplegia
- Paresthesia (an early sign)

Other neurologic abnormalities

- Lhermitte's sign: Neck flexion results in an electric shock-like feeling in the torso or extremities.
- Paralysis, spasticity, and hyperreflexia, due to upper motor neuron dysfunction from involvement of the lateral corticospinal tracts
- Decreased joint position and vibration sense, due to involvement of the dorsal columns.
- Cerebellar signs (e.g., Charcot triad of dysarthria, ataxia, and tremor)
- Psychiatric disorder (5–10%): depression, paranoia, or dementia

Acute disseminated encephalitis

- Pathophysiologically and radiographically identical to multiple sclerosis
- Characterized by acute onset of sensory, cranial nerve, motor, and cerebellar abnormalities with encephalopathy and altered mentation or personality change, progressing to coma and eventual death in 30%

Four clinical types

1. Relapsing-remitting (70%): acute exacerbations with full or partial remissions
2. Primary progressive
3. Relapsing-progressive: features of both relapsing-remitting and primary progressive types
4. Secondary progressive: patients with relapsing-remitting type progress over time

---

Pathogenesis and Pathology

Multiple sclerosis is most likely an autoimmune disease, with the autoantigen being one of several myelin proteins, such as proteolipid protein, myelin oligodendrocyte glycoprotein, or myelin basic protein. The pathologic hallmark of the disease is multicentric, multiphasic central nervous system inflammation and demyelination.

Eye Movement Abnormalities in Multiple Sclerosis

Internuclear ophthalmoplegia (common) ▸▸
- Usually bilateral
- Often manifested as slow adducting saccades, with or without normal range of adduction (i.e., adduction lag)

Cerebellar eye signs
- Gaze-evoked nystagmus (common)
- Upbeat, downbeat, or torsional nystagmus
- Positional nystagmus (see section 7.5.6)

Acquired pendular nystagmus (common)

Saccadic oscillations, such as ocular flutter

Saccadic dysmetria

Impaired smooth pursuit and combined eye-head tracking (VOR cancellation)

Impaired optokinetic responses

Other abnormalities
- Horizontal and vertical gaze palsies
- Gaze-evoked blepharoclonus
- Superior oblique myokymia
- Convergence spasm
- Oculomotor, trochlear, or abducens palsies

Workup

MRI

Demyelination plaques on T2 images

- Commonly found in periventricular area, internal capsule, corpus callosum, pons, and brachium pontis
- May also appear throughout the myelinated white matter and not uncommonly in the gray matter

Cerebrospinal fluid analysis

- Elevated cell count (up to 50/mm^3)
- Elevated protein (up to 0.1 g/L)

- Normal glucose level
- Selective increase in IgG (e.g., oligoclonal bands, free κ chains), or an abnormal colloidal gold curve

Evoked potentials

Abnormal visual, auditory, or somatosensory evoked potentials are present in patients with multiple sclerosis.

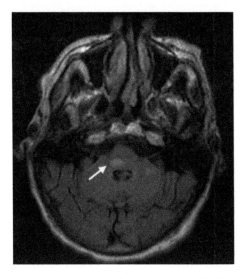

Axial MRI showing a demyelinating lesion (arrow) in the right pons.

Treatment

Acute attacks

For acute attacks (e.g., optic neuritis, transverse myelitis), use corticosteroids. They do not affect the course of multiple sclerosis over time, but they may reduce the duration and severity of attacks.

The Optic Neuritis Treatment Trial (ONTT) showed that

- Treatment with high-dose intravenous methylprednisolone (1 g/day) for three days accelerates visual recovery but has no long-term visual benefit.
- Intravenous methylprednisolone reduces the development of multiple sclerosis over two years, but has no additional beneficial effect after two years.
- Oral prednisone (1 mg/kg/day) is contraindicated because it is associated with an increased rate of new attacks of optic neuritis in the same or in the fellow eye.

Relapsing-remitting multiple sclerosis

For relapsing-remitting multiple sclerosis, use β-interferon or Copolymer I

β-interferon

- Three forms: Avonex, Betaseron, and Rebif
- Reduces the number of exacerbations and may slow progression of the disease
- Acute attacks tend to be shorter and less severe.
- The Controlled High-Risk Avonex Multiple Sclerosis Trial (CHAMPS trial) showed that β-interferon 1A reduces conversion to multiple sclerosis in high-risk patients by about 50% over three years. The inclusion criteria were:

  1. Age 18–50 years
  2. Acute, isolated demyelinating event involving either the optic nerve, brainstem or cerebellum, or spinal cord
  3. At least two MRI lesions that are 3 mm in size; one of which must be periventricular or ovoid in shape

Copolymer I (Copaxone) is a synthetic form of myelin basic protein. It reduces the relapse rate by about 33%.

Chronic and advanced multiple sclerosis and spasticity

For chronic and advanced disease, use Novantrone (mitoxantrone), an immunosuppressant. Muscle relaxants and tranquilizers such as baclofen, tizanidine, diazepam, clonazepam, and dantrolene are indicated for spasticity.

9.5.4 **Wernicke's Encephalopathy**

Wernicke's encephalopathy is a neurologic disorder of acute onset caused by thiamine (vitamin B_1) deficiency. It is characterized by a triad of ophthalmoplegia, ataxia, and global confusional state.

Etiology of Wernicke's Encephalopathy
Chronic alcoholism (most common)
Malnutrition
Chronic renal failure
Hyperalimentation

Eye Movement Abnormalities in Wernicke's Encephalopathy
Horizontal or vertical gaze palsies that may progress to total ophthalmoplegia[1]
Internuclear ophthalmoplegia[2]
Abduction deficits[3]
Gaze-evoked nystagmus[4]
Impaired VOR[4]
Central positional vertical nystagmus (usually upbeat)

1. Horizontal gaze palsy results from involvement of the abducens nucleus; total ophthalmoplegia is due to involvement of all three ocular motor nerve nuclei (oculomotor, trochlear, and abducens).

2. Internuclear ophthalmoplegia results from involvement of the medial longitudinal fasciculus (MLF)

3. Abduction deficits result from involvement of the abducens nerve

4. Gaze-evoked nystagmus and impaired VOR result from involvement of the vestibular nucleus (i.e., medial vestibular nucleus-nucleus prepositus hypoglossi [MVN-NPH] region).

Workup

Workup consists of neuroimaging to rule out focal neurologic disease.

Treatment

Treatment is with intravenous thiamine, 100 mg daily, until normal diet is resumed.

Prognosis

- Symptoms (including ocular motor) are reversible with thiamine treatment.
- Mortality is 10–20%.
- **Korsakoff psychosis** is a complication that occurs in 80% of patients:

  1. Characterized by severe and enduring memory loss
  2. Ocular motor symptoms may persist, including gaze-evoked nystagmus, slow and inaccurate saccades, and impaired pursuit
  3. Only 20% of patients with Korsakoff psychosis have complete recovery.

Neurodegenerative Diseases

	Eye movement abnormalities	Other features	Genetics
Lysosomal storage disorders			
Tay-Sachs disease (GM₂ gangliosidosis or hexosaminidase A deficiency)	Combined horizontal and vertical gaze palsy	Cherry-red spot in the macula; recurrent seizures; mental retardation	Autosomal recessive, 15q23-q24
Adult variant of Tay-Sachs disease (GM₂ gangliosidosis or hexosaminidase A deficiency)	Vertical gaze palsy	Proximal muscle weakness; cerebellar and bulbar dysarthria; progressive gait ataxia	Autosomal recessive, 15q23-q24
Niemann-Pick disease, type C (sphingomyelinase deficiency)	Vertical gaze palsy (initially vertical saccadic palsy)	Part of DAF syndrome,[a] cerebellar gait and limb ataxia, dystonia, dysarthria, spasticity, decreased intellect	Autosomal recessive, 18q11-q12
Gaucher's disease, juvenile neurono-pathic form (glucocerebroside β-glucosidase deficiency)	Horizontal gaze palsy (initially horizontal saccadic palsy); ocular motor apraxia	Splenomegaly; thrombocytopenia with easy bruising; seizures	Autosomal recessive, 1q21
GM₁ gangliosidosis (acid β-galactosidase deficiency)	Ocular motor apraxia	Cherry-red spot in the macula; coarse facial features; hepatosplenomegaly; progressive neurologic deterioration	Autosomal recessive, 3p21.33
Krabbe's infantile leukodystrophy (β-galactosidase deficiency)	Ocular motor apraxia	Optic atrophy; cherry-red spot in the macula; spasticity, seizures, bulbar signs, deafness	Autosomal recessive, 14q31
Aminoacidopathies			
Maple syrup urine disease (deficiency of branched-chain α-keto acid dehydrogenase complex)	Adduction and upgaze palsy; combined horizontal and vertical gaze palsy; internuclear ophthalmoplegia	Poor feeding; metabolic acidosis; alternating muscular hypotonia and hypertonia, dystonia, seizures	Unknown; 19q13.1-q13.2, 7q31-q32

continued

	Eye movement abnormalities	Other features	Genetics
Glutaric aciduria (deficiency of glutaryl-CoA dehydrogenase)	Gaze palsy	Macrocephaly, seizures, hypotonia, opisthotonos, dystonia, and choreoathetosis; gliosis and neuronal loss in the basal ganglia	Autosomal recessive, 19p13.2
Disorders of metal metabolism *Wilson's disease (hepatolenticular degeneration)*	*Slow vertical saccades; gaze distractibility*	Kayser-Fleischer rings in the cornea (accumulation of copper); sunflower cataract; optic neuropathy; Parkinsonian symptoms (rigidity, bradykinesia)	Autosomal recessive, 13q14.3-q21.1

ᵃDAF sydrome: *downgaze palsy, ataxia/athetosis, foam* cells in the bone marrow.

The eye movement abnormalities, features, and genetics of some neurodegenerative diseases are listed in the table above. Other neurodegenerative diseases include:

- Peroxisomal assembly disorders, which may cause ocular motor apraxia

- Mitochondrial encephalopathies, such as chronic progressive external ophthalmoplegia, the syndrome of mitochondrial encephalomyopathy, lactic acidosis, and strokelike episodes (MELAS), the syndrome of mitochondrial neuro-gastrointestinal encephalomyopathy (MNGIE), the syndrome of sensory ataxic neuropathy, dysarthria, and ophthalmoplegia (SANDO), and Leigh's syndrome (see section 14.1.2)

- Others

  Abetalipoproteinemia (see sections 12.6.3 and 10.4.3)

  Ataxia telangiectasia (see section 10.4.3)

  Wernicke's encephalopathy (see section 9.5.4)

  Pelizaeus-Merzbacher disease (see section 11.3.5)

  Kernicterus (acute bilirubin encephalopathy) which may cause vertical gaze palsy.

9.5.6 Dementia

Alzheimer's disease

- Most common cause of dementia
- Most cases are sporadic, with familial forms accounting for <7% of all cases.
- Four major loci: amyloid precursor protein gene on chromosome 21, presenilin I gene on chromosome 14, presenilin II gene on chromosome 1, and candidate markers on chromosomes 12 and 19

Clinical Features of Alzheimer's Disease

Insidious onset of progressive memory loss
Language disorders (e.g., anomia, progressive aphasia)
Impaired visuospatial skills
Impaired executive functions

Eye Movement Abnormalities in Alzheimer's Disease

Frontal lobe involvement: large saccadic intrusions (i.e., anticipatory saccades) due to a distracting stimulus or impaired ability to suppress inappropriate saccades to a novel visual stimulus (i.e., visual grasp reflex)
Parietal lobe involvement:
- Inability to shift visual attention (mimics Balint's syndrome)
- Increased latency of visually guided saccades
Involvement of secondary visual areas in parietal cortex: impaired smooth pursuit with catchup saccades

Pathology

Alzheimer's disease is characterized by neurofibrillary tangles and senile plaques in the cerebral cortex, predominantly involving the association regions and particularly the medial aspect of the temporal lobe.

Treatment

- No clinically proven treatment to prevent it or slow its progression
- May use psychotropic medications and behavioral interventions, cholinesterase inhibitors, N-methyl-D-aspartate (NMDA) antagonists, antidepressants and avoid centrally acting anticholinergic medications

Creutzfeldt-Jakob Disease

Creutzfeldt-Jakob disease (CJD) accounts for 85% of all human prion disease (which also includes Kuru, fatal insomnia, and Gerstmann-Sträussler-Scheinker disease, which has cerebellar eye signs). The four types of CJD are sporadic, familial, iatrogenic, and variant CJD.

Sporadic CJD

- Most common type of CJD, with an incidence of about 1 case per million
- Mean age of onset: 62 years; death in about 8 months
- Caused by spontaneous conversion of normal cellular proteinaceous infectious particle (PrP^c) to scrapie proteinaceous infectious particle (PrP^{sc}) or by somatic mutation

---

Clinical Features of CJD

Classic triad:
1. Rapidly progressive dementia
2. Myoclonic jerks
3. Typical electroencephalographic changes

Variable constellation of pyramidal, extrapyramidal, and cerebellar signs

Heidenhain variant of sporadic CJD: sudden onset of homonymous hemianopia or cortical blindness with normal neuroimaging, before the development of dementia or myoclonus

---

Eye Movement Abnormalities in CJD

Slow horizontal and vertical saccades
Periodic alternating nystagmus
Centripetal nystagmus
Gaze deviation
Skew deviation
Balint's syndrome (see section 11.3.2)
Supranuclear paralysis of eyelid closure
Lithium or bismuth overdose may lead to syndromes that mimic CJD

The pathology of sporadic CJD includes spongiform change (vacuolation of neuropils and neurons), amyloid plaques, neuronal loss, and gliosis primarily in the gray matter (10% have amyloid plaques in the cerebellum or cerebral hemispheres).

Electroencephalography (EEG) shows characteristic periodic or pseudoperiodic paroxysms of high-voltage slow (1–2 Hz) and sharp wave complexes on an increasingly slow and low-voltage background.

There is no effective treatment.

Familial CJD

Familial CJD is autosomal dominant and accounts for 10% of all CJD; caused by mutations in the *PrP* gene.

Iatrogenic CJD

Many cases of iatrogenic CJD have been reported. This type of the disease is caused by infection from prion-containing material (e.g., dura mater, EEG electrode, corneal transplant).

Variant CJD

- Fewer than 200 reported cases
- Younger patients (mean age of onset, 28 years)
- Caused by infection from ingestion of beef products contaminated with bovine spongiform encephalopathy ("mad cow disease")
- Psychiatric abnormalities and sensory symptoms are more common at presentation.
- Pathology: presence of florid amyloid plaques

AIDS Dementia Complex

AIDS dementia complex is made up of neurologic complications that arise from primary HIV infection (other neurologic complications of the infection include HIV encephalopathy, vacuolar myelopathy, peripheral neuropathies, and polymyositis).

Clinical Features of AIDS Dementia Complex

Usually develop in advanced AIDS when $CD4^+$ lymphocyte counts fall below 200 cells/mm^3
- Cognitive changes such as psychomotor slowing, memory loss, and word-finding difficulties
- Motor disturbances such as imbalance, clumsiness, and weakness
- Behavioral changes

With the advent of highly active antiretroviral therapy, a less severe dysfunction called minor cognitive motor disorder (MCMD), has become more common than AIDS dementia complex.

Eye Movement Abnormalities in AIDS Dementia Complex

Frontal lobe involvement

Increased latency of saccades, especially vertical
Increased fixation instability
Increased error on antisaccade task
Acquired ocular motor apraxia

Brainstem or cerebellar involvement

Gaze-evoked nystagmus
Dissociated nystagmus
Slow saccades
Ocular flutter
Decreased or asymmetric slow pursuit gain

MRI

- Diffuse cortical atrophy and ventricular enlargement
- Hyperintense lesions in the periventricular subcortical white matter and centrum semiovale on T2-weighted images

Treatment

AIDS patients are treated with highly active antiretroviral therapy, which decreases the incidence of AIDS dementia complex and induces remission.

9.5.7 Vergence Disorders

Divergence Paralysis (Divergence Insufficiency)

Divergence paralysis is relatively uncommon.

Eye Movement Abnormalities in Divergence Paralysis or Insufficiency

- Comitant esotropia that is present at distance but not at near
- Full ductions and versions, with normal saccadic velocities on abduction
- Must be differentiated from
  1. Bilateral sixth nerve palsy (incomitant esotropia on lateral gaze, same degree of esotropia at distance and at near, decreased amplitude or velocity on abduction)
  2. Decompensated esophoria (same degree of esotropia at distance and at near)
  3. Decompensated monofixation esotropia (sensory and motor findings of monofixation syndrome, such as binocular peripheral fusion, monocular central suppression, esotropia of 8 prism diopters or smaller on cover/uncover test)

Etiology of Divergence Paralysis or Insufficiency

Raised intracranial pressure
Midbrain tumor
Miller Fisher syndrome (initial sign)
Diazepam intoxication
Head trauma
Intracranial hypotension (low-pressure syndrome)
Cerebellar lesions (e.g., Arnold-Chiari malformation, cerebellar degeneration, spinocerebellar ataxia type 3)

Treatment

Treat divergence palsy with base-out prisms or by unilateral or bilateral lateral rectus resection.

Divergence Excess

Divergence excess is an exotropia that is greater at distance than at near (at least 10 prism diopters difference). It must be differentiated from pseudo-divergence excess (which is more common) by

- Using +3.00 lenses (to suspend accommodative vergence): In pseudo-divergence excess, the deviations at distance and at near equalize with the use of +3.00 lenses, whereas in true divergence excess, the difference between distance and near deviations remain.
- Forty-five-minute patch test/monocular occlusion (to suspend fusional vergence): In pseudo-divergence excess, the deviations at distance and at near equalize with the patch test, whereas in true divergence excess, the difference between distance and near deviations remains.

Treatment

Treat divergence excess with base-in prisms or by bilateral lateral rectus recession.

Convergence insufficiency

Convergence insufficiency is a common condition. It is an exotropia that is greater at near than at distance (at least 10 prism diopters difference).

Symptoms

- Asthenopia
- Visual fatigue
- Blurred vision or intermittent diplopia when reading

Etiology of Convergence Insufficiency
Occurs in teenagers, college students, the elderly, or in patients after a mild head trauma
Parkinson's disease or progressive supranuclear palsy: impaired or absent vergence, together with vertical gaze abnormalities
Cerebral lesions (especially lesions of the nondominant cerebral hemisphere or the parietal lobe): impaired stereopsis and poor fusional vergence

Treatment

1. Orthoptic exercise ("pencil push-ups")—most responsive when the deviation is less than 8 prism diopters
2. Surgery

Convergence Spasm (Spasm of the Near Triad) ▸▸

Convergence spasm is intermittent convergence, usually accompanied by accommodation and pupillary miosis.

Etiology of Convergence Spasm
Functional (most common)
Diseases at the diencephalic–mesencephalic junction, such as thalamic hemorrhage ("thalamic esotropia"), pineal tumors, and midbrain stroke
Encephalitis
Wernicke-Korsakoff syndrome
Occipitoatlantal instability with vertebrobasilar ischemia
Arnold-Chiari malformation
Multiple sclerosis
Metabolic disturbances
Phenytoin intoxication

Convergence and Saccadic Oscillations

- **Convergence-retraction nystagmus** (saccades): seen in pretectal syndrome (see section 9.4.3)
- **Pretectal pseudo-bobbing**: downward and convergent jerks, slow return to mid-position (see section 8.3.1)
- **Voluntary flutter**: often seen in normal individuals in association with convergence effort (see section 8.2.4)

Vergence Oscillations

Oculomasticatory myorhythmia (see section 9.4.4)

- Smooth, pendular, convergent-divergent movements occurring at a frequency of about 1 Hz
- Pathognomonic for Whipple's disease (also associated with vertical saccadic palsy)

Divergence nystagmus (nystagmus with divergent quick phase)

- In downbeat nystagmus (e.g., Arnold-Chiari malformation), an upward and inward slow phase (i.e., divergent quick phase)
- In upbeat nystagmus, a downward and inward slow phase (i.e., divergent quick phase)

Repetitive divergence

- Divergence movements characterized by slow divergence to extreme abducted position, followed by quick return to mid-position
- Seen in comatose patients with hepatic encephalopathy and in neonates with seizures

Chapter 10

Ocular Motor Disorders Caused by Lesions in the Cerebellum

10.1 Lesions in the Vestibulocerebellum

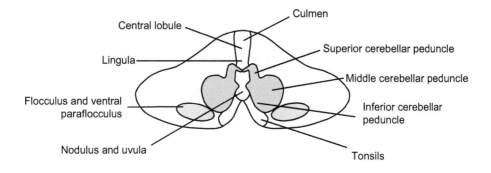

The Cerebellum (inferior anterior surface)

Central lobule

Culmen

Lingula

Superior cerebellar peduncle

Middle cerebellar peduncle

Flocculus and ventral
paraflocculus

Inferior cerebellar
peduncle

Nodulus and uvula

Tonsils

The vestibulocerebellum consists of the flocculus, ventral paraflocculus, nodulus, and uvula.

10.1.1 Flocculus and Ventral Paraflocculus

- The flocculus receives inputs from the vestibular nucleus and nerve, nucleus prepositus hypoglossi (NPH), inferior olivary nucleus, cell groups of the paramedian tracts (PMT), nucleus reticularis tegmenti pontis (NRTP), and mesencephalic reticular formation.

- The ventral paraflocculus receives inputs from contralateral pontine nuclei.

- Project to ipsilateral superior and medial vestibular nuclei, and the y-group

Eye Movement Abnormalities in Flocculus and Ventral Paraflocculus Lesion

Impaired ipsilateral gaze-holding (i.e., horizontal gaze-evoked, centripetal, and rebound nystagmus)

Downbeat nystagmus, which worsens on looking laterally and downward

Impaired smooth pursuit in all directions (horizontal and vertical)

Impaired eye–head tracking (VOR cancellation)

Impaired ability to suppress caloric nystagmus by fixating on a stationary target

Impaired VOR adaptation

Postsaccadic drift (a pulse-step mismatch)

10.1.2 Nodulus and Uvula

The Cerebellum (mid-sagittal section)

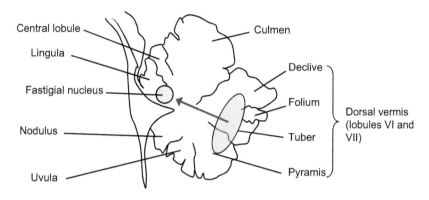

- Receive input from the medial and inferior vestibular nuclei, vestibular nerve, NPH, and inferior olivary nucleus
- Project to the vestibular nuclei

Eye Movement Abnormalities in Nodulus and Uvula Lesion

- Abnormal velocity storage mechanism of the VOR (see section 3.13)
  1. Increased duration of vestibular response (i.e., increased velocity storage)
  2. Periodic alternating nystagmus in the dark (also present in light if the flocculus and paraflocculus are lesioned such that visual fixation is impaired)
  3. Loss of ability to suppress postrotational nystagmus by tilting of the head (loss of tilt dumping/suppression). Normally, tilting of the head (e.g., head pitch) reduces postrotational nystagmus
  4. Loss of habituation (see section 3.12)
- Downbeat nystagmus in primary position
- Positional downbeat nystagmus (see section 7.5.6)

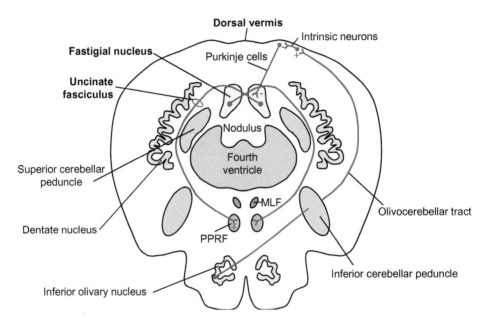

Schemata of projections from the inferior olivary nucleus, through the inferior cerebellar peduncle, to the dorsal vermis where Purkinje cells inhibit the fastigial nucleus. The fastigial nucleus projects via the uncinate fasciculus to excite the contralateral PPRF. Redrawn from Sharpe JA, Morrow MJ, Newman NJ, et al. Continuum: Neuro-ophthalmology. Baltimore, MD: Williams and Wilkins; 1995. With permission of Lippincott, Williams & Wilkins.

10.2.1 The Dorsal Vermis (Oculomotor Vermis)

- The oculomotor vermis consists of parts of the declive, folium, tuber, and pyramis.
- Receives inputs from the inferior olivary nucleus, vestibular nuclei, NPH, paramedian pontine reticular formation (PPRF), NRTP, and dorsolateral and dorsomedial pontine nuclei
- Projects to the caudal fastigial nucleus
- Stimulation of the Purkinje cells in the dorsal vermis elicits contralaterally directed saccades and smooth pursuit

Eye Movement Abnormalities in Dorsal Vermis Lesion
Hypometric ipsilesional saccades and mild hypermetric contralesional saccades
Impaired ipsilesional smooth pursuit to target moving toward the side of lesion
Tonic gaze deviation away from the side of lesion

10.2.2 The Fastigial Nucleus

- Receives inputs from the dorsal vermis, inferior olivary nucleus, and NRTP
- Decussates and projects via the uncinate fasciculus of the brachium conjunctivum to the contralateral PPRF, rostral interstitial nucleus of the medial longitudinal fasciculus, nucleus of the posterior commissure, omnipause neurons in nucleus raphe interpositus, the mesencephalic reticular formation, and superior colliculus
- Neurons in the fastigial oculomotor region (FOR) fire during both ipsilateral and contralateral saccades.
  1. The contralateral FOR neurons burst before the onset of saccade, and the onset of firing is not correlated with any property of the saccade.
  2. Conversely, the time of onset for neurons in the ipsilateral FOR varies, with bursts occurring later for larger saccades.
  3. Thus, the difference in time of onset between contralateral and ipsilateral FOR activity encodes the amplitude of saccades (i.e., the larger the difference in time of onset, the larger the saccade amplitude).

Eye Movement Abnormalities in Fastigial Nucleus Lesion

- Similar effects as seen in lateral medullary syndrome
  1. "Ipsipulsion" of saccades (i.e., hypermetric ipsilesional and hypometric contralesional saccades)
  2. Impaired contralesional smooth pursuit to target moving away from the side of lesion
  3. Tonic gaze deviation toward the side of lesion (lateropulsion)
- Disinhibition of fastigial nucleus may cause opsoclonus

10.2.3. The Uncinate Fasciculus

Eye movement abnormalities in uncinate fasciculus lesion include hypometric ipsilesional saccades and hypermetric contralesional saccades ("contrapulsion").

10.3 Developmental Anomalies of the Hindbrain and Cerebellum

10.3.1 Arnold-Chiari Malformation

Arnold-Chiari malformation is a malformation of the medullary–spinal junction with herniation of intracranial contents through the foramen magnum. The three types are illustrated in the figure below.

Type I	Type II	Type III
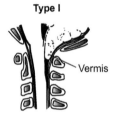	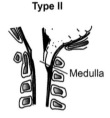	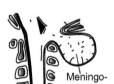
Herniation of cerebellar vermis (symptoms usually occur in adulthood)	Herniation of cerebellar vermis, medulla & fourth ventricle (symptoms usually occur in childhood)	Part of medulla & cerebellum lie within a cervico-occipital meningomyelocele (symptoms occur in infancy)

Redrawn from Lindsay KW. Neurology and Neurosurgery Illustrated. 3rd ed. New York: Churchill Livingstone; 1997. With permission from Elsevier.

Eye Movement Abnormalities in Arnold-Chiari Malformation

Downbeat nystagmus, worse on lateral gaze, occasionally with torsional component

Other types of nystagmus
- Gaze-evoked and rebound nystagmus (including torsional rebound)
- Horizontal unidirectional nystagmus (present in central position)
- Periodic alternating nystagmus
- Seesaw nystagmus
- Divergence or convergence nystagmus
- Positional nystagmus

Internuclear ophthalmoplegia

Strabismus
- Divergence paralysis
- Skew deviation

Saccadic dysmetria

Impaired pursuit and VOR cancellation

Abnormal VOR
- Increased VOR gain
- Decreased VOR time constant and impaired tilt suppression

Impaired optokinetic nystagmus with slow buildup of eye velocity in response to constant-velocity stimuli

---

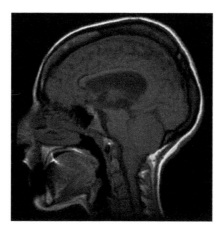

Sagittal MRI showing Arnold-Chiari malformation type II with herniation of the cerebellar vermis and medulla through the foramen magnum.

10.3.2 Dandy-Walker Malformation

Clinical Features of Dandy-Walker Malformation

Triad of:
1. Complete or partial agenesis of the vermis
2. Cystic dilation of the fourth ventricle
3. Enlarged posterior fossa with upward displacement of lateral sinuses, tentorium, and torcular herophili

Developmental delay

Difficulty with balance, spasticity, and poor fine motor control

Enlarged head circumference

Signs and symptoms of hydrocephalus (70–90%)

Eye Movement Abnormalities in Dandy-Walker Malformation

Mild saccadic dysmetria

Nystagmus and strabismus (also seen in patients with agenesis of vermis or hypoplasia of the entire cerebellum)

Differential diagnosis of posterior fossa cystic malformations

Dandy-Walker complex (a spectrum of anomalies):

- Dandy-Walker malformation: the classic triad
- Dandy-Walker variant: hypoplasia of the vermis and cystic dilation of the fourth ventricle without enlargement of the posterior fossa
- Mega cisterna magna: enlarged posterior fossa, secondary to an enlarged cisterna magna, but a normal cerebellar vermis and fourth ventricle

Retrocerebellar arachnoid cyst, which results in anterior displacement of the fourth ventricle and cerebellum

10.3.3 Walker-Warburg Syndrome

Walker-Warburg syndrome, aslo known as HARD +/− E syndrome, is a congenital condition characterized by *h*ydrocephalus, *a*gyria, *r*etinal *d*ysplasia, with or without *e*ncephalocele. It is usually lethal within the first few months of life.

Clinical Features of Walker-Warburg Syndrome

Eye manifestations

Retinal dysplasia (100%)

Microphthalmia (53%)

Coloboma (24%)

CNS manifestations

Type II lissencephaly (100%): argyria, macrogyria, polymicrogyria

Hypoplasia of cerebellar vermis (100%)

Ventriculomegaly and hydrocephalus (95%)

Dandy-Walker malformation (53%)

Other manifestations

Congenital muscular dystrophy (100%)

Genital anomalies (65%)

10.4 Hereditary Ataxias

10.4.1 Episodic Ataxias

Clinical feature	Episodic ataxia type 1	Episodic ataxia type 2	Benign recurrent vertigo
Age of onset	2–20 years	2–30 years	2–50 years
Male to female ratio	1:1	1:1	1:2
Duration of attacks	Seconds to minutes	Hours	Minutes to hours
Triggers	Stress, exercise, startle	Stress, exercise, caffeine	Stress, sleep deprivation, hormones
Migraine	Unknown	50%	75%
Interictal signs	Myokymia in periorbital muscles and fingers, EMG evidence in mild cases	Mild ataxia; nystagmus (gaze-evoked, rebound, and downbeat); dysmetric saccades with normal velocity; impaired pursuit, OKN, and VOR cancellation; increased VOR gain	Vestibulopathy: vertigo, nausea or vomiting, peripheral vestibular nystagmus
Acetazolamide response[a]	50%	90% (may also try a calcium channel blocker such as flunarizine)	70%
Genetics	Autosomal dominant, 12q13; KCNA1 (a potassium channel gene)	Autosomal dominant, 19p; CACNA1A (a calcium channel gene)	Unknown
Location of gene product	Brain (Purkinje, basket, and granular cells in the cerebellum); peripheral nerves (juxtaparanodal regions of nodes of Ranvier)	Brain (especially the cerebellum); neuromuscular junction	Unknown
MRI findings	Normal	May have midline cerebellar atrophy	Normal

EMG, electromyograph; OKN, optokinetic nystagmus; VOR, vestibulo-ocular reflex.

[a]Acetazolamide: 250 mg orally per day; increase by 250 mg every 3 days to maximum daily dosage of 3 g. Acetazolamide alters the pH in cerebellum, thereby stabilizing the mutated calcium channels.

10.4.2 Spinocerebellar Ataxias (SCA) with Eye Movement Abnormalities

Current name (alternative name)	Eye movement abnormalities	Other features	Genetics
SCA1	Hypermetric and mildly slow saccades; gaze-evoked and rebound nystagmus; decreased VOR gain	Optic nerve pallor; pyramidal tract signs; dysphagia	Autosomal dominant (AD), 6p23 (CAG triplet repeats)
SCA2 (olivopontocerebellar atrophy)	Very slow saccades, especially horizontal	Dysarthria; decreased tendon reflexes	AD, 12q24 (CAG triplet repeats)
SCA3 (Machado-Joseph disease)	Dysmetric saccades; gaze-evoked and rebound nystagmus; square wave jerks; decreased VOR gain; strabismus	Faciolingual myokymia; dystonia; Parkinsonism	AD, 14q24.3-q31 (CAG triplet repeats)
SCA6 (Holmes type; ADCA3 of Harding)	Dysmetric saccades with normal velocity; downbeat nystagmus; gaze-evoked and rebound nystagmus; square wave jerks; increased or decreased VOR gain	Late onset; "pure" cerebellar atrophy with loss of Purkinje cells	AD, 19p13.13 (CAG triplet repeats)
SCA7 (ADCA2 of Harding)	Slow saccades; supranuclear ophthalmoplegia	Pigmentary maculopathy; hearing loss; extrapyramidal signs	AD, 3p21.1-p12 (CAG triplet repeats)
SCA8	Dysmetric saccades; gaze-evoked nystagmus; square wave jerks; impaired pursuit	Dysarthria; atrophy of cerebellar vermis and hemispheres	AD, 13q21 (CGT triplet repeats)
SCA20	Hypermetric saccades; square wave jerks; impaired pursuit	Dysarthria; palatal tremor; dentate nucleus calcification	AD, 11p13-q11
Dentatorubral pallidoluysian atrophy (Haw River syndrome)	Slow saccades	Epilepsy; myoclonus; choreoathetosis; dementia	AD, 12p (CAG triplet repeats)

VOR, vestibulo-ocular reflex.

10.4.3 Recessive Ataxias

Current name (alternative name)	Eye movement abnormalities	Other features	Genetics
Friedreich's ataxia (classic and atypical forms)	Square wave jerks; decreased VOR gain	Onset before 20 years; sensory loss; areflexia; Babinski responses; cardiomyopathy; diabetes mellitus	Autosomal recessive, 9q
Hereditary vitamin E deficiency (α-tocopherol transfer protein gene) and abetalipoproteinemia (see section 12.6.3)	Progressive ophthalmoplegia; slow saccades; dissociated nystagmus (adduction faster than abduction); internuclear ophthalmoplegia	Friedreich-like picture; retinitis pigmentosa	Autosomal recessive, 8q
Ataxia telangiectasia (Louis-Bar syndrome)	Ocular motor apraxia; gaze-evoked nystagmus; square wave jerks; periodic alternating nystagmus	Oculocutaneous telangiectasia; radiosensitivity; immunological disorders; cancer; elevated α-fetoprotein	Autosomal recessive, 11q
Spinocerebellar ataxia with saccadic intrusions (SCASI)	Hypermetric saccades; saccadic intrusions; macrosaccadic oscillations; large saccades have higher speed than normal	Sensorimotor neuropathy; pyramidal tract signs with increased reflexes and extensor plantar responses; myoclonic jerks, fasciculations	Autosomal recessive, 1p36
Ataxia-oculomotor apraxia 1 (AOA1)	Oculomotor apraxia; external ophthalmoplegia	Onset 2–10 years; peripheral axonal neuropathy; chorea; hypoalbuminemia	Autosomal recessive, 9p13.3
Ataxia-oculomotor apraxia 2 (AOA2)	Oculomotor apraxia; gaze-evoked nystagmus; impaired smooth pursuit	Onset 11–20 years; sensorimotor neuropathy; increased serum α-fetoprotein	Autosomal recessive, 9p34

10.5 Cerebellar Infarction

10.5.1 Superior Cerebellar Artery Syndrome

The superior cerebellar artery supplies the superior surface of the cerebellar hemisphere, vermis, and superior cerebellar peduncle. Superior cerebellar artery syndrome is the most common type of cerebellar infarction.

Eye Movement and Neurologic Abnormalities in Superior Cerebellar Artery Syndrome
Saccadic contrapulsion: hypermetric contralesional saccades and hypometric ipsilesional saccades Ipsilateral ataxia of gait and limbs Dysarthria (common in rostral cerebellar lesion) Ipsilateral Horner's syndrome Contralateral pain and temperature loss in trunk and limbs; contralateral fourth nerve palsy. Vertigo (less common; more characteristic of posterior inferior cerebellar artery syndrome)

10.5.2 Posterior Inferior Cerebellar Artery Syndrome

The posterior inferior cerebellar artery supplies the lateral medulla, inferior cerebellar peduncle, the nodulus, and uvula.

Eye Movement and Neurologic Abnormalities in Posterior Inferior Cerebellar Artery Syndrome
One of the following three patterns is seen: 1. Classic lateral medullary syndrome (see section 9.2.1) 2. Isolated vertigo and nystagmus (often misdiagnosed as inner ear disease; therefore, look for gaze-evoked nystagmus, which is usually prominent) 3. Vertigo, ipsilateral axial lateropulsion, dysmetria or unsteadiness

10.5.3 Anterior Inferior Cerebellar Artery Syndrome

Anterior inferior cerebellar artery syndrome is uncommon. The anterior inferior cerebellar artery supplies portions of the vestibular nuclei, adjacent dorsolateral brainstem, labyrinthine artery, and inferior lateral cerebellum, including the flocculus. This syndrome is often misdiagnosed as lateral medullary syndrome.

Eye Movement and Neurologic Abnormalities in Anterior Inferior Cerebellar Artery Syndrome

In addition to those abnormalities seen in lateral medullary syndrome (see section 9.2.1), the following abnormalities may be seen:

- Gaze-evoked nystagmus
- Horizontal gaze palsy due to involvement of the abducens nucleus
- Ipsilateral facial motor palsy (seventh cranial nerve)
- Deafness (eighth cranial nerve)

Chapter 11

Ocular Motor Disorders Caused by Lesions in the Cerebrum

11.1 Ocular Motor Syndromes Caused by Lesions in the Thalamus

Nuclei of the thalamus

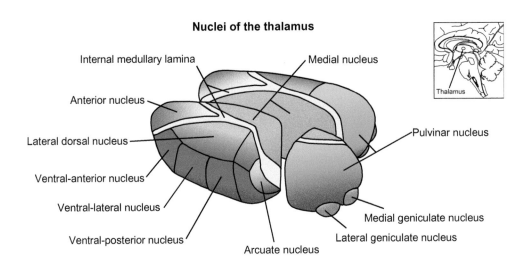

Internal medullary lamina

Medial nucleus

Anterior nucleus

Lateral dorsal nucleus

Pulvinar nucleus

Ventral-anterior nucleus

Ventral-lateral nucleus

Ventral-posterior nucleus

Medial geniculate nucleus

Lateral geniculate nucleus

Arcuate nucleus

Thalamus

Eye Movement Abnormalities in Thalamus Lesion

"Wrong-way deviation": conjugate gaze deviation away from the side of the lesion[1]

Sustained downward deviation of the eyes[2], with convergence and miosis ("peer at the nose")

"Thalamic esotropia" (due to a caudal thalamic lesion)[3] ▸▸

Less common findings

- Tilt of subjective visual vertical ipsilaterally or contralaterally (due to posterolateral thalamic infarction)
- Paralysis of downgaze[4]: Seen in caudal thalamus infarction, as a result of occlusion of the proximal portion of the posterior cerebral artery, or its perforator branch, the posterior thalamosubthalamic paramedian artery
- Impairment of horizontal gaze[5]
- Difficulties in shifting gaze into the contralateral hemifield, decrease in spontaneous scanning, and loss of stereoacuity[6]

---

1. May be an irritative phenomenon; electrical stimulation of the internal medullary lamina (IML) elicits saccades directed away from the site of stimulation.

2. Due to compression on structures responsible for upgaze located in the pretectal area of the midbrain.

3. May be due to disturbance of convergence inputs to the oculomotor nuclei; combined lesions of the thalamus and midbrain may impair convergence unilaterally.

4. May be due to involvement of the adjacent riMLF or its immediate premotor inputs.

5. May be due to disturbance of the mesencephalic reticular formation or of descending pathways.

6. Due to involvement of the pulvinar.

11.2 Ocular Motor Syndromes Caused by Lesions in the Basal Ganglia

11.2.1 Lesions in the Caudate Nucleus and Substantia Nigra Pars Reticulata

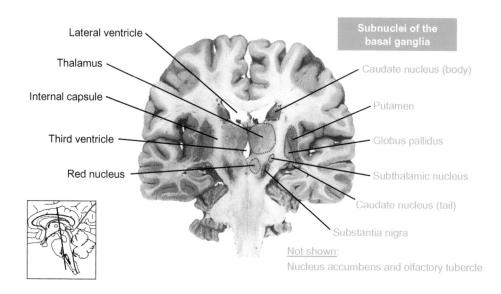

Lateral ventricle
Thalamus
Internal capsule
Third ventricle
Red nucleus

Subnuclei of the basal ganglia

Caudate nucleus (body)
Putamen
Globus pallidus
Subthalamic nucleus
Caudate nucleus (tail)
Substantia nigra

Not shown:
Nucleus accumbens and olfactory tubercle

Caudate nucleus

- Receives inputs from the frontal eye field (FEF), supplementary eye field (SEF), dorsolateral prefrontal cortex (DLPC), internal medullary lamina of the thalamus, and substantia nigra pars compacta (SNpc, the dopaminergic portion)
- Projects to substantia nigra pars reticulata (SNpr) and the globus pallidus

Eye Movement Abnormalities in Caudate Nucleus Lesion
Hypometric and slow contralateral memory-guided saccades with increased latency Gaze preference toward the ipsilesional hemifield

Substantia nigra pars reticulata

- Receives inhibitory inputs from the caudate nucleus
- Sends inhibitory signals to intermediate layers of the superior colliculus

Eye Movement Abnormalities in Substantia Nigra Pars Reticulata Lesion
Saccadic intrusions directed contralateral to the side of lesion

11.2.2 Parkinson's Disease

Parkinson's disease is a progressive neurodegenerative disorder that affects about 1% of adults over 60 years of age.

Clinical Features of Parkinson's Disease

Resting tremor (about 4 Hz)
- "Pill-rolling" motion of the hand
- Decreases with movement and disappears in sleep

Rigidity
- Increased resistance to passive movement about a joint
- The resistance can either be constant (lead pipe) or intermittent (cogwheeling) throughout the range of motion.

Bradykinesia
- Difficulty with rapid alternating movement (e.g., opening and closing fist)
- Masklike facies
- Micrographia (affecting fine finger movement)

Postural instability (leading to falls) and stooped posture
Shuffling gait with decreased arm swing
Autonomic symptoms: urinary frequency, constipation
Other features: depression (20–30%), cortical dementia (10–15%), slowness of thought and response

Pathophysiology

1. Loss of pigmented dopaminergic neurons in the SNpc
2. Presence of Lewy bodies (not specific for Parkinson's disease)
3. Decreased dopamine reaching the striatum causes increased inhibitory output from the globus pallidus internal segment and SNpr, thereby inhibiting movement

The basal ganglia motor circuit

GPi = Globus pallidus internal segment
GPe = Globus pallidus external segment
SNpr = Substantia nigra pars reticulata

Square-wave jerks

Saccades

- Early stage: hypometric horizontal and vertical, especially upward, saccades with normal velocity (in contrast, progressive supranuclear palsy is characterized by slow downward saccades with normal range of motion)
- Advanced stage: slow saccades

Smooth pursuit: impaired both horizontally and vertically

Vestibulo-ocular reflex (VOR): normal for natural head movements (decreased gain in dark and during low-frequency rotation)

Combined eye–head tracking (VOR cancellation): abnormal, due to impaired smooth pursuit

Convergence insufficiency (common)

Oculogyric crisis

- Common causes: side effect of neuroleptic agents (most common), postencephalitic parkinsonism, striatocapsular infarction, bilateral putaminal hemorrhage
- Typical attack: feelings of fear or depression, which give rise to obsessive fixation on a thought; eyes deviate upward, and sometimes laterally (movements of the eyes in the upper field of gaze appear nearly normal)—may reflect an imbalance of the vertical gaze-holding mechanism (neural integrator)
- Treatment: anticholinergic drugs

Lid abnormalities: decreased blink, lid retraction on looking straight ahead, lid lag on downgaze, apraxia of eyelid opening

Treatment

1. Standard therapy: levadopa and carbidopa (a peripheral decarboxylase inhibitor to reduce motor fluctuations and dyskinesia) e.g., such as Sinemet or Sinemet CR

2. Monoamine oxidase-β inhibitor (e.g., Selegiline); may have neuroprotective effect

3. Dopamine agonist (e.g., bromocriptine, a D2 agonist, and apomorphine, a D1 and D2 agonist)

4. Anticholinergics (e.g., Benzhexol)

5. Amantadine (seldom used)

6. Surgery
   - Thalamotomy or thalamic deep brain stimulation of the ventral lateral nucleus to reduce medically refractory tremor. The mechanism of action is unknown; these procedures may destroy autonomous neural activity (synchronous bursts) that has the same frequency as the limb tremor.
   - Pallidotomy or pallidal stimulation to reduce contralateral dyskinesia (e.g., bradykinesia, rigidity, and tremor).
   - Subthalamotomy (because the subthalamic nucleus is hyperactive in Parkinson's disease)
   - Transplantation of dopamine-producing cells (e.g., fetal nigral cells)

11.2.3 Eye Movement Abnormalities in Parkinsonism

Disease	Clinical features	Distinctive eye movement abnormalities	Pathology	Causes
Parkinson's disease	Resting tremor; rigidity; akinesia/ bradykinesia	Hypometric vertical saccades, especially upward (see section 11.2.2)	Presence of Lewy bodies and loss of pigmented dopaminergic neurons in substantia nigra	Idiopathic (most common); familial toxic; vascular; postinfectious
Progressive supranuclear palsy (PSP)	More common in males; prominent akinesia; truncal rigidity; subcortical dementia	Slow vertical saccades, especially downward; vertical gaze palsy in advanced stage (see section 9.4.4)	Neurofibrillary tangles and neuronal loss in subcortical and brainstem areas	Idiopathic
Lytico-Bodig (amyotrophic lateral sclerosis/ Parkinsonism- dementia complex)	Predominantly rigidity and akinesia with little or no tremor; dementia; amyotrophic lateral sclerosis; found in Guam	Vertical gaze palsy; impaired pursuit; abnormal VOR cancellation; abnormal convergence; abnormal OKN; nystagmus; saccadic palsy; abnormal fixation	Neurofibrillary tangles (similar to those found in PSP); no Lewy bodies; no Alzheimer plaques	Unknown: may be due to toxin (e.g., B-methylamino-L- alanine in cycad plants); virus (postencephalitic, slow virus or prion); genetic mutation
Corticobasal ganglionic degeneration	Asymmetric, rapidly progressive akinesia and rigidity; resistant to levadopa; cortical signs: dementia, alien limb syndrome, limb apraxia, reflex myoclonus	Vertical gaze palsy; markedly delayed visually guided saccades with normal velocity	Enlarged achromatic neurons in cortical areas; nigral and striatal neuronal loss	Unknown

Disease	Clinical features	Distinctive eye movement abnormalities	Pathology	Causes
Lewy bodies disease	Either predominantly Parkinsonism (tremor, rigidity) or predominantly dementia; abnormal response to neuroleptics	Vertical gaze palsy	Lewy bodies in cerebral cortex; density of Lewy bodies correlated with severity of dementia	Unknown
Multiple system atrophy (MSA)	Three clinical presentations: ■ Shy-Drager syndrome: autonomic and urinary dysfunction predominate ■ Striatonigral degeneration (MSA-P): Parkinsonism predominates ■ Sporadic olivo-pontocerebellar atrophy (MSA-C): cerebellar dysfunction predominates	Hypometric vertical saccades	Glial cytoplasmic inclusions, cell loss, and gliosis in spinal cord, basal ganglia, cerebellum, and pyramidal tracts	Unknown

VOR, vestibulo-ocular reflex; OKN, optokinetic nystagmus.

11.2.4 Huntington's Disease

Huntington's disease is an incurable, adult-onset, autosomal dominant disorder associated with cell loss within the striatum (caudate nucleus and putamen) in the basal ganglia and in the cortex. It results from a defect of the *IT15* gene on chromosome 4, causing increased CAG triplet repeat length and production of the "huntingtin" protein.

Clinical Features of Huntington's Disease

Chorea

- Initially, chorea may appear as uncontrollable flailing of the extremities (ballism).
- As the disease progresses, chorea coexists with and is gradually replaced by dystonia (sustained muscle contractions causing twisting and abnormal posture) and parkinsonism (bradykinesia, rigidity, and postural instability).
- In advanced stages, patients present with akinetic-rigid syndrome with minimal or no chorea.

Dementia

Depression

Eye Movement Abnormalities in Huntington's Disease

Saccades

- Acquired ocular motor apraxia[1] (i.e., difficulties initiating saccades to command, often facilitated by a head thrust or a blink)
- Difficulties suppressing reflexive saccades to novel visual stimuli, especially during the antisaccade task[2]
- Slow saccades, especially vertical[3]

Impaired smooth pursuit

Preservation of VOR and gaze-holding

Saccadic intrusions[4]

---

1. Involvement of either the frontal lobes or the caudate nucleus (which inhibits the substantia nigra pars reticulata or SNpr) may lead to difficulties in initiating voluntary saccades that require learned or predictive behavior.

2. Due to excessive distractibility resulting from involvement of the SNpr which normally inhibits the superior colliculus to suppress reflexive saccades to visual stimuli.

3. Involvement of saccadic burst neurons or prenuclear inputs such as the superior colliculus or frontal eye fields.

4. Due to excessive distractibility during attempted fixation (SNpr involvement).

Treatment

For severe chorea: benzodiazepines, valproic acid, dopamine-depleting agents (reserpine or tetrabenazine), or neuroleptics

For Parkinsonism: levodopa or dopamine agonists

For depression: antidepressants (e.g., selective serotonin reuptake inhibitors)

11.2.5 Other Basal Ganglia Diseases

Disorder	Eye movement abnormalities	Clinical features
Bilateral lesions in the lentiform nucleus (putamen and globus pallidus)	Abnormal predictive and memory-guided saccades (both are internally generated); normal visually guided saccades and antisaccades (both are externally triggered by a visual target)	Dystonia; infrequently causes behavioral disturbances such as abulia (apathy, loss of initiative, loss of spontaneous thought and emotional responses)
Spasmodic torticollis	Abnormal VOR, including torsional VOR; tilt of subjective visual vertical	Slow contraction of cervical and nuchal musculature against antagonist resistance, with turning movement of the head
Essential blepharospasm	Generally, eye movements are normal; saccadic latencies may be increased in certain visually guided and memory-guided saccade tasks	Recurrent, spasmodic contraction of the orbicularis oculi muscles; causes blindness during the spastic phase when eyelids are closed; a subgroup of patients cannot open their flaccid, closed eyelids, and this type of blepharospasm is called lid-opening apraxia
Tardive dyskinesia	Increased saccade distractibility	Induced by prolonged use of neuroleptics; stereotypic chewing, licking, and smacking movements
Sydenham's chorea (chorea minor)	Saccade hypometria	Sudden, usually rapid, distal, brief, irregular involuntary movements; hypotonia
Tourette's syndrome	Intermittent involuntary gaze deviations; impaired sequencing of memory-guided saccades; increased latency and decreased peak velocity of antisaccades; normal fixation and pursuit	Blepharospasm and eye tics
Lesch-Nyhan disease	Impaired ability to make voluntary saccades and increased errors in antisaccade task; intermittent gaze deviations similar to Tourette's syndrome	Hyperuricemia, recurrent self-injurious behavior, and extrapyramidal features; blepharospasm

VOR, vestibulo-ocular reflex.

11.3.1 Lesions in the Frontal Lobe

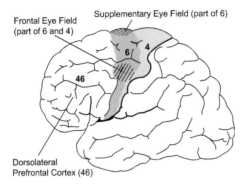

* Numbered areas denote corresponding Brodmann areas

Frontal Eye Field

The human homologue lies around the lateral part of the precentral sulcus, in adjacent areas that include part of the precentral gyrus, middle frontal gyrus, and superior frontal gyrus (portions of Brodmann areas 6 and 4).

- Receives inputs from posterior visual cortical areas, contralateral frontal eye field (FEF), supplementary eye field (SEF), dorsolateral prefrontal cortex (DLPC), inferior parietal cortex, intralaminar thalamic nuclei, substantia nigra pars reticulata (SNpr), superior colliculus, and dentate nucleus in the cerebellum
- Projects to the contralateral FEF, SEF, posterior visual cortical areas, superior colliculus (both directly and indirectly via the caudate and SNpr), nucleus reticularis tegmenti pontis (NRTP), and nucleus raphe interpositus (rip)
- Contributes to all voluntary and visually guided saccades, to smooth pursuit, and to vergence

Eye Movement Abnormalities in Frontal Eye Field Lesion

Acutely, ipsilesional gaze deviation

Chronically, subtle saccade abnormalities

- Increased latency of predictive saccades, memory-guided saccades, antisaccades, and saccades generated using the "overlap" paradigm (see section 4.1)
- Hypometria of saccades made to targets (visual or remembered) located contralateral to the side of the lesion
- Impaired ability to suppress inappropriate saccades to a novel visual stimulus

Impaired smooth pursuit and optokinetic nystagmus for targets moving toward the side of the lesion

Supplementary Eye Field

The human homologue lies in the posteriomedial portion of the superior frontal gyrus (portion of Brodmann area 6).

- Receives inputs from the FEF, prefrontal, cingulate, parietal, and temporal cortex, as well as the thalamus and claustrum
- Projects to the FEF, to the prefrontal, cingulate, parietal, and temporal cortex, and to the thalamus, claustrum, caudate nucleus, superior colliculus, NRTP, and rip
- Important for planning saccades to both visual and nonvisual cues as part of learned or complex behaviors

Eye Movement Abnormalities in Supplementary Eye Field Lesion

Inaccurate memory-guided saccades if gaze shifts during the memory period

Loss of ability to make a remembered sequence of saccades to an array of visual targets (especially with left-sided SEF lesions)

Normal visually guided saccades

Dorsolateral Prefrontal Cortex

The human homologue lies in the middle frontal gyrus and adjacent cortex (Brodmann areas 46 and 9).

- Receives inputs from the FEF, SEF, posterior parietal cortex and limbic cortex (including parahippocampal and cingulate cortex), thalamus, and medial pulvinar
- Projects to the FEF, SEF, posterior parietal and limbic cortex, caudate and putamen, superior colliculus and paramedian pontine reticular formation
- Important for programming memory-guided saccades and antisaccades

Eye Movement Abnormalities in Dorsolateral Prefrontal Cortex Lesion

Impaired predictive and memory-guided saccades toward contralesional targets

Impaired antisaccades

11.3.2 Lesions in the Parietal Lobe

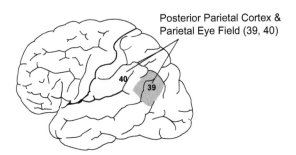

Posterior Parietal Cortex &
Parietal Eye Field (39, 40)

40   39

* Numbered areas denote corresponding Brodmann areas

Posterior Parietal Cortex (Area 7a in monkeys)

The human homologue lies in the inferior parietal lobule (portions of Brodmann areas 39 and 40).

- Receives inputs from medial superior temporal visual area (MST), superior colliculus, cingulate cortex, pulvinar, and the intralaminar thalamic nuclei
- Projects to the FEF, DLPC, and cingulate gyrus
- Important for directing visual attention in extrapersonal space

Parietal Eye Field

The human homologue lies in the intraparietal sulcus, the superior part of the angular gyrus, and the supramarginal gyrus (portions of Brodmann areas 39 and 40).

- Receives input from secondary visual areas
- Projects to the FEF and the superior colliculus
- Important for triggering visually guided saccades

Eye Movement Abnormalities in Parietal Lobe Lesion

Unilateral lesions

Ipsilesional gaze deviation

Contralesional inattention (especially with right-sided lesion)

Increased latency for visually guided saccades

Impaired smooth pursuit if target moves across a textured background

Bilateral lesions: Balint's syndrome (psychic paralysis of gaze)

Difficulty in making visually guided saccades (increased latency and decreased accuracy; e.g., impaired ability to perform visual search)

Peripheral visual inattention (simultanagnosia)

Inaccurate arm pointing (optic ataxia)

11.3.3 Lesions in the Posterior Cortical Areas

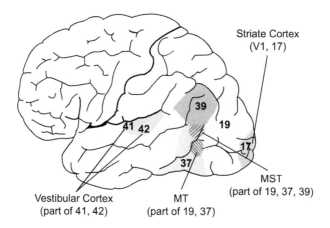

Striate Cortex
(V1, 17)

Vestibular Cortex
(part of 41, 42)

MT
(part of 19, 37)

MST
(part of 19, 37, 39)

* Numbered areas denote corresponding Brodmann areas

Primary Visual Cortex (Striate Cortex, V1)

The human homologue lies in Broderman area 17. The primary visual cortex receives input from the lateral geniculate nucleus.

Eye Movement Abnormalities in Primary Visual Cortex Lesion
Impaired ability to generate saccades or smooth pursuit in response to visual stimuli presented in the blind hemifield

Middle Temporal Visual Area (MT or V5)

The human homologue lies at the occipital-temporal-parietal junction (junction of Brodmann areas 19, 37, and 39).

- Receives inputs from primary visual cortex (V1)
- Projects to medial superior temporal visual area (MST), other cortical areas concerned with visual motion, FEF, and dorsolateral pontine nuclei

Eye Movement Abnormalities in Middle Temporal Visual Area Lesion: Scotoma of Motion
Retinotopic defect of motion (scotoma of motion): decreased smooth pursuit speed and dysmetric saccades in all directions in the contralesional hemifield (see section 5.3)

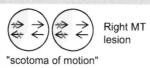

Right MT lesion

"scotoma of motion"

Medial Superior Temporal Visual Area (MST)

The human homologue lies close to middle temporal visual area (MT) at the occipital-temporal-parietal junction (junction of Brodmann areas 19, 37, and 39).

- Receives visual inputs from MT, and receives vestibular and ocular motor signals
- Projects to the FEF and other cortical areas concerned with visual motion and to dorsolateral pontine nuclei

---

Eye Movement Abnormalities in Medial Superior Temporal Visual Area Lesion: Directional Pursuit Defects

Decreased smooth pursuit speed toward the side of lesion, regardless of the hemifield where the target lies (see section 5.3)

Saccades are not affected.

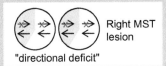

"directional deficit"

Right MST lesion

Posterior Temporal Lobe/Insula (Vestibular Cortex)

The human homologue lies in the posterior aspect of the superior temporal gyrus, which is part of the vestibular cortex (i.e., the parieto-insular-vestibular cortex; Brodmann areas 41 and 42).

Eye Movement Abnormalities in Posterior Temporal Lobe/Insula Lesion

Tilt of subjective visual vertical contralateral to the side of the lesion

Abolishment of circularvection (sense of self-rotation) during optokinetic stimulation

---

11.3.4 Eye Movement Abnormalities in Chronic Extensive Hemispheric Lesions

Eye Movement Abnormalities in Chronic Large Hemispheric Lesions

Fixation
- In darkness, eyes drift away from the side of the lesion.
- Square-wave jerks

Forced eyelid closure: Cogan's "spasticity of conjugate gaze"—conjugate eye deviation away from the side of the lesion

Saccades
- Slow horizontal saccades in both directions, especially contralesional saccades
- Dysmetric saccades (hypometric and hypermetric) into the blind hemifield
- Vertical saccades may have inappropriate horizontal component.

Smooth pursuit: decreased pursuit gain toward the side of the lesion

Vestibular
- During sinusoidal head rotation in dark, VOR gain may be slightly asymmetric, with higher gain during eye movements away from the side of the lesion. During attempted fixation of a stationary target, the asymmetry is increased.
- No response asymmetry during rapid head turns

Optokinetic
- Decreased gain for stimuli directed toward the side of the lesion
- Impaired optokinetic after-nystagmus

11.3.5 Ocular Motor Apraxia

Acquired Ocular Motor Apraxia

Acquired ocular motor apraxia is caused by acute bilateral frontal or frontoparietal lesions, such as found with bihemispheric infarcts, Huntington's disease, and AIDS-related dementia.

Eye Movement Abnormalities in Acquired Ocular Motor Apraxia

Loss of voluntary saccades and smooth pursuit[1]
   Example: Inability to make saccades (horizontal and vertical) to command or to follow a target
Use combined eye-head movements, often with a blink, to shift gaze
Preservation of reflexive eye movements (reflexive saccades, VOR)
   Example: Preserved VOR slow and quick phases; ability to initiate reflexive saccades to novel visual stimuli
Spasm of fixation: inability to shift gaze using voluntary eye movement when a target is continuously present (gaze shift occurs when the target disappears)

---

1. Due to disruption of descending pathways from *both* the frontal eye field (FEF) and the parietal cortex, so that cortical inputs cannot reach the superior colliculus and brainstem to generate voluntary saccades and smooth pursuit.

Congenital Ocular Motor Apraxia ▸▸

Congenital ocular motor apraxia can be idiopathic (i.e. Cogan's type) or associated with other systemic diseases.

Eye Movement Abnormalities in Congenital Ocular Motor Apraxia (Idiopathic or Cogan's Type)

Abnormal horizontal saccades
 ■ Increased latency and hypometric voluntary and reflexive horizontal saccades, including VOR quick phases (in contrast, reflexive saccades are not affected in acquired form)
 ■ Horizontal saccades have normal velocity
 ■ Normal vertical saccades (in contrast, vertical saccades are affected in acquired form)
Impaired smooth pursuit with low gain and catch-up saccades
Head thrust
 ■ In young patients, the head thrust is compensatory: the head is thrust in the direction of the eccentric target so that the eyes are driven in the opposite direction by the VOR. The head then overshoots the target to allow the contraversively rotated eyes to fixate the target. Once fixation is achieved, the head slowly resumes its central position to allow a direct, straight gaze.
 ■ In older patients, the head thrust is used as a trigger to generate saccades.
 ■ Usually improves with age

Usually can be distinguished from the idiopathic (Cogan's) type when vertical saccades are additionally affected and when saccades are slow. Differential diagnosis include:

Idiopathic (Cogan's type)

Joubert's syndrome[1]

Ataxia telangiectasia

Ataxia-oculomotor apraxia type 1 and 2

Gaucher's disease

GM_1 gangliosidosis

Krabbe's leukodystrophy

Peroxisomal assembly disorder

Pelizaeus-Merzbacher disease[2]

Proprionic acidemia

Lesch-Nyhan disease

Bardet-Biedl syndrome

Cornelia de Lange syndrome

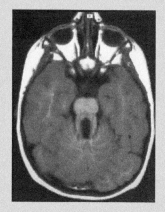

Axial MRI showing molar tooth sign in Joubert's syndrome.

---

1. **Joubert's syndrome** (Joubert-Bolthauser syndrome, or cerebellooculorenal syndrome)
- Sporadic or autosomal recessive (5 loci mapped: 9q34.3, 11q12-q13, 6q23, 2q13, and 12q21.32)
- Characterized by:
  1. Hypoplastic or aplastic cerebellar vermis
  2. Ocular motor apraxia
  3. Episodic tachypnea and apnea, rhythmic protrusion of the tongue, ataxia, hypotonia, psychomotor retardation, retinal dystrophy, cystic dysplastic kidneys, juvenile nephronophthisis, duodenal atresia, and liver fibrosis
  4. Other ocular motor findings: alternating skew deviation, torsional nystagmus, seesaw and pendular nystagmus, and fibrosis of extraocular muscles
- Neuroimaging: "Molar tooth sign"
  1. Abnormally deep posterior interpeduncular fossa
  2. Thickened, elongated and reoriented superior cerebellar peduncles
  3. Hypoplastic or aplastic cerebellar vermis

2. **Pelizaeus-Merzbacher disease** (Sudanophilic leukodystrophy)
- X-linked recessive
- A disorder of central myelin
- A fairly characteristic clinical picture:
  1. Present in infancy with a combination of elliptical pendular and upbeat nystagmus, and intermittent head-shaking, simulating spasmus nutans
  2. Followed by loss of developmental milestones, choreiform and athetoid movements, ocular motor apraxia, saccade dysmetria and other cerebellar signs including truncal titubation
  3. Late findings include seizures, pyramidal signs, spasticity, optic atrophy and retinal degeneration
  4. Preserved intellectual function despite neurological deterioration
  5. Death ensues between 5 and 7 years of age.

Part IV *Nuclear and Infranuclear Ocular Motor Disorders, Disorders of Neuromuscular Transmission, and Extraocular Muscle Myopathies*

Nuclear and infranuclear ocular motor disorders are caused by lesions in the oculomotor, trochlear, or abducens nerves that may be located anywhere from the ocular motor nuclei to the termination of the nerves in the extraocular muscles. These disorders are common causes of diplopia. When examining a patient with diplopia, the physician should first establish whether the diplopia is monocular (present during viewing with one eye) or binocular (present during viewing with both eyes). Although exceptions do occur, as a general rule, monocular diplopia is usually caused by ocular diseases (which require a detailed ophthalmologic examination to rule out any abnormalities in the cornea, lens, and retina), whereas binocular diplopia is usually caused by strabismus.

If a patient experiences binocular diplopia, the physician should then establish whether the diplopia is comitant (same degree of diplopia in different gaze) or incomitant (diplopia that varies with gaze). Comitant strabismus is common in childhood strabismus with no underlying neurologic abnormalities and is sometimes seen in patients with longstanding incomitant strabismus that secondarily becomes comitant over time due to spread of comitance. Incomitant strabismus, in contrast, is usually caused by either an innervational or mechanical abnormality. Innervational disorders can be further classified as those caused by supranuclear or internuclear lesions, such as skew deviation and internuclear ophthalmoplegia, and those caused by nuclear or infranuclear lesions, including ocular motor nerve palsy, peripheral neuropathy, disorders of neuromuscular junctions, and disorders affecting the extraocular muscles. Likewise, mechanical abnormalities causing incomitant strabismus can be further classified as those caused by a restrictive process (such as Brown's syndrome), and those caused by other inflammatory, infectious, neoplastic, iatrogenic, and traumatic processes (see section 12.1 for an approach to diplopia).

In this part, nuclear and infranuclear eye movement disorders are discussed, including oculomotor, trochlear, and abducens nerve palsy (chapter 12), peripheral neuropathy such as Guillain-Barré and Miller Fisher syndromes (chapter 12), disorders of neuromuscular junctions such as myasthenia gravis and botulism (chapter 13), and disorders affecting the extraocular muscles (chapter 14). Although congenital fibrosis of extraocular muscles is traditionally believed to be a primarily mechanical or fibrotic process affecting the extraocular muscles, recent evidence suggests that fibrosis of extraocular muscles belongs to a group of congenital neuromuscular disorders caused by developmental errors in innervation. These congenital neuromuscular disorders are discussed in section 12.2.3.

12.1 An Approach to Diplopia

Is the Diplopia Monocular or Binocular?

Binocular diplopia is usually caused by strabismus, whereas monocular diplopia is usually caused by ocular diseases.

Differential Diagnosis of Monocular Diplopia

Anterior segment abnormalities (e.g., refractive error, astigmatism, corneal opacities, cataract)

Retinal abnormalities (e.g., retinal hemorrhage, retinal folds)

Central causes

- Palinopsia (perseveration of a visual image over time i.e. inability to erase cortical images)
- Polyopia (perseveration of a visual image in space)

If the Diplopia Is Binocular, Is It Comitant or Incomitant?

Incomitant diplopia is usually caused by an acquired strabismus resulting from abnormal innervation or mechanical restriction.

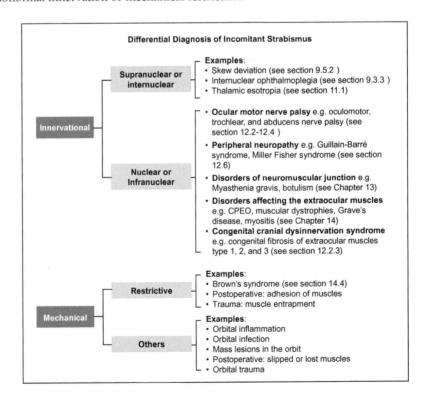

Differential Diagnosis of Incomitant Strabismus

Innervational

Supranuclear or internuclear
Examples:
- Skew deviation (see section 9.5.2)
- Internuclear ophthalmoplegia (see section 9.3.3)
- Thalamic esotropia (see section 11.1)

Nuclear or Infranuclear
- **Ocular motor nerve palsy** e.g. oculomotor, trochlear, and abducens nerve palsy (see section 12.2-12.4)
- **Peripheral neuropathy** e.g. Guillain-Barré syndrome, Miller Fisher syndrome (see section 12.6)
- **Disorders of neuromuscular junction** e.g. Myasthenia gravis, botulism (see Chapter 13)
- **Disorders affecting the extraocular muscles** e.g. CPEO, muscular dystrophies, Grave's disease, myositis (see Chapter 14)
- **Congenital cranial dysinnervation syndrome** e.g. congenital fibrosis of extraocular muscles type 1, 2, and 3 (see section 12.2.3)

Mechanical

Restrictive
Examples:
- Brown's syndrome (see section 14.4)
- Postoperative: adhesion of muscles
- Trauma: muscle entrapment

Others
Examples:
- Orbital inflammation
- Orbital infection
- Mass lesions in the orbit
- Postoperative: slipped or lost muscles
- Orbital trauma

12.2 Oculomotor Nerve Palsy

The oculomotor (third) nerve:

- Innervates the medial rectus, superior rectus, inferior rectus, inferior oblique, and levator palpebrae muscles
- Carries parasympathetic fibers to the iris sphincter and the ciliary body.
- Common causes of third nerve palsy:

Adults: aneurysms, vascular disease (including ischemia, diabetes, hypertension, and inflammatory arteritis), trauma, migraine

Children: birth trauma, accidental trauma, neonatal hypoxia, migraine

Clinical Features of Oculomotor Nerve Palsy

Complete palsy

- Limitation of adduction, elevation, and depression due to involvement of the medial, superior, and inferior rectus muscles
- Globe incyclotorted and exotropic due to unopposed action of the unaffected superior oblique and lateral rectus muscles
- Ptosis due to involvement of the levator palpebrae muscle
- Dilated, poorly reactive pupil due to involvement of the iris sphincter
- Loss of accommodation due to involvement of the ciliary body

Incomplete palsy: any combination of ophthalmoparesis, ptosis, and dilated, poorly reactive pupil

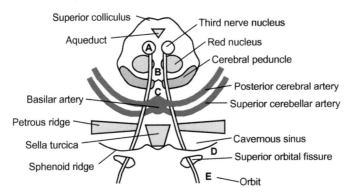

Superior colliculus
Aqueduct
Third nerve nucleus
Red nucleus
Cerebral peduncle
Posterior cerebral artery
Superior cerebellar artery
Basilar artery
Petrous ridge
Sella turcica
Sphenoid ridge
Cavernous sinus
Superior orbital fissure
Orbit

Redrawn with permission from Bajandas FJ, Kline LB. The seven syndromes of the III nerve (oculomotor). In Bajandas FJ, Kline LB, eds. Neuro-Ophthalmology Review Manual. 5th ed. Thorougfare, NJ: SLACK Inc.; 2004:98.

Anatomy of the third nerve

The oculomotor nucleus

The third nerve originates from the oculomotor nucleus complex, which lies at the ventral border of the periaqueductal gray matter in the midbrain.

The oculomotor nerve fascicle

The nerve fascicle passes ventrally through the medial longitudinal fasciculus, the tegmentum, the red nucleus, and the substantia nigra, and finally emerges from the cerebral peduncle to form the oculomotor nerve trunk, which lies between the superior cerebellar and posterior cerebral arteries.

The subarachnoid space

The nerve then passes through the subarachnoid space, running beneath the free edge of the tentorium. It continues lateral to the posterior communicating artery and below the temporal lobe uncus, where it runs over the petroclinoid ligament. It pierces the dura mater at the top of the clivus to enter the cavernous sinus.

The cavernous sinus

Within the cavernous sinus, the nerve runs along the lateral wall of the sinus together with the trochlear nerve and the ophthalmic (V_1) and maxillary (V_2) divisions of the trigeminal nerve.

As it leaves the cavernous sinus, it divides into the superior and inferior divisions, which pass through the superior orbital fissure, and enters the orbit within the annulus of Zinn.

The orbit

Within the orbit, the smaller superior division runs lateral to the optic nerve and ophthalmic artery and supplies the superior rectus and levator palpebrae muscles. The larger inferior division supplies the medial rectus, inferior rectus, and inferior oblique muscles, as well as the iris sphincter and ciliary body.

12.2.1 Topographical Diagnosis of Acquired Oculomotor Nerve Palsy

Lesions of the oculomotor nerve nucleus

The Oculomotor Nucleus Complex

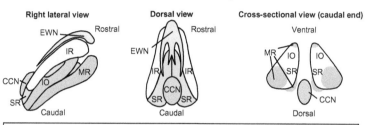

CCN = central caudal nucleus; EWN = Edinger-Westphal nucleus; SR = superior rectus subnucleus
IR = inferiors rectus subnucleus; MR = medial rectus subnucleus; LR = lateral rectus subnucleus
SO = superior oblique subnucleus; IO = inferior oblique subnucleus

Redrawn from Büttner-Ennever JA, Akert K. Medial rectus subgroups of the oculomotor nucleus and their abducens internuclear input in the monkey. J Comp Neurol. 1981; 197:17–27. With permission of John Wiley & Sons.

The oculomotor nucleus complex lies in the midbrain and consists of:

1. A midline unpaired structure called the central caudate nucleus that supplies the levator palpebrae muscle on both sides

2. Four lateral paired subnuclei that innervate the superior, inferior, and medial rectus, as well as the inferior oblique muscles

3. The Edinger-Westphal nucleus, which contains preganglionic, parasympathetic neurons whose axons project to the ciliary ganglion and ultimately control pupillary constriction and accommodation.

Third nerve palsy caused by a nuclear lesion is rare. When it occurs, it produces specific deficits in both eyes because of the anatomy of the nucleus complex:

1. Superior rectus subnucleus: Axons from one superior rectus (SR) subnucleus cross and pass through the opposite SR subnucleus; thus, a lesion of one SR subnucleus results in bilateral superior rectus palsy.

2. Central caudal nucleus:
   - Unpaired and supplies both levator palpebrae muscles; thus, a lesion in the nucleus causes bilateral ptosis
   - Located in the most caudal part of oculomotor nuclear complex, so it may be selectively affected (i.e., bilateral ptosis may be the only manifestation of a nuclear third nerve palsy), or it may be selectively spared

3. Medial rectus subnuclei: lie in three different locations; thus, an isolated medial rectus palsy (unilateral or bilateral) without other muscle involvement cannot be a nuclear third nerve palsy

4. Edinger-Westphal nucleus: spread throughout the rostral half of the oculomotor nucleus complex; thus, the pupil may be spared in lesions affecting the caudal half of the complex, but when the pupil is involved, both pupils are affected (i.e., bilateral internal ophthalmoplegia)

Eye Movement Abnormalities in Nuclear Third Nerve Palsy

Obligatory nuclear lesions
- Unilateral third nerve palsy with bilateral superior rectus palsy and bilateral ptosis
- Bilateral third nerve palsy with normal levator function (sparing of the central caudal nucleus) or normal pupils (sparing of Edinger-Westphal nucleus), or both

Possible nuclear lesions
- Bilateral total third nerve palsy
- Bilateral ptosis (affecting the central caudal nucleus only)
- Isolated weakness of any single muscle except the levator, superior rectus, and medial rectus

Not nuclear lesions
- Unilateral third nerve palsy with normal contralateral superior rectus function
- Unilateral internal ophthalmoplegia
- Unilateral ptosis
- Isolated unilateral or bilateral medial rectus palsy

Etiology of Nuclear Third Nerve Palsy

Ischemia (most common cause)
- From embolic or thrombotic occlusion of small, dorsal perforating branches of the mesencephalic portion of the basilar artery
- Less often from occlusion of the distal portion of the basilar artery (top of the basilar syndrome)

Hemorrhage

Infiltration or tumor

Inflammation

Compression

Others (rare): cephalic tetanus, amyotrophic lateral sclerosis, Kugelberg-Welander disease

Lesions of the oculomotor nerve fascicle

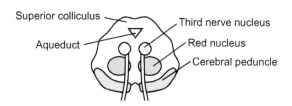

The Oculomotor Nerve Fascicle

Superior colliculus — Third nerve nucleus

Aqueduct — Red nucleus

Cerebral peduncle

Lesions of the oculomotor nerve fascicle can present as an isolated complete or incomplete palsy.

- A fascicular lesion can cause isolated dysfunction of either the superior or inferior division because anatomic separation into superior and inferior divisions begins in the brainstem. However, dysfunction of either the superior or inferior division is more likely to be caused by a lesion in the posterior orbit than a lesion in the fascicle.

- Lesions of the oculomotor nerve fascicle usually present in association with other neurologic signs due to involvement of other midbrain structures:

1. **Weber's syndrome:** ipsilateral third nerve palsy, plus contralateral hemiparesis including the lower face and tongue due to involvement of the cerebral peduncle

2. **Benedikt's syndrome:** ipsilateral third nerve palsy, plus contralateral tremor due to involvement of the red nucleus

3. **Nothnagel's syndrome:** ipsilateral third nerve palsy, plus ipsilateral cerebellar ataxia due to involvement of the superior cerebellar peduncle

4. **Claude's syndrome:** Benedikt's plus Nothnagel's syndrome due to involvement of the red nucleus and superior cerebellar peduncle

Etiology of Fascicular Third Nerve Palsy
Ischemia (most common) due to occlusion of the basilar artery or occlusion of the perforating or medial interpeduncular branches of the posterior cerebral artery
Hemorrhage
Infiltration
Inflammation
Compression
Trauma
Demyelination

Lesions in the subarachnoid space

Lesions in the subarachnoid space can be located anywhere between the ventral surface of the midbrain where the nerve exits and the posterior clinoid process where the nerve enters the cavernous sinus. There are three presentations: (a) isolated dilated, and poorly reactive pupil with normal motility and lid position; (b) third nerve palsy with pupillary involvement; and (c) third nerve palsy with pupillary sparing.

Causes of isolated, dilated, and poorly reactive pupil with normal motility and lid position (extremely rare)

1. Intracranial aneurysms (most common)
   - Aneurysm at the junction of internal carotid and the posterior communicating arteries: other signs usually develop within a few hours
   - Basilar artery aneurysm: other signs develop in days or weeks
2. Supratentorial expanding mass (e.g., hematoma). Herniation of the uncus across the tentorial edge may compress the third nerve and lead to Hutchinson pupil (patient is usually comatose).
3. Cysts in the interpeduncular cistern
4. Intrinsic lesion of the nerve (e.g., schwannomas or cavernous angiomas)
5. Infection (e.g., basal meningitis from tuberculosis or syphilis)

Causes of third nerve palsy with pupillary involvement

1. Intracranial aneurysms (most common): aneurysm at the junction of internal carotid and the posterior communicating arteries, basilar artery aneurysm, or aneurysm at the junction of the basilar and superior cerebellar arteries
2. Trauma (e.g., from aneurysm surgery)
3. Ischemia (20% of cases)
4. Carotid-cavernous fistula (especially posterior draining, low-flow, spontaneous dural type)
5. Supratentorial mass or compressive lesion in the interpeduncular cistern
6. Intrinsic lesion of the nerve (e.g., schwannomas or cavernous angiomas)
7. Infection (e.g., basal meningitis)

Causes of third nerve palsy with pupillary sparing

1. Ischemia (most common)
   - Diabetes mellitus, hypertension, migraine, lupus, and temporal arteritis
   - Pupillomotor fibers travel in the outer layers of the third nerve and are closer to the blood supply; therefore, pupil is spared in 80% of cases from ischemic cause, whereas pupil is involved in 95% of cases from compressive lesions.
2. Compressive lesions (e.g., intracranial aneurysms, acute subdural hematoma)
   - Often cause incomplete palsy with ocular or orbital pain
   - Patients with a painful, incomplete pupil-sparing third nerve palsy should have a MRI and computed tomography/magnetic resonance angiography.

- Both ischemic and compressive lesions cause ocular or orbital pain because sensory fibers from V_1 join the nerve within the lateral wall of the cavernous sinus and run proximally along the nerve bundles to enter the brainstem.
3. Inflammation
4. Others: monoclonal gammopathy, lymphoma, leukemia

Lesions in the cavernous sinus and superior orbital fissure

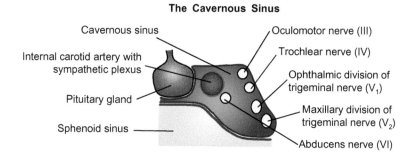

The Cavernous Sinus

Cavernous sinus

Internal carotid artery with sympathetic plexus

Pituitary gland

Sphenoid sinus

Oculomotor nerve (III)

Trochlear nerve (IV)

Ophthalmic division of trigeminal nerve (V_1)

Maxillary division of trigeminal nerve (V_2)

Abducens nerve (VI)

Lesions in the cavernous sinus and superior orbital fissure may present as an isolated third nerve palsy, or, more often, a cranial polyneuropathy. Because it is difficult to determine whether a lesion involves the sinus, the fissure, or both, damage in this region is often considered as a single entity, the sphenocavernous syndrome.

Sphenocavernous syndrome

- Involvement of third, fourth, and sixth cranial nerves
- Involvement of the ophthalmic (V_1) and maxillary (V_2) divisions of the trigeminal nerve
- Sympathetic paralysis (e.g., eyelid edema, conjunctival chemosis)
- Poorly reactive pupil that is small or in mid-position is pathognomonic. The poorly reactive pupil is due to combined involvement of parasympathetic fibers (which travel with nerve and cause pupillary constriction) and oculosympathetic plexus (which is located within the cavernous sinus and causes pupillary dilation).

Causes

1. Vascular lesion (e.g., aneurysm of the internal carotid artery, cavernous sinus thrombosis, carotid-cavernous fistula)
2. Tumors (e.g., meningioma, pituitary tumor, craniopharyngioma, nasopharyngeal carcinoma, metastatic tumors, lymphoma)
3. Infection (e.g., syphilis)
4. Ischemia (e.g., diabetes, temporal arteritis)
5. Inflammation (e.g., Tolosa-Hunt syndrome, lupus, rheumatoid arthritis)
6. Trauma (e.g., skull fracture, iatrogenic)

Lesions within the orbit

- Orbital lesions may selectively involve either the superior division, which innervates the superior rectus and levator palpebrae muscles, or the inferior division, which innervates the medial rectus, inferior rectus, inferior oblique muscles, and carries parasympathetic fibers to iris sphincter and ciliary muscle.
- Associated optic neuropathy or proptosis is usually present.
- Orbital lesions include inflammation, ischemia, infiltration, compression, or trauma.

Pathologic processes of uncertain or variable location

Examples of pathologic processes of uncertain or variable location include nerve infarction (associated with hypertension, diabetes, arteritis), idiopathic, infections, following immunization, ophthalmoplegic migraine, and side effects of drugs.

12.2.2 Congenital Oculomotor Nerve Palsy

Congenital oculomotor nerve palsy accounts for almost half of the third nerve palsy seen in children. It is most often unilateral and sporadic, and there are no other neurologic or systemic abnormalities. It is characterized by ptosis, ophthalmoparesis, and pupillary involvement. The pupil is usually miotic, rather than dilated, because of aberrant regeneration. Causes of congenital oculomotor nerve palsy are:

1. Absent or incomplete development of the nucleus, nerve, or both

2. Trauma (e.g., amniocentesis, birth injury)

Other congenital syndromes involving the oculomotor nerve are described below.

Congenital adduction palsy with synergistic divergence

- Unilateral adduction deficit
- Simultaneous bilateral abduction on attempted adduction of the affected eye
- Pathogenesis: absent innervation of the affected medial rectus muscle with anomalous oculomotor innervation to the lateral rectus

Vertical retraction syndrome

- Limited elevation and depression of the affected eye, with retraction of the globe and narrowing of palpebral fissure on attempted vertical movement
- Pathogenesis: anomalous oculomotor innervation of the vertical muscles in the affected eye

Oculomotor paresis with cyclic spasms (cyclic oculomotor palsy) ▸▸

- Usually unilateral, present at birth, and persists unchanged for life
- Two alternating phases:
  1. Paretic phase—ptosis, ophthalmoparesis, mydriasis, and reduced accommodation for about 2 min, followed by
  2. Spastic phase—the ptotic eyelid elevates, the globe adducts, the pupil constricts, and accommodation increases for 10–30 sec
- Present during sleep (with reduced rate and amplitude)
- Voluntary eye movement efforts may influence the cycle (e.g., the paretic phase may be prolonged with abduction effort, or the spastic phase may be prolonged with adduction or accommodation-convergence efforts).
- Causes: congenital trauma or infections, posterior fossa tumor in acquired cases (very rare)
- Pathogenesis: injury to intracranial portion of the nerve results in retrograde degeneration, such that the oculomotor nucleus contains two populations of neurons:
  1. Normal neurons that are not injured or recovered completely. They transmit remnants of physiological movements.
  2. Neurons that have been damaged but remain alive. They produce abnormal cyclic spasms by summation of subthreshold stimuli and rhythmic mass discharges.

12.2.3 Congenital Cranial Dysinnervation Syndrome

Congenital cranial dysinnervation syndrome is a group of congenital neuromuscular disorders caused by developmental errors in innervation. These disorders are present at birth and are usually nonprogressive. They have an autosomal inheritance pattern, but may occur sporadically. They may result from failed or misguided development of neurons (i.e., primary dysinnervation), or they may result from aberrant innervation during development (i.e., secondary dysinnervation). This syndrome includes:

1. Congenital fibrosis of the extraocular muscles (CFEOM1, CFEOM2, and CFEOM 3)
2. Duane's syndrome (see section 12.4.2)
3. Möbius syndrome (see section 12.4.2)
4. Horizontal gaze palsy with progressive scoliosis (HGPPS) (see section 12.4.2)
5. Congenital facial palsy
6. Congenital ptosis

Congenital fibrosis of the extraocular muscles type 1 (CFEOM1)

- Most common form of CFEOM (previously known as congenital fibrosis syndrome, congenital external ophthalmoplegia with or without co-contraction)
- Autosomal dominant; mutation on chromosome 12 (12p11.2-q12) or chromosome 16 (16q24.2-q24.3)
- Bilateral
- Clinical features
  1. Ptosis
  2. Severely limited vertical ductions; variable limitation of horizontal ductions
  3. Eyes infraducted 20–30° below horizontal with a chin-up position.
  4. Esotropia, exotropia, or orthotropia
  5. Significant hyperopic refractive error with astigmatism
- Pathogenesis: primary maldevelopment of the superior division of the oculomotor nerve

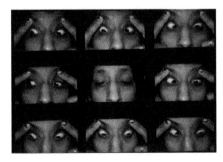

CFEOM1. Note bilateral ptosis, infraducted position of the eyes, and limited duction, especially vertical. Photograph courtesy of Dr. Stephen Kraft.

Congenital fibrosis of the extraocular muscles type 2 (CFEOM2)

- Previously known as strabismus fixus
- Autosomal recessive; mutation of *PHOX2a* gene on chromosome 11 (11q13.2)
- Bilateral
- Clinical features
  1. Ptosis
  2. Limited horizontal and vertical ductions
  3. Eyes fixed in an abducted position with large exotropia (80–100 prism diopters)
- Pathogenesis: primary maldevelopment of both the oculomotor and trochlear nuclei

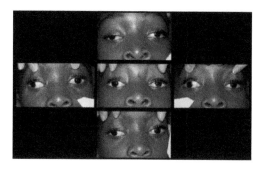

CFEOM2. Note bilateral ptosis, large exotropia, and limited duction.
Photograph courtesy of Dr. Stephen Kraft.

Congenital fibrosis of the extraocular muscles type 3 (CFEOM3)

- Autosomal dominant; mutation on chromosome 16 (16q24.2-q24.3)
- Bilateral or unilateral
- Variable phenotype within a family
- Clinical features
  1. Ptosis
  2. Variable limitation of horizontal and vertical ductions
  3. Eyes fixed in an infraducted (or supraducted) and abducted position
- Pathogenesis: variable defect in the development of the oculomotor nuclei

12.2.4 Oculomotor Nerve Synkinesis

In oculomotor nerve synkinesis, axons regenerating within the proximal end of the severed branch of the oculomotor nerve become misdirected and innervate muscles for which they are not originally matched. In acquired palsy, synkinesis usually appears about nine weeks after injury, but it can be delayed until three to six months afterward; in congenital palsy, it appears about one to six months after birth.

As a general rule, synkinesis does not occur after ischemic injury. Thus, in a patient who has a presumed ischemic palsy, the development of synkinesis requires further investigation to rule out other causes, such as compression or inflammation.

Eye Movement Abnormalities in Oculomotor Nerve Synkinesis

Pseudo-Graefe sign: retraction and elevation of the eyelid on attempted downgaze (misdirection of fibers for inferior rectus to levator palpebrae)

Horizontal gaze-eyelid synkinesis: elevation of eyelid on attempted adduction (misdirection of fibers for medial rectus to levator palpebrae)

Adduction on attempted elevation or depression (misdirection of fibers for superior or inferior rectus to medial rectus)

Limited vertical movement with occasional retraction of the globe on attempted vertical movement (due to simultaneous contraction of elevators and depressors)

Pseudo-Argyll Robertson pupil: light-near dissociation of the pupil. The pupil does not react to light stimulation, but constricts on adduction (misdirection of fibers for medial rectus to pupillary sphincter muscles).

Etiology of Oculomotor Nerve Synkinesis

Secondary oculomotor nerve synkinesis

Seen after partial recovery of the third nerve

Causes

1. Intracranial aneurysm
2. Trauma (e.g., basal skull fracture)
3. Tumors
4. Syphilis
5. Basal meningitis

Primary oculomotor nerve synkinesis (without apparent preexisting third nerve palsy)

Lesions grow so slowly that mild damage to the nerve is not recognized, which allows regeneration to occur

Causes

1. Intracavernous meningioma or trigeminal schwannoma
2. Intracavernous aneurysm
3. Aneurysm in the subarachnoid space

12.2.5 Workup and Treatment of Oculomotor Nerve Palsy

Workup

Investigations for third nerve palsy should be guided by clinical findings and suspected location of the lesion. Suggested workup for five clinical scenarios is listed below:

Dilated and poorly reactive pupil with no ophthalmoplegia or ptosis

- Extremely rare
- Usually occurs in a comatose or obtunded patient with an expanding supratentorial mass (Hutchinson pupil)
- In alert patients, more likely to be caused by a tonic pupil or pharmacological blockade
- Order MRI and magnetic resonance (MR) or computed tomography (CT) angiography to rule out basilar tip aneurysm or other mass lesion.

Complete or incomplete ophthalmoplegia, ptosis, and dilated, poorly reactive pupil

- Occurs with a lesion at any point along the course of the third nerve, but aneurysm should be suspected, especially if there is associated orbital pain or headache
- Order MRI and MR or CT angiography and conventional angiography (if suspicion is high).

Complete or incomplete ophthalmoplegia, ptosis, but pupil is spared

- Most common cause is ischemia, but may also occur with compressive lesion or inflammation
- Also need to consider myopathic or neuromuscular disease (e.g., myasthenia gravis)
- In complete, pupil-sparing palsy in patients over 50 years of age (most likely ischemia), measure blood pressure, serum glucose and erythrocyte sedimentation rate (ESR); if no improvement within 4 months, order MRI and MR or CT angiography.
- In incomplete, pupil-sparing palsy and in patients under 50 years of age, order MRI and MR or CT angiography, lumbar puncture, plus blood pressure, serum glucose, and ESR.

Ophthalmoplegia, ptosis, and a pupil that is small or in mid-position

- Pathognomonic for a lesion in the cavernous sinus
- Order MRI and MR or CT angiography.

Third nerve palsy with synkinesis (aberrant regeneration)

- Primary synkinesis is commonly caused by a slow-growing lesion in the cavernous sinus or subarachnoid space.
- Order MRI and MR or CT angiography.

Treatment

1. Occlusion
2. Prisms
3. Botulinum to lateral rectus muscle (in acute phase of partial third nerve palsy or isolated medial rectus palsy) to eliminate horizontal deviation in primary position and prevent contracture of the lateral rectus (the medial rectus antagonist)
4. Strabismus surgery
5. Ptosis surgery

12.3 Trochlear Nerve Palsy

The trochlear (fourth) nerve innervates the superior oblique muscle, which incyclotorts, depresses, and abducts the globe. Fourth nerve palsy is the most common cause of acquired vertical strabismus. Common causes of fourth nerve palsy are congenital or trauma.

Clinical Features of Trochlear Nerve Palsy

Hypertropia and excyclotorsion of the affected eye

Diplopia
- Can be vertical, diagonal, or torsional
- Greatest on downgaze

Overaction of the ipsilateral inferior oblique muscle (antagonist of the affected superior oblique) over time

Abnormal head posture
- Contralateral head tilt to minimize the diplopia (most common)
- Paradoxical ipsilateral head tilt to maximize the diplopia so that the second image can be ignored (rare)
- In bilateral case, chin-down position to compensate for the induced V-pattern on downgaze

Facial asymmetry
- Characteristic of congenital palsy
- Consists of shallowing of the midfacial region between the lateral canthus and the edge of the mouth

Anatomy of the fourth nerve

The trochlear nucleus

The trochlear nerve originates from the trochlear nucleus, which is located at the ventral border of the periaqueductal gray matter at the level of the inferior colliculus. It lies at the dorsal margin of the medial longitudinal fasciculus.

The trochlear nerve fascicle

The fascicle crosses the midline at the anterior medullary velum (anterior floor of the fourth ventricle) before exiting the brainstem; thus, the right fourth nerve fascicle becomes the left fourth nerve, which innervates the left superior oblique muscle.

The trochlear nerve is the only cranial nerve that exits from the dorsal surface of the brainstem, and it has the longest intracranial course (75 mm).

The subarachnoid space

The nerve curves around the lateral surface of the upper pons, passing between the superior cerebellar and posterior cerebral arteries to reach the prepontine cistern. It then runs forward on the free edge of the tentorium for 1–2 cm before penetrating the dura of the tentorial attachment and entering the cavernous sinus.

The cavernous sinus

Within the lateral wall of the cavernous sinus, the nerve lies below the oculomotor nerve and above the ophthalmic division (V_1) of the trigeminal nerve. It then crosses over the oculomotor nerve and receives filaments from the carotid sympathetic plexus.

The orbit

The nerve enters the orbit through the superior orbital fissure above the annulus of Zinn in company with the frontal and lacrimal branches of the ophthalmic division of the trigeminal nerve. It divides into several small fascicles that innervate the superior oblique muscle.

12.3.1 Topographical Diagnosis of Acquired Trochlear Nerve Palsy

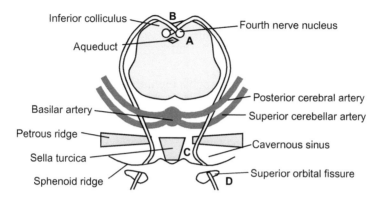

Redrawn with permission from Bajandas FJ, Kline LB. The five syndromes of the IV nerve (trochlear). In: Bajandas FJ, Kline LB, eds. Neuro-Ophthalmology Review Manual. 5th ed. Thoroughfare, NJ: SLACK Inc.; 2004:108.

Lesions of the Trochlear Nucleus/Fascicle

Because of the short course of the fascicle, distinguishing a nuclear from a fascicular lesion is virtually impossible. There are two common associated signs, described below.

Contralateral (to the side of the palsy) Horner's syndrome

Horner's syndrome is caused by damage to descending sympathetic fibers from the hypothalamus in the dorsal brainstem (i.e., first-order neurons).

- For example, a right-sided midbrain lesion causes damage to the right trochlear nucleus (resulting in a left fourth nerve palsy) and damage to descending sympathetic fibers (resulting in a right Horner's syndrome).
- If the lesion affects the fascicle after it crosses the midline, then the Horner's syndrome is on the same side of the fourth nerve palsy.

Ipsilateral (to the side of the palsy) relative afferent pupillary defect

Relative afferent pupillary defect (RAPD) is caused by damage to pupillary light fibers that leave the optic tract and travel via the brachium of the superior colliculus to synapse in the pretectal nucleus.

- For example, a right-sided midbrain lesion causes damage to the right trochlear nucleus (resulting in a left fourth nerve palsy) and damage to pupillary light fibers originating from the right optic tract (resulting in a left RAPD) (see section 9.4.3).
- If the lesion affects the fascicle after it crosses the midline, then the RAPD is on the opposite side of the fourth nerve palsy.

Causes

1. Trauma (most common), particularly contusion and hemorrhage of the tegmentum at the junction of the midbrain and pons

---

2. Ischemia

3. Primary and metastatic tumors

4. Vascular malformation

5. Inflammation/demyelination

Lesions in the Subarachnoid Space

The fourth nerve is particularly susceptible to injury or compression as it emerges from the dorsal surface of the brainstem. Both nerves are often affected. Causes of lesions in the subarachnoid space are:

1. Trauma (most common), including minor head injury and iatrogenic cause

2. Aneurysm (e.g., at the junction of the basilar and superior cerebellar arteries)

3. Basal meningitis (e.g., syphilis, tuberculosis, sarcoidosis, Lyme disease)

4. Intrinsic lesion of the nerve (e.g., schwannomas, cavernous angiomas)

5. Carotid-cavernous fistula (posterior draining, low-flow, spontaneous dural type)

6. Arteriovenous malformation

7. Ischemia

8. Increased intracranial pressure

Lesions in the Cavernous Sinus and Superior Orbital Fissure

Lesions in the cavernous sinus and superior orbital fissure are associated with paresis of the third nerve, the sixth nerve, and the ophthalmic (V_1) and maxillary (V_2) divisions of the trigeminal nerve, as well as with sympathetic paralysis.

Lesions within the orbit

Lesions within the orbit are associated with paresis of the third nerve, the sixth nerve, and the ophthalmic (V_1) and maxillary (V_2) divisions of the trigeminal nerve, plus orbital signs (e.g., loss of vision, proptosis, chemosis).

Pathologic processes of uncertain or variable location

Example of pathologic processes of uncertain or variable location include nerve infarction (associated with hypertension, diabetes, arteritis), idiopathic, ophthalmoplegic migraine, tetanus, Sjögren's syndrome, and familial periodic ataxia.

12.3.2 Congenital Trochlear Nerve Palsy

Congenital trochlear nerve palsy accounts for 75% of all fourth nerve palsies. Many cases do not present until adulthood. Most are sporadic, but autosomal-dominant transmission occurs occasionally. Most patients are neurologically normal, but some have cerebral palsy. Causes are:

1. Unknown

2. Aplasia or hypoplasia of the trochlear nerve nucleus

3. Lax and abnormally long superior oblique tendon, or the tendon may be misdirected or absent (which may be due to a primary defect or secondary to denervation atrophy)

Clinical Features of Congenital Trochlear Nerve Palsy

Contralateral head tilt to minimize the diplopia

Large vertical fusional amplitude ranging from 10 to 25 prism diopters (normal range: 3–6 prism diopters)

May develop diplopia from decompensation of the palsy after a minor head trauma or without any antecedent event. Review old photographs and measure vertical fusional amplitude to differentiate a decompensated congenital palsy from an acquired palsy.

May be bilateral

Facial asymmetry (75% cases)

12.3.3 Workup, Differential Diagnosis, and Treatment of Trochlear Nerve Palsy

Workup

The Three-Step Test

Example: Right fourth nerve palsy

Right eye

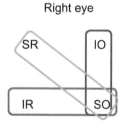

Left eye

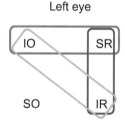

| SR = superior rectus |
| IR = inferior rectus |
| SO = superior oblique |
| IO = inferior oblique |

Step 1. Determine the side of hypertropia in primary position

Example: If there is a right hypertropia (HT) in primary position, then the depressors of the right eye (inferior rectus [IR] and superior oblique [SO]) or the elevators of the left eye (superior rectus [SR] and inferior oblique [IO]) are weak (these muscles are outline in red in the figure above).

- The vertical rectus muscles (SR and IR) have their greatest vertical action when the eye is abducted.

- The oblique muscles (SO and IO) have their greatest vertical action when the eye is adducted.

- Example: If a right HT increases on left gaze, then the oblique muscles of the right eye (SO and IO), or the vertical rectus muscles of the left eye (SR and IR) are involved (outlined in blue in the figure).

Step 3. Determine whether the hypertropia increases on right or left head tilt
(Bielschowsky's head tilt test)

- During right head tilt, the right eye incyclotorts (SO and SR), and left eye excyclotorts (IO and IR).

- During left head tilt, the right eye excyclotorts (IO and IR), and left eye incyclotorts (SO and SR).

- Example: If a right HT increases on right head tilt, then the incyclotorters of the right eye (SO and SR) or the excyclotorters of the left eye (IO and IR) are involved (outlined in green in the figure). Because the right SO is outlined in all three steps, the diagnosis is right fourth nerve palsy.

The three-step test is useful for the diagnosis of fourth nerve palsy; however, it is not reliable in diagnosing palsy of other cyclovertical muscles. Why does the hypertropia increase on right head tilt in right fourth nerve palsy (i.e., step 3)?

- During right head tilt, the otolith–ocular reflex (ocular counterroll) is activated, such that the right eye incyclotorts (SO and SR) and the left eye excyclotorts (IO and IR)

- The primary action of SO is incyclotorsion, and its secondary action is depression, whereas the primary action of SR is elevation, and its secondary action in incyclotorsion. Thus, normally, during right head tilt, the net movement of the right eye is incyclotorsion with minimal vertical movement because the vertical action of SO and SR cancels each other out.

- In right fourth nerve palsy, the elevating action of SR is unopposed by the palsied SO; thus, the hypertropia increases during right head tilt.

Torsion

Torsion is assessed subjectively using a double Maddox rod and assessed objectively using ophthalmoscopy or photography. Characteristics of torsion are:

- Congenital palsy: often has very little or no measurable subjective torsion.

- Acquired palsy: usually has a measurable degree of torsion.

- Bilateral palsy: is often present with a complaint of torsional diplopia or measurable excyclotorsion greater than 10°.

Bilateral superior oblique palsy

Bilateral superior oblique palsy should be suspected when patients present with:

1. Closed-head injury
2. Subjective complaints of torsion
3. Objective torsion greater than 10°
4. Positive Bielschowsky's head tilt test on each side (i.e., right hypertropia on right head tilt and left hypertropia on left head tilt)
5. V-pattern esotropia
6. Chin-down head posture.

Differential Diagnosis

1. Skew deviation
2. Thyroid-related ophthalmopathy
3. Brown's syndrome
4. Primary inferior oblique overaction

Treatment

1. Occlusion
2. Prisms
3. Surgery (performed only after the palsy has been stable for at least six months), using one or a combination of the following procedures:
   - Weakening of the ipsilateral inferior oblique (the antagonist of the affected superior oblique)
   - Weakening of the contralateral inferior rectus (the yoke muscle of the affected superior oblique)
   - Strengthening the affected superior oblique.

12.4 Abducens Nerve Palsy

The abducens nerve innervates the lateral rectus muscle, which abducts the globe. Sixth nerve palsy causes limitation of abduction and esotropia.

Anatomy of the Sixth Nerve

The abducens nucleus

The abducens nucleus lies in the floor of the fourth ventricle, at the level of the lower pons, and contains three populations of neurons:

1. Abducens motoneurons, which innervate the ipsilateral lateral rectus muscle
2. Abducens internuclear neurons, which project to the contralateral medial rectus subnucleus of the oculomotor nucleus via the medial longitudinal fasciculus.
3. Neurons that project to the cerebellar flocculus.

The genu of the facial nerve curves over the dorsal and lateral surface of the nucleus, while the medial longitudinal fasciculus (MLF) lies medial to each nucleus.

The abducens nerve fascicle

During its passage in the pons, the fascicle is adjacent to the motor nucleus and fascicle of the facial nerve, the motor nucleus of the trigeminal nerve, the spinal tract of the trigeminal nerve, the superior olivary nucleus, the central tegmental tract, and the corticospinal tract.

The subarachnoid space

The nerve emerges from the brainstem between the pons and the medulla, lateral to the pyramidal prominence. It then runs upward along the ventral surface of the pons, lateral to the basilar artery, and passes between the pons and the anterior inferior cerebellar artery to ascend through the subarachnoid space along the clivus. It then pierces the dura mater, courses around or through the inferior petrosal sinus, and passes under the petroclinoid (Gruber's) ligament in Dorello's canal to enter the cavernous sinus.

The cavernous sinus

The nerve bends laterally around the intracavernous carotid artery and runs medial and parallel to the ophthalmic division (V_1) of the trigeminal nerve. The oculosympathetic fibers leave the internal carotid artery and join briefly with the abducens nerve before joining the ophthalmic division (V_1) of the trigeminal nerve. Unlike the oculomotor and trochlear nerves, the abducens nerve does not lie within the lateral wall of the sinus, but rather it runs within the body of the sinus.

The orbit

The nerve enters the orbit through the superior orbital fissure, passes through the annulus of Zinn, and innervates the lateral rectus.

12.4.1 Topographical Diagnosis of Acquired Abducens Nerve Palsy

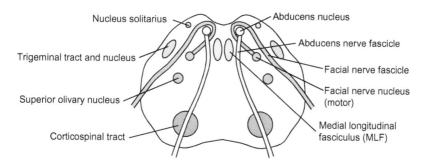

Redrawn with permission from Bajandas FJ, Kline LB. The six syndromes of the VI nerve (abducens). In: Bajandas FJ, Kline LB, eds. Neuro-Ophthalmology Review Manual. 5th ed. Thoroughfare, NJ: SLACK Inc.; 2004:98.

Lesions of the abducens nucleus

1. Horizontal conjugate gaze palsy (ipsilateral): affects saccades, smooth pursuit, and vestibulo-ocular reflex (VOR)

2. One-and-a-half syndrome: involves abducens nucleus and MLF, causing a horizontal (ipsilateral) conjugate gaze palsy, and adducting deficit in the eye ipsilateral to the MLF lesion

3. Horizontal conjugate gaze palsy and ipsilateral, peripheral, facial nerve palsy: involves the facial nerve fascicle, which loops around the abducens nucleus before exiting the brainstem

4. Causes of lesions of abducens nerve nucleus: ischemia, infiltration, compression, inflammation, and trauma

Lesions of the abducens nerve fascicle

Causes of abducens fascicle include ischemia, infiltration, compression, inflammation, demyelination, and infection. Three syndromes are seen:

1. **Raymond-Cestan syndrome** (lesion in ventral paramedian pons)

   - Ipsilateral sixth nerve palsy
   - Contralateral hemiplegia (due to involvement of the corticospinal tract)

2. **Millard-Gubler syndrome** (lesion in ventral paramedian pons)

   - Ipsilateral sixth nerve palsy
   - Contralateral hemiplegia (due to involvement of the corticospinal tract)
   - Ipsilateral, peripheral facial (seventh) nerve palsy

3. **Foville's fasciculus syndrome** (lesion in pontine tegmentum [i.e., dorsal pons])

   - Ipsilateral sixth nerve palsy or horizontal gaze palsy due to involvement of the sixth nerve nucleus/fascicle
   - Ipsilateral peripheral facial nerve (seventh nerve) palsy due to involvement of the facial nerve fascicle
   - Loss of taste of anterior two-thirds of the tongue due to involvement of the nucleus solitarius, a sensory nucleus of the facial (seventh) nerve
   - Ipsilateral analgesia of the face due to involvement of the trigeminal tract and nucleus (fifth nerve)
   - Ipsilateral peripheral deafness due to involvement of the superior olivary nucleus, where second-order cochlear fibers (eighth nerve) synapse
   - Ipsilateral central Horner's syndrome due to involvement of the descending sympathetic fibers from the hypothalamus in the lateral part of the tegmentum

Lesions in the subarachnoid space

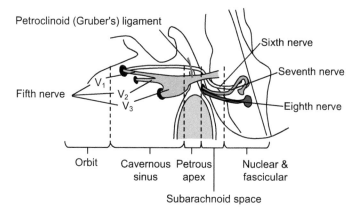

Redrawn with permission from Bajandas FJ, Kline LB. The six syndromes of the VI nerve (abducens). In: Bajandas FJ, Kline LB, eds. Neuro-Ophthalmology Review Manual. 5th ed. Thoroughfare, NJ: SLACK Inc.; 2004:91.

Causes of lesions in the subarachnoid space are

1. Aneurysm, atherosclerosis, or dolichoectasia of the anterior inferior cerebellar artery, posterior inferior cerebellar artery, or basilar artery (associated with severe headache)

2. Space-occupying lesion above the tentorium (transtentorial herniation) or in the posterior fossa

3. Trauma (e.g., descent of brainstem from vertex blows, iatrogenic [neurosurgical], or blunt, closed-head injury)

4. Arnold-Chiari malformation

5. Meningitis (often bilateral palsy; e.g., bacterial, spirochetal, viral, or neoplastic)

6. Basal tumors (e.g., meningioma, chordoma, trigeminal schwannoma, vestibular schwannoma [acoustic neuroma])

7. Intrinsic tumor of the abducens nerve (e.g., schwannoma, cavernous angioma)

8. Increased intracranial pressure (unilateral or bilateral palsy) due to compression of the abducens nerve between the pons and the basilar artery or clivus, or due to stretching of the nerve along the sharp edge of the petrous temporal bone.

9. After lumbar puncture, shunting for hydrocephalus, or spinal anesthesia (usually unilateral palsy)

10. Spontaneous intracranial hypotension

11. Dural, posterior draining, carotid-cavernous sinus fistula

Lesions at the petrous apex (petrous apex syndrome)

Characteristics of petrous apex syndrome are

- Ipsilateral sixth nerve palsy
- Ipsilateral facial pain due to involvement of the Gasserian ganglion
- Ipsilateral facial paralysis due to involvement of the seventh cranial nerve
- Ipsilateral deafness due involvement of the eighth cranial nerve.

Causes of the syndrome are

1. Severe mastoiditis extending to the tip of the petrous bone, causing localized inflammation of the meninges (Gradenigo's syndrome)
2. Aneurysm of the intrapetrosal segment of the internal carotid artery
3. Tumors
4. Basal skull or petrous bone fracture (other signs: hemotympanum, Battle's sign, cerebrospinal fluid otorrhea)
5. Nasopharyngeal carcinoma (extending from the sphenopalatine/pterygopalatine fossa)
6. Lateral sinus thrombosis or phlebitis that extends into the inferior petrosal sinus
7. Jugular vein ligation during radical neck surgery

Lesion in the cavernous sinus and superior orbital fissure

Three typical presentations

1. Isolated sixth nerve palsy, caused by:
   - Intracavernous vascular lesion (e.g., aneurysm of the internal carotid artery, or carotid-cavernous fistula)
   - Tumors that infiltrate or compress the cavernous sinus (e.g., meningioma, metastasis, nasopharyngeal carcinoma, Burkitt's lymphoma, pituitary adenoma with or without apoplexy, craniopharyngioma)
   - Ischemia (e.g., diabetes, temporal arteritis, lupus, migraine)
   - Inflammation, either granulomatous (e.g., tuberculosis, sarcoidosis, Tolosa-Hunt syndrome) or nongranulomatous (e.g., sphenoid sinus abscess or idiopathic hypertrophic pachymeningitis)
2. Isolated sixth nerve palsy and ipsilateral postganglionic Horner's syndrome (due to involvement of oculosympathetic fibers that leave the internal carotid artery and join briefly with the abducens nerve before joining the ophthalmic division of the trigeminal nerve).
3. Sixth nerve palsy in association with paresis of the third nerve, the fourth nerve, and the ophthalmic (V_1) and maxillary (V_2) divisions of the trigeminal nerve, as well as sympathetic paralysis.

Lesions within the orbit

Lesions within the orbit are associated with paresis of the third nerve, the fourth nerve, and the ophthalmic (V_1) and maxillary (V_2) divisions of the trigeminal nerve, plus orbital signs (e.g., loss of vision, proptosis, chemosis).

Pathologic processes of uncertain or variable location

Examples of pathologic processes of uncertain or variable location include nerve infarction (associated with hypertension, diabetes, arteritis), idiopathic, infections, following immunization, ophthalmoplegic migraine, transient isolated sixth nerve palsy in newborns, and side effects of drugs.

12.4.2 Congenital Abducens Palsy

Duane's syndrome ▸▸

Clinical features

1. Marked limitation of abduction and variable limitation of adduction. Three types:

   Duane's type I: limited abduction

   Duane's type II: limited adduction

   Duane's type III: limited abduction and adduction

2. Narrowing of palpebral fissure and globe retraction on attempted adduction (due to abnormal innervation of the lateral rectus by branches from the third nerve)

3. Usually bilateral, occurs more frequently in females and in the left eye

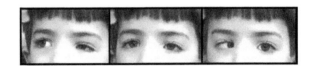

Duane's syndrome type I in the left eye. Photograph courtesy of Dr. Lawrence Tychsen.

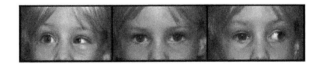

Duane's syndrome type III in the right eye. Photograph courtesy of Dr. Lawrence Tychsen.

Etiology

Environmental: a teratogenic event between the fourth and eighth weeks of gestation

Genetic: most cases are sporadic and are autosomal dominant in 5–10% of patients. Genetic defects have been identified in chromosomes 2q31 or 8q13.

Pathogenesis

Duane's syndrome may be caused by primary maldevelopment of the abducens nucleus, abducens nerve, and the lateral rectus muscle.

Systemic association

Thirty to fifty percent of patients exhibit systemic associations including:

1. Deafness (10%)

2. Wildervanck's syndrome (cervico-oculo-acoustic syndrome): consists of Duane's syndrome, a cervical malformation called Klippel-Feil anomaly, and deafness

3. Goldenhar syndrome (oculo-auricular-vertebral dysplasia): consists of epibulbar dermoids, preauricular appendages, auricular abnormalities, vertebral anomalies, and hemifacial microsomia

4. Duane's syndrome with radial ray anomalies (defects in chromosome 20q13.13-q13.2)

   ▪ Also known as Duane/radial dysplasia syndrome, Okihiro syndrome, or DR syndrome (for *D*uane anomaly, *d*eafness, *r*adial dysplasia, *r*enal dysplasia)

   ▪ Autosomal dominant

   ▪ Radial dysplasia ranges from hypoplasia of the thenar eminence (base of thumb) with or without weakness of thumb abduction and apposition, hypoplasia or absence of the thumb, hypoplasia or absence of the radial and ulnar bones, to absence of forearm.

   ▪ Other variable features: hearing loss, dysmorphic facies, and renal, vertebral, and cardiac (Holt-Oram syndrome) anomalies

5. Bosley-Salih-Alorainy syndrome

   ▪ Mutation of *HOXA1* gene on chromosome 7 (7p15.3-p14.3)

   ▪ Bilateral Duane's type III, leading to horizontal gaze palsy

   ▪ Bilateral sensorineural hearing loss due to absent cochlea and vestibule

   ▪ Hypoplasia or agenesis of internal carotid artery

   ▪ Other variable features: central hypoventilation, facial weakness, swallowing difficulties, vocal cord paresis, conotruncal heart defects, skull and craniofacial abnormalities, external ear defects, autism spectrum disorder, and mental retardation

Möbius syndrome

Clinical features

1. Involvement of the face: facial nerve palsy, masklike facies with the mouth constantly held open, and facial asymmetry

2. Bilateral horizontal gaze palsy

3. A sporadic condition; defects in chromosome 13q12.2-q13

Etiology

Peripheral theory: primary damage in the peripheral muscles or nerves, with retrograde degeneration of cranial nerve nuclei

Central theory: primary damage in cranial nerve nuclei

Systemic associations

1. Limb malformations (e.g., brachydactyly, syndactyly, congenital amputation)

2. Hypoplasia or absence of branchial musculature, particularly the pectoralis muscle (Poland anomaly) and atrophy of the tongue

3. Cardiovascular anomalies (e.g., dextrocardia, patent ductus arteriosus, ventricular septal defects)

4. Others: deafness, mental retardation, micrognathia

Horizontal gaze palsy and progressive scoliosis ▶▶

Horizontal gaze palsy and progressive scoliosis is an autosomal recessive condition resulting from a mutation on chromosome 11q23-q25.

Clinical features

1. Congenital absence of horizontal conjugate eye movements (including absence of horizontal VOR), with preservation of vertical eye movement and convergence

2. Progressive scoliosis: 2–10 years of age

Pathogenesis

- Maldevelopment of dorsomedial pontine structures, including the abducens nuclei and MLF

- Selective damage to the brainstem including the gracile nucleus, lateral vestibular nucleus, and the superior colliculus, which may lead to kyphoscoliosis

12.4.3 **Workup and Treatment of Abducens Nerve Palsy**

Workup

1. Isolated sixth nerve palsy in patients with known ischemic risk factors or over 50 years of age:
   - Conservative management, including blood pressure, serum glucose, ESR, antinuclear antibody test, and screening and confirmatory tests for syphilis
   - If no improvement within four months, order MRI with contrast, with attention to basal skull

2. Isolated sixth nerve palsy in patients without ischemic risk factors or less than 50 years of age:
   - Order MRI with contrast, with attention to basal skull.
   - Measure blood pressure and order serum glucose, ESR, antinuclear antibody test, and screening and confirmatory tests for syphilis

3. Sixth nerve palsy with other neurologic signs or cranial nerve involvement: Order MRI, magnetic resonance or computed tomography angiography, lumbar puncture, or cerebral angiography.

Treatment

1. Occlusion
2. Prisms
3. Surgery (performed only after the palsy has been stable for at least six months)
   - Incomplete palsy: medial rectus recession (weakening) and lateral rectus resection (strengthening)
   - Complete palsy: partial or full transposition of the superior and inferior rectus muscles toward the insertion of the lateral rectus muscle

12.5.1 Differential Diagnosis of Acquired Ophthalmoplegia

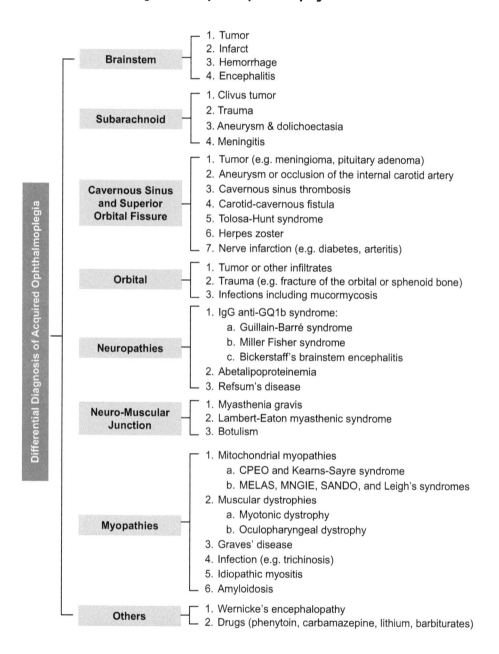

Differential Diagnosis of Acquired Ophthalmoplegia

Brainstem
1. Tumor
2. Infarct
3. Hemorrhage
4. Encephalitis

Subarachnoid
1. Clivus tumor
2. Trauma
3. Aneurysm & dolichoectasia
4. Meningitis

Cavernous Sinus and Superior Orbital Fissure
1. Tumor (e.g. meningioma, pituitary adenoma)
2. Aneurysm or occlusion of the internal carotid artery
3. Cavernous sinus thrombosis
4. Carotid-cavernous fistula
5. Tolosa-Hunt syndrome
6. Herpes zoster
7. Nerve infarction (e.g. diabetes, arteritis)

Orbital
1. Tumor or other infiltrates
2. Trauma (e.g. fracture of the orbital or sphenoid bone)
3. Infections including mucormycosis

Neuropathies
1. IgG anti-GQ1b syndrome:
    a. Guillain-Barré syndrome
    b. Miller Fisher syndrome
    c. Bickerstaff's brainstem encephalitis
2. Abetalipoproteinemia
3. Refsum's disease

Neuro-Muscular Junction
1. Myasthenia gravis
2. Lambert-Eaton myasthenic syndrome
3. Botulism

Myopathies
1. Mitochondrial myopathies
    a. CPEO and Kearns-Sayre syndrome
    b. MELAS, MNGIE, SANDO, and Leigh's syndromes
2. Muscular dystrophies
    a. Myotonic dystrophy
    b. Oculopharyngeal dystrophy
3. Graves' disease
4. Infection (e.g. trichinosis)
5. Idiopathic myositis
6. Amyloidosis

Others
1. Wernicke's encephalopathy
2. Drugs (phenytoin, carbamazepine, lithium, barbiturates)

12.5.2 Cavernous Sinus and Superior Orbital Fissure Syndrome (Sphenocavernous Syndrome)

The Cavernous Sinus

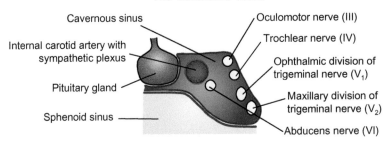

- Cavernous sinus
- Internal carotid artery with sympathetic plexus
- Pituitary gland
- Sphenoid sinus
- Oculomotor nerve (III)
- Trochlear nerve (IV)
- Ophthalmic division of trigeminal nerve (V₁)
- Maxillary division of trigeminal nerve (V₂)
- Abducens nerve (VI)

The Orbital Apex

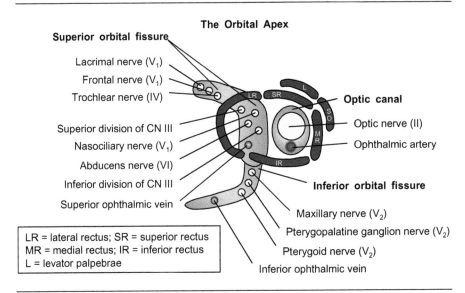

- Superior orbital fissure
- Lacrimal nerve (V₁)
- Frontal nerve (V₁)
- Trochlear nerve (IV)
- Superior division of CN III
- Nasociliary nerve (V₁)
- Abducens nerve (VI)
- Inferior division of CN III
- Superior ophthalmic vein
- Optic canal
- Optic nerve (II)
- Ophthalmic artery
- Inferior orbital fissure
- Maxillary nerve (V₂)
- Pterygopalatine ganglion nerve (V₂)
- Pterygoid nerve (V₂)
- Inferior ophthalmic vein

LR = lateral rectus; SR = superior rectus
MR = medial rectus; IR = inferior rectus
L = levator palpebrae

Anatomy of the cavernous sinus

The cavernous sinus is a plexus of various sized veins that divide and coalesce. It contains:

1. The oculomotor (III), trochlear (IV), and the ophthalmic (V₁) and maxillary divisions (V₂) of the trigeminal nerves, which lie along the lateral wall of the sinus

2. The abducens nerve, internal carotid artery, and sympathetic plexus, which lie within the body of the sinus

Because it is difficult to determine whether a lesion involves the cavernous sinus, the fissure, or both, damage in this region is often considered as a single entity, the sphenocavernous syndrome.

Involvement of third, fourth, and sixth cranial nerves

Involvement of the ophthalmic (V_1) and maxillary (V_2) divisions of the trigeminal nerve

Sympathetic paralysis (e.g., eyelid edema, conjunctival chemosis)

Poorly reactive pupil that is small or in mid-position (pathognomonic) due to combined involvement of parasympathetic fibers (which travel with third nerve and cause pupillary constriction) and oculosympathetic plexus (which is located within the cavernous sinus and causes pupillary dilation)

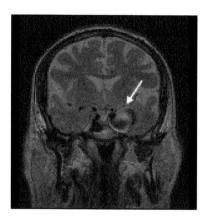 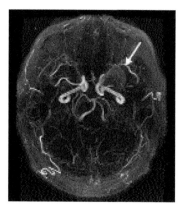

Coronal MRI (A) and magnetic resonance angiogram (B) showing a giant intracavernous aneurysm of the internal carotid artery.

Etiology of Sphenocavernous Syndrome

Vascular lesions (e.g., aneurysm of the internal carotid artery, cavernous sinus thrombosis, carotid-cavernous fistula)

Tumors (e.g., meningioma, pituitary tumor, craniopharyngioma, nasopharyngeal carcinoma, metastatic tumors, lymphoma)

Infection (e.g., syphilis, tuberculosis)

Ischemia (e.g., diabetes, temporal arteritis)

Inflammation (e.g., Tolosa-Hunt syndrome, lupus, rheumatoid arthritis)

Trauma (e.g., skull fracture, iatrogenic)

To differentiate a sphenocavernous syndrome from an orbital apex lesion:

- Sphenocavernous syndrome is characterized by a painful ophthalmoplegia (due to involvement of the trigeminal nerve), and the patient generally has normal vision and no protopsis.

- A lesion in the orbital apex causes ophthalmoplegia that may or may not be painful, but it is usually associated with protopsis and visual loss from optic neuropathy.

12.5.3 Cavernous Sinus Thrombosis

Cavernous sinus thrombosis is usually a late complication of an infection of the central face or paranasal sinuses in an otherwise healthy individual. The condition is associated with high rates of morbidity and mortality. Causative agents are *Staphylococcus aureus* (70%), *Streptococcus pneumoniae*, gram-negative bacilli, anaerobes, and fungi, including *Aspergillus* and *Rhizopus*.

Clinical Features of Cavernous Sinus Thrombosis

Sinusitis or a mid-face infection (most commonly a furuncle infection from manipulation such as squeezing, or surgical incision)

Headache, fever, and malaise preceding the onset of ocular involvement

Ocular findings

- Periorbital edema and chemosis
- Proptosis
- Increased intraocular pressure
- Incomplete or complete ophthalmoplegia involving the oculomotor, trochlear, or abducens nerves
- Spread of infection to the contralateral cavernous sinus and the fellow eye (through communicating veins) is pathognomonic

Meningeal signs (e.g., nuchal rigidity, Kernig and Brudzinski signs)

Signs of sepsis (late findings; e.g., chills, fever, shock, delirium, and coma)

Workup

Computed tomography will reveal increased density of the cavernous sinus.

Treatment

1. Aggressive broad-spectrum antibiotic therapy
2. Anticoagulation with heparin to prevent further thrombosis and reduce incidence of septic emboli
3. Corticosteroids (as adjunctive therapy) to reduce inflammation and edema
4. Drainage of primary source of infection (e.g., sphenoid sinusitis, facial abscess)

Prognosis

- Without antibiotics, the mortality rate is 100% due to sepsis or central nervous system infection.
- With aggressive management, the mortality rate is 30%.
- Complete recovery is rare: 50% of patients have residual cranial nerve deficits, and about 25% have residual visual impairment.

12.5.4 Carotid-Cavernous Fistula

Carotid-cavernous fistulas are abnormal communications between the carotid artery and the cavernous sinus. They can be classified according to their location (anterior vs. posterior drainage) or their hemodynamic qualities (direct vs. indirect fistula).

Clinical Features of Carotid-Cavernous Fistula

Anterior drainage (anterior to superior orbital vein) = *red* eye
- Corkscrew conjunctival veins (arterialization) (86–100%)
- Proptosis (71–85%)
- Orbital bruit (57–85%)
- Increased intraocular pressure (38–71%)
- Dilated retinal veins (32–41%)
- Extraocular muscle paresis, neurogenic or myogenic (from vascular congestion)

Posterior drainage (posterior to petrosal sinus) = *white* eye: ocular motor nerve palsy

---

Direct fistula	Indirect fistula
High flow, high pressure	Low flow, low pressure
Associated with head trauma (basal skull fracture)	Usually occurs spontaneously, especially in women
Fed by intracavernous internal carotid artery	Fed by dural branches (e.g., internal maxillary artery or meningohypophyseal artery)
Spontaneous recovery uncommon	Spontaneous recovery common
Complications: visual loss (75%); cortical venous drainage, leading to hemorrhagic stroke, or subarachnoid hemorrhage	Complications: cortical venous drainage, leading to hemorrhagic stroke, or subarachnoid hemorrhage
Require urgent treatment	Observation

Workup

1. Digital subtraction angiography to identify the vessels supplying the fistula
2. MRI shows distended superior ophthalmic vein (anterior drainage) and enhancement of cavernous sinus

Treatment

1. For indirect fistulas, prognosis is usually good without treatment.
2. For direct fistulas or those that threaten vision:
   - Neuro-endovascular surgery to block the flow through the fistula using coils (thrombogenic), balloon (direct mechanical occlusion), or cyanoacrylate glue or particles
   - Ligation of internal carotid artery
   - Carotid compression is usually ineffective
   - Craniotomy for direct surgery on cavernous sinus is associated with high morbidity.

12.5.5 Tolosa-Hunt Syndrome

Tolosa-Hunt syndrome is a painful ophthalmoplegia caused by nonspecific inflammation (noncaseating granulomatous or nongranulomatous) of the cavernous sinus or superior orbital fissure. It affects middle-aged or elderly patients and its course is usually one of spontaneous remission and relapse.

Clinical Features of Tolosa-Hunt Syndrome

Acute onset of severe, steady, retro-orbital or periorbital pain and diplopia
Involvement of optic nerve and trigeminal nerve (V_1 and rarely V_2)
Incomplete or complete ophthalmoplegia involving the oculomotor, trochlear, or abducens nerves
Pupillary involvement:
  - Dilated if parasympathetic fibers, which travel via the oculomotor nerve, are affected
  - Constricted if the sympathetic plexus around the internal carotid artery is affected, causing Horner's syndrome (i.e., Raeder's paratrigeminal syndrome, which is a combination of painful palsies of the ocular motor nerves associated with Horner's syndrome)
Ptosis

Workup

1. An MRI will reveal soft tissue infiltration in the cavernous sinus without erosion of bone. The infiltrate is either hypointense on T1- and isointense on T2-weighted images or hyperintense on T1- and intermediate-weighted images.

2. Exclude other infiltrating, infectious, or neoplastic causes.

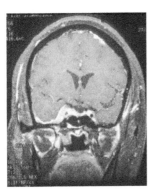

Coronal MRI with contrast demonstrating right cavernous sinus fullness consistent with Tolosa-Hunt syndrome. The imaging features are nonspecific and must be placed within the clinical context to differentiate the diagnosis from other infiltrating, infectious, or neoplastic processes in the cavernous sinus.

Treatment

Treat the patient with corticosteroids.

Prognosis

- Usually good response to corticosteroids
- Relapse rate 30–40%
- Because tumors in the cavernous region may also respond to corticosteroids, caution is required in making a diagnosis of Tolosa-Hunt syndrome, especially in relapsing cases.

12.6 Neuropathies Causing Ophthalmoplegia

12.6.1 Guillain-Barré Syndrome

Guillain-Barré syndrome is an acute, inflammatory, demyelinating polyradiculoneuropathy that is the most frequent cause of acute paralysis in adults and children. It affects 2 in every 100,000 persons, and it affects males more than females. Some patients are HLA-B35 positive (if associated with *Campylobacter jejuni* infection). Guillain-Barré syndrome is associated with:

- Respiratory or gastrointestinal infections, such as *Campylobacter jejuni* (in 40% cases), viruses, and mycoplasma, which usually occur one to three weeks before disease onset in 60% of patients
- Vaccination, surgery, and medications such as lithium.

Clinical Features of Guillain-Barré Syndrome

Progressive motor weakness of more than one limb: asymmetric, progresses from lower to upper limbs, and peaks by four weeks after onset in 98% of patients

Areflexia

Neuro-ophthalmic findings:

- Ptosis
- Ophthalmoplegia (the abducens nerve is most frequently involved)
- Dilated, nonreactive pupil
- Accommodation paralysis
- Optic neuritis
- Papilledema (increased protein causing decreased cerebrospinal fluid resorption and, consequently, increased intracranial pressure)

Pathogenesis and pathology

Guillain-Barré syndrome is an acquired immune-mediated disorder. Pathology shows perivenular inflammation with mononuclear cell infiltrate and segmental demyelination with preservation of axons.

Workup

1. Lumbar puncture: increased protein (peak by four weeks after onset due to inflammation of nerve roots), and mild pleocytosis in cerebrospinal fluid (CSF)
2. Electromyography (EMG): primary demyelination.
3. Nerve conduction study: slow or blocked in 80% of patients

Treatment

1. Supportive
2. Plasmapheresis or intravenous immunoglobulin

Prognosis

Patients attain complete recovery in the majority of cases; mortality is 10%, and 20% have residual disability.

12.6.2 Miller Fisher Syndrome

Miller Fisher syndrome is a subtype of Guillain-Barré syndrome, characterized by a rapidly progressive triad of areflexia, ataxia, and ophthalmoplegia. Males are affected more than females, with a 2:1 ratio. Some patients are HLA-B39 positive. Miller Fisher syndrome is associated with recent gastrointestinal infection (e.g., *Campylobacter jejuni*).

Clinical Features of Miller Fisher Syndrome

Areflexia
Ataxia: truncal ataxia, difficulty with tandem gait, and positive Romberg test
Ophthalmoplegia
- Symmetric and complete
- Affects upgaze first, then horizontal and downgaze
Other ocular motor findings:
- Internuclear ophthalmoplegia
- One-and-a half syndrome
- Pretectal syndrome
- Spasm of near reflex
- Divergence paralysis
Other neuro-ophthalmic findings: ptosis (20%); dilated, nonreactive pupil (50%); optic neurits (rare); cranial nerve palsies, especially facial nerve palsy.

Workup

1. IgG anti-GQ1b ganglioside antibodies
   - Present in 90% of patients with Guillain-Barré syndrome, Miller Fisher syndrome, and Bickerstaff's brainstem encephalitis (characterized by ophthalmoplegia, ataxia, pyramidal and sensory tract signs, and CSF pleocytosis)
   - Caused by cross-reactivity between *Campylobacter jejuni* surface epitope and neural tissue
   - The antibodies cause a neuropathy, as well as a decrease of acetylcholine release from the motor endplate, resulting in a neuromuscular conduction defect.
2. Lumbar puncture: increased protein in CSF
3. EMG: primary demyelination
4. Nerve conduction study: slow conduction
5. Imaging: usually normal

Treatment

1. Supportive
2. Plasmapheresis or intravenous immunoglobulin

Prognosis

Patients attain complete recovery within 8–12 weeks in the majority of cases; mortality is rare.

12.6.3 Abetalipoproteinemia (Bassen-Kornzweig Syndrome)

Abetalipoproteinemia is a rare congenital disorder characterized by a complete absence of apolipoprotein B, causing malabsorption of all fat-soluble vitamins, including A, D, E, and K. The disorder is autosomal recessive, caused by mutations in the microsomal triglyceride transfer protein gene.

Other diseases that cause vitamin E deficiency have similar clinical findings (e.g., in adults with bowel disease that causes fat malabsorption, or in familial vitamin E deficiency, which is caused by mutations in the α-tocopherol transfer protein gene on chromosome 8q13).

Clinical Features of Abetalipoproteinemia

Steatorrhea

Cerebellar ataxia

Areflexia

Loss of proprioception

Pigmentary retinopathy

Ocular motor findings:

- Ophthalmoplegia and ptosis
- Slow saccades
- Dissociated nystagmus on lateral gaze, characterized by fast adduction with a limited range of motion and slow abduction with a full range of motion
- Internuclear ophthalmoplegia

Workup

1. Blood smear: acanthocytes (i.e., red blood cells with spiny projections of the membrane)
2. Lipid profile
3. Small-intestine biopsy showing characteristic lipid deposits in mucosal cells

Treatment

Treat patients with oral or intravenous vitamin A, E, and K, as well as iron supplements.

12.6.4 Refsum's Disease

Refsum's disease is an extremely rare disorder caused by a defect in the metabolism of phytanic acid, leading to accumulation of phytanic acid in plasma and tissues. It is an autosomal recessive disorder, caused by deficient activity of phytanoyl-CoA hydroxylase, a peroxisomal enzyme catalyzing the first step of phytanic acid alpha-oxidation. The disorder is usually diagnosed during childhood or early adulthood.

Clinical Features of Refsum's Disease

Neurologic manifestations: peripheral neuropathy, cerebellar ataxia
Ocular manifestations: cataract, pigmentary retinopathy, visual filed constriction
Ophthalmoplegia
Cardiomyopathy
Sensorineural deafness
Ichthyosiform desquamation

Workup

Blood tests reveal an increased serum level of phytanic acid.

Treatment

Prescribe a diet low in phytanic acid and phytol diet (i.e., a diet low in milk products, animal fats, and green, leafy vegetables).

12.7 Ocular Motor Nerve Hyperactivity

12.7.1 Superior Oblique Myokymia

Superior oblique myokymia is a dyskinesia caused by spontaneous discharge of the trochlear nerve.

Clinical Features of Superior Oblique Myokymia

Intermittent uniocular microtremor consisting of spasms of torsional–vertical rotations, causing diplopia, monocular oscillopsia, or tremulous sensation of the eye

Lasts for seconds and occurs in clusters

May be triggered by

- Blinking
- Titling the head toward the side of the affected eye
- Downgaze

Usually no underlying disease, but cases have been reported after trochlear nerve palsy, mild head trauma, brainstem stroke or demyelination, cerebellar tumor, and vascular compression at the root exit zone of the trochlear nerve by a branch of the superior cerebellar artery or a branch of the posterior cerebral artery.

Pathogenesis

- Neuronal damage and subsequent regeneration, leading to desynchronized contractions of muscle fibers
- Vascular compression at the root exit zone of the trochlear nerve, causing ephaptic transmission (i.e., similar to trigeminal neuralgia and hemifacial spasm)

Workup

Thin-slice MRI: Consider enhanced spoiled gradient recalled acquisition in the steady state (SPGR) and flow imaging using steady acquisition (FIESTA) to rule out vascular compression at the root exit zone.

Treatment

1. May resolve spontaneously
2. Medications: carbamazepine, gabapentin, baclofen or propanolol (topical or systemic)
3. Surgery
   - Superior oblique tenotomy with ipsilateral inferior oblique recession
   - For cases caused by vascular compression at the root exit zone, vascular decompression using a Teflon pad placed between the compressing artery and trochlear nerve

---

12.7.2 Ocular Neuromyotonia

Clinical Features of Ocular Neuromyotonia

A rare disorder characterized by episodes of diplopia caused by involuntary, sometimes painful, contractions of extraocular muscles innervated by the oculomotor, trochlear or abducens nerves

- Usually unilateral, but bilateral cases occur
- May be precipitated by holding the eyes in eccentric gaze, often during sustained adduction
- In most cases, it involves contraction of one or more muscles innervated by a single ocular motor nerve.

Etiology

After radiation therapy to the parasellar region or skull base

Idiopathic

Pathogenesis

The pathogenesis is unknown; potential mechanisms include:

- Ephaptic neural transmission
- Changes in the pattern of neuronal transmission following denervation
- Axonal hyperexcitability due to dysfunction of potassium channels (similar to systemic neuromyotonia).

Workup

Order an MRI, and pay particular attention to suprasellar region and the posterior fossa,

Treatment

Carbamazepine is often effective.

Chapter 13

Disorders of Neuromuscular Transmission

13.1 Myasthenia Gravis

Myasthenia gravis is the most common disorder affecting the neuromuscular junction (incidence: 5 per 100,000). Ocular involvement accounts for initial complaints in 75% of patients. Of patients presenting with ocular myasthenia, 50–80% eventually develop generalized myasthenia, usually within two years of onset.

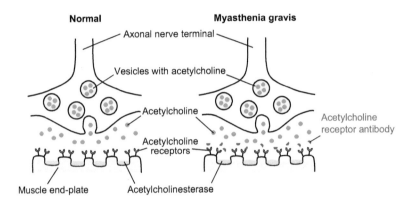

Clinical Features of Myasthenia Gravis

Variable ptosis, diplopia, and muscle weakness, including proximal limb muscles (e.g., triceps, deltoids), muscles of facial expression, mastication and speech, and neck extensors; worse at the end of the day and on exertion.

Ptosis

- Lid fatigue: Ptosis worsens on sustained upgaze.
- Enhancement of ptosis (the curtain sign): Manual elevation of one eyelid in bilateral ptosis leads to worsening of ptosis in the fellow eye (i.e., follows Hering's law).
- Cogan's lid-twitch sign: When the patient to looks down for about 15 sec and then refixates rapidly back to primary position, an upward overshoot of the lid occurs, followed by a slow droop or several twitches before the lid settles back to its ptotic position.
- Spontaneous eyelid retraction: Eyelid retraction usually occurs when the eye returns from upgaze to primary position due to post-tetanic facilitation of the levator palpebrae.

External ophthalmoparesis

- Extraocular muscle involvement with no set pattern; pupils are not involved
- Variable measurement of phoria or tropia during the same or different examinations

Orbicularis weakness: Sustained eyelid closure leads to fatigue of orbicularis and widening of palpebral fissure (the "peek sign" or "peekaboo sign").

Gaze-evoked centripetal drift or "fatigue nystagmus" (due to fatigue on sustained lateral gaze)[1]

Abnormal saccades

- Hypermetria of small saccades[2]
- Hypometria of large saccades[3]
- Quivering eye movements consisting of an initial small saccadic movement, followed by a rapid backward drift[4]
- "Hyperfast" saccades[5]

Diplopia: single or multiple extraocular muscle involvement that may mimic oculomotor, trochlear, abducens, or multiple ocular motor nerve palsies, internuclear ophthalmoplegia, one-and-a-half syndrome, or gaze palsy

Tensilon (edrophonium) injection

- Saccade hypermetria[6]
- Macrosaccadic oscillations[6]

---

1. The "fatigue nystagmus" differs from gaze-evoked nystagmus caused by cerebellar disease, which often diminishes with sustained lateral gaze

2. Hypermetria of small saccades results from central adaptation which, in an attempt to overcome the weakness from myasthenia, increases the saccadic pulse such that small saccades become hypermetric

3. For large saccades, the eye starts off with normal velocity. Due to intra-saccadic fatigue, however, the pulse is unsustained causing the eye to slow down in mid-flight, such that large saccades become hypometric. The eye then reaches the target slowly by a step of innervation

4. The global fibers (predominantly fast-twitch) of the agonist muscle start the saccade with a normal pulse, but then they rapidly fatigue, aborting the pulse and the eye stops. The orbital fibers (predominantly tonic) also fatigue during the saccade, aborting the step. Then the mechanical forces of the orbit rapidly pull the eye toward the central position, causing a glissade. The combination of aborted saccade and oppositely directed glissade constitutes the quivering movement

5. A saccade may appear to be "hyperfast" because the pulse is originally programmed for a larger amplitude saccade which is aborted in mid-flight due to fatigue

6. Tensilon injection unmasks the effects of central adaptation and exposes the increased saccadic innervation, resulting in saccade hypermetria and macrosaccadic oscillations

Pathophysiology

Myasthenia gravis is an autoimmune disease caused by the presence of antibodies against acetylcholine receptors, which leads to decreased number of available receptors (usually less than one-third that of normal). It is associated with other autoimmune diseases, including thymoma, dysthyroidism, sarcoidosis, pernicious anemia, aplastic anemia, and collagen vascular diseases (e.g., rheumatoid arthritis, lupus, ankylosing spondylitis, ulcerative colitis, Sjögren's syndrome).

Workup

Tensilon (edrophonium chloride) test

- Side effects: cholinergic (e.g., bradycardia, angina, bronchospasm)
- Steps for performing Tensilon test:

  1. Prepare 10 mg/mL Tensilon in a tuberculin syringe, 0.6 mg atropine in a tuberculin syringe, and 10 mL normal saline.
  2. Establish intravenous access using butterfly needle; flush with 1 mL normal saline.
  3. Inject 0.2 mL Tensilon, flush with 1 ml normal saline, and wait 1 min for possible side effects.
  4. Inject 0.6 mL Tensilon, flush with 1 mL normal saline, then attach atropine syringe.
  5. Wait 3 min; improvement of ptosis or diplopia constitutes a positive test.

Ice test

Improvement of ptosis after application of ice for 2 min on the ptotic eyelid constitutes a positive test. The ice test is especially useful for very young, elderly, or ill patients.

Sleep test

Improvement of ptosis or ocular alignment after 30–45 min of sleep constitutes a positive test.

Electromyography

- Repetitive nerve stimulation with supramaximal stimuli delivered at 2–3 Hz: Rapid decrement of the amplitude of compound muscle action potentials (CMAPs) ≥10–15% confirms the diagnosis in 95% of cases.
- Single-fiber electromyography (EMG; e.g., frontalis muscle) is highly sensitive (88–99% sensitivity). A positive test consists of increased jitter (increased latency between nerve stimulation and action potential of muscle fibers) and increased blockage (response failure).

Acetylcholine receptor antibody

Acetylcholine receptor antibody is not detectable in about 15% of patients.

Muscle-specific kinase

Muscle-specific kinase is detected in 20% patients who have no acetylcholine receptor antibody and is usually detected in patients with generalized myasthenia gravis.

Computed tomography of the chest

Computed tomography of the chest should be conducted to rule out thymoma, which occurs in about 10% of patients.

Other blood tests

Blood tests should include complete blood count, erythrocyte sedimentation rate, antinuclear antibody, and thyroid function tests to rule out other associated autoimmune diseases.

Treatment

1. Patching or prisms for diplopia
2. Mestinon (pyridostigmine bromide, a cholinesterase inhibitor). Cholinergic side effects (e.g., diarrhea, tearing, and fasciculations) are common with this drug.
3. Thymectomy (limited transcervical or endoscopic transcervical approach or median sternotomy) is indicated for:

   - Any patients with thymoma
   - Patients <50 years old whose condition is not controlled by Mestinon.

   Benefits of thymectomy:

   - Clinical improvement in 85%
   - Drug-free remission in 35%
   - Reduced medication requirement in 50%
4. Immunosuppressive agents: corticosteroids, azathioprine, or cyclosporine
5. Plasmapheresis or intravenous immunoglobulin, especially in myasthenic crisis (i.e., acute respiratory insufficiency or dysphagia)

13.2 Pediatric Myasthenia Gravis

13.2.1 Juvenile Myasthenia Gravis

Juvenile myasthenia gravis is similar to adult myasthenia in presentation, pathogenesis, clinical course, and response to therapy, except that it frequently improves with age. The optimal age for thymectomy and the use of immunosuppression in the juvenile form of the disease is controversial.

13.2.2 Neonatal Myasthenia Gravis

Neonatal myasthenia gravis is a transient disorder that results from the passive transfer of acetylcholine receptor antibodies from myasthenic mothers to their babies. It may occur anytime in the first 72 h of life and abates spontaneously after 2–3 weeks as the antibodies are cleared, with no adverse sequelae after resolution. Symptoms include:

- Hypotonia, a feeble cry, feeding difficulty, facial paralysis, and mild respiratory distress
- Ptosis, ophthalmoplegia, and orbicularis weakness in 15%.

Treatment consists of administering cholinesterase inhibitors and supporting vital functions.

13.2.3 Congenital Myasthenic Syndromes

Congenital myasthenic syndromes comprise a group of hereditary neuromuscular transmission disorders differentiated from neonatal myasthenia by the persistence of symptoms (neonatal myasthenia has a transient monophasic course). They are not autoimmune-related (i.e., absence of anti-acetylcholine receptor antibodies). The Tensilon test is usually negative because it relies on intact acetylcholinesterase and normal channel opening time. Congenital myasthenic syndromes are classified into those that are primarily presynaptic or primarily postsynaptic.

Presynaptic Congenital Myasthenia Syndromes

Familial infantile myasthenia gravis

- Autosomal recessive
- Clinical features: hypotonia at birth, fluctuating ptosis, feeding difficulties, episodic apnea following crying
- Pathophysiology: defect in acetylcholine synthesis, mobilization, and packaging
- Responds to neostigmine, but not to corticosteroids, and improves with age

Postsynaptic Congenital Myasthenia Syndromes

Congenital acetylcholinesterase deficiency

- Autosomal recessive
- Clinical features: fatigability, weakness, atrophy, ophthalmoparesis, and abnormally slow pupillary light response

- Pathophysiology: absent acetylcholinesterase
- EMG
  1. Repetitive nerve stimulation shows decremental responses to 2-Hz stimulation, postactivation facilitation, and postactivation exhaustion.
  2. Reduplicated CMAPs to single stimuli are most characteristic.
  3. Miniature endplate potentials (MEPPs) show prolonged delay.
- Unresponsive to cholinesterase inhibitors or corticosteroids

Primary acetylcholine receptor deficiency

- Autosomal recessive
- Clinical features: ptosis and poor feeding in the neonatal period, eventually developing generalized fatigue and complete external ophthalmoplegia by adolescence
- Pathophysiology: deficient acetylcholine receptors
- EMG: severe reduction in MEPPs
- Responds to Mestinon

Slow-channel syndrome

- Autosomal dominant
- Unlike all other congenital myasthenia syndromes that present in infancy, it usually becomes apparent in adolescence.
- Clinical features: ophthalmoparesis, ptosis, and prominent muscle atrophy
- Pathophysiology
  1. Excessively prolonged opening time of cation channels of acetylcholine receptors
  2. Cationic cellular toxicity causes a fixed vacuolar myopathy and muscle atrophy
- EMG: reduplicated CMAP responses to single stimuli; prolonged MEPPs and endplate potentials with decreased amplitude
- Unresponsive to cholinesterase inhibitors

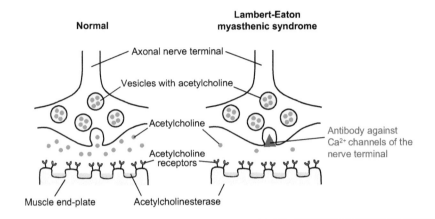

Lambert-Eaton myasthenic syndrome is a rare, presynaptic disorder of neuromuscular transmission in which quantal release of acetylcholine is impaired. Two-thirds of all cases are paraneoplastic. Of this type:

- Most cases occur in men.
- Small-cell cancer of the lung is associated in 80% of cases.
- The syndrome is usually present before the the malignancy is discovered.

One-third of all cases are autoimmune. Of this type:

- Most cases occur in women
- The syndrome may be associated with other autoimmune diseases such as pernicious anemia, thyroid disease, and Sjögren's syndrome.

Clinical Features of Lambert-Eaton Myasthenic Syndrome

Weakness and fatigability
- Muscles in proximal leg and the pelvic girdle are most severely affected
- Mild bulbar muscle weakness and ptosis may also occur.

Hyporeflexia, but muscle wasting is infrequent

Autonomic dysfunction (e.g., dry mouth, loss of pupillary reflex, decreased sweating, erectile dysfunction)

Pathophysiology

- Normally, an action potential arriving at the nerve terminal induces an influx of calcium into the terminal, which then leads to the release of acetylcholine into the synaptic cleft.

- In Lambert-Eaton myasthenic syndrome, antibodies against voltage-gated calcium channels in the nerve terminal cause impaired release of acetylcholine (i.e., a presynaptic disorder).
- In paraneoplastic Lambert-Eaton syndrome, small-cell lung cancer expresses voltage-gated calcium channels that act as an antigen and stimulate production of antibodies against calcium channels in nerve terminals.

Electromyography

- Repetitive nerve stimulation: decremental responses at 2 Hz but marked facilitation of CMAP at 50-Hz stimulation or after brief exercise
- Single-fiber EMG: increased jitter and blockage that improve as units fire at higher rates

Treatment

1. Identify and treat underlying malignancy; may lead to partial remission if treated.
2. Medications
   - 3,4-Diaminopyridine is the drug of choice; it increases calcium influx.
   - Cholinesterase inhibitors have a weak effect; they are usually used as adjunctive therapy.
   - Immunotherapy (e.g., corticosteroids or azathioprine)
3. Plasmapheresis
4. Intravenous immunoglobulin therapy

13.4 **Botulism**

Botulism is caused by *Clostridium botulinum*. There are three forms:

1. Food-borne botulism: from ingestion of contaminated food (e.g., tainted canned food)
2. Wound botulism: from a contaminated wound
3. Infantile botulism: from toxins produced by *C. botulinum* that colonize the intestine (e.g., history of honey ingestion or soil eating)

There are eight types of *C. botulinum* (A, B, Cα, Cβ, D, E, F and G), with types A, B, and E being the most common types found in North America.

Clinical Features of Botulism

- Nausea, vomiting, dysphagia, and weakness of proximal muscles
- Ptosis, ophthalmoplegia, dilated nonreactive pupil (i.e., internal ophthalmoplegia)
- Quivering eye motions consisting of hypometric multistep saccades followed by backward drifts
- In infantile botulism: hypotonia, hyporeflexia, constipation, poor feeding, dry mouth, ptosis, internal and external ophthalmoplegia, muscle weakness, and decreased respiratory function

Pathophysiology

Botulinum toxins interfere with the release of acetylcholine vesicles after stimulus-induced influx of calcium into the nerve terminal (i.e., a presynaptic disorder).

Electromyography

Results of EMG are similar to those of Lambert-Eaton myasthenic syndrome:

- Repetitive nerve stimulation: decremental responses at 2 Hz but marked facilitation of CMAP at 50 Hz stimulation
- Single-fiber EMG: increased jitter and blockage that improve as units fire at higher rates

Treatment

1. Cholinesterase inhibitors are ineffective in botulism.
2. Treat with bivalent (A and B) or trivalent (A, B, and E) antitoxin, 20,000–40,000 units, 2–3 times per day.
3. For food-borne botulism, remove stomach and intestinal content, and administer antitoxin.
4. For wound botulism, debride wound and administer antitoxin and penicillin.

Chapter 14

Disorders Affecting the Extraocular Muscles

14.1.1 Chronic Progressive External Ophthalmoplegia and Kearns-Sayre Syndrome ▸▸

Chronic progressive external ophthalmoplegia (CPEO) occurs in 90% of patients with mitochondrial myopathy. It is characterized by a slowly progressive ptosis and ophthalmoplegia. The ophthalmoplegia is usually preceded by ptosis for months to years, and downgaze is usually intact.

Kearns-Sayre Syndrome is a subtype of chronic progressive external ophthalmoplegia. Most cases are sporadic and associated with single deletions of mitochondrial DNA.

Clinical Features of Kearns-Sayre Syndrome

Severe CPEO before age 20

Pigmentary retinopathy

- The retinopathy in CPEO affects mainly the posterior pole initially with a salt-and-pepper appearance and causes mild night blindness and electroretinogram (ERG) changes
- This is in contrast to retinitis pigmentosa, which affects the peripheral and mid-peripheral retina initially with bony spicules pigmentation and causes severe night-blindness and ERG changes

In addition to the above two criteria, patients have to exhibit at least one of the following abnormalities:

- Cardiac: heart block
- Neurologic: increased protein in cerebrospinal fluid, cerebellar ataxia, deafness, dementia
- Endocrine: short stature, hypoparathyroid (tetany), gonadal dysfunction, diabetes mellitus
- Muscular: facial muscle weakness (especially the orbicularis and frontalis)

Pathology

Ragged-red fibers are seen on light microscopy (using modified Gomori trichrome stain).

- Due to accumulation of enlarged mitochondria under the sarcolemma of affected muscles
- Found in skeletal muscles, orbicularis, and extraocular muscles
- On electron microscopy, the mitochondria contain paracrystalline ("parking lot") inclusions and disorganized cristae that are sometimes arranged concentrically.

Workup

1. Muscle biopsy (e.g., deltoid)
2. ERG

3. Electrocardiogram (EKG)

4. Genetic testing

Treatment

There is no effective treatment for CPEO. Maintaining a high-lipid, low-carbohydrate diet, taking co-enzyme Q10, biotin, or thiamine, and avoiding medications such as valproate and phenobarbital may be helpful.

14.1.2 Other Mitochondrial Myopathies Causing Ophthalmoplegia

MELAS syndrome

- MELAS stands for mitochondrial encephalomyopathy, lactic acidosis, and strokelike episodes.
- Maternally inherited; caused by point mutations of mitochondrial DNA (A3243G mutation accounts for about 80% of all cases)
- Clinical features
  1. Strokelike episodes before age 40 (hallmark feature)
  2. Encephalopathy characterized by developmental delay, seizures, or dementia
  3. Mitochondrial dysfunction manifested as lactic acidosis or ragged-red fibers
  4. Ophthalmoplegia
  5. Optic atrophy and pigmentary retinopathy
  6. Diabetes mellitus and hearing loss

MNGIE syndrome

- MNGIE stands for mitochondrial neuro-gastrointestinal encephalomyopathy.
- Autosomal recessive; caused by mutations in the nuclear gene *ECGF1*, resulting in thymidine phosphorylase deficiency, which in turn causes deletions, duplications, and depletion of mitochondrial DNA
- Clinical features: ophthalmoplegia, peripheral neuropathy, leukoencephalopathy, and gastrointestinal symptoms (recurrent nausea, vomiting, or diarrhea) with intestinal dysmotility

SANDO syndrome

SANDO stands for sensory ataxic neuropathy, dysarthria, and ophthalmoplegia. It is sporadic and is caused by multiple deletions of mitochondrial DNA.

Mitochondrial DNA-associated Leigh's syndrome (subacute necrotizing encephalomyelopathy)

Genetics of Leigh's syndrome

- Mitochondrial (i.e. maternal) inheritance (10–30% cases): caused by mutations of mitochondrial DNA, resulting in deficiency of enzymes in the respiratory chain, which leads to lactic acidosis
- Autosomal recessive (70–90% cases): caused by mutations of nuclear DNA

Clinical features

1. Onset typically between 3 and 12 months of age, with about 75% of patients dying by 2–3 years of age, most often as a result of respiratory or cardiac failure
2. Developmental delay, hypotonia, respiratory disturbances (e.g., apnea, episodic hyperventilation), weakness, spasticity, poor feeding, failure to thrive, seizures, ataxia, and hypertrophic cardiomyopathy
3. Ophthalmic findings: optic atrophy and retained cell nuclei in lens cortex
4. Ocular motility findings: gaze-evoked nystagmus, seesaw nystagmus, upbeat nystagmus, ocular tilt reaction, horizontal and vertical gaze palsies that may progress to total ophthalmoplegia

14.2 Muscular Dystrophies

14.2.1 Myotonic Dystrophy

Myotonic dystrophy is the most common adult-onset muscular dystrophy (prevalence = 5 per 100,000). It is autosomal dominant and results from amplification of a trinucleotide CTG repeat in the gene that encodes myotonin-protein kinase on chromosome 19. Myotonic dystrophy exhibits "anticipation" (i.e., increased severity of the disease in successive generations of an affected family) due to increased number of CTG repeats in successive generations.

Clinical Features of Myotonic Dystrophy

- Myotonia of skeletal muscles (involuntary delayed relaxation following a contraction; e.g., after sustained handgrip)
- Progressive weakness of the distal muscles
- Typical facies: frontal balding, hollowing of temporalis and masseter muscles, facial weakness, slackened mouth, long face, and thin neck (wasting of sternomastoid muscle)
- Other systemic features: cardiac conduction defect (90%), intellectual impairment, testicular atrophy, respiratory muscle weakness, and gastrointestinal dysmotility
- Ptosis and ophthalmoplegia
- Other ophthalmic features: cataract ("Christmas tree cataract" or spokelike opacity in 100% of patients), epithelial dystrophy of the cornea, sluggish miotic pupils, iris neovascularization, and pigmentary retinopathy

Pathology

- Variation in diameter and shape of skeletal muscle fibers, myofiber degeneration and regeneration, as well as ringed fibers ("ringbinden")
- Increased number of sarcolemmal nuclei, which are centrally located

Workup

1. Slit-lamp examination to rule out the presence of cataract
2. Electromyography (EMG): waxing and waning in amplitude and frequency of motor unit potentials, as well as myopathic changes
3. Electrocardiography (EKG): bradycardia with prolonged PR interval
4. Muscle biopsy
5. Genetic testing

Treatment

1. Phenytoin for myotonia
2. Cataract surgery

3. Pacemaker for cardiac conduction defect

4. Ptosis surgery

5. Prisms for diplopia

14.2.2 Oculopharyngeal Dystrophy

Oculopharyngeal dystrophy results from the expansion of a GCG trinucleotide repeat in the *PABP2* gene on chromosome 14q11. Oculopharyngeal dystrophy can be autosomal dominant (8 to 13 GCG repeats) or recessive (7 GCG repeats). Many patients are of French-Canadian descent, and symptoms and signs usually present late in life.

Clinical Features of Oculopharyngeal Dystrophy

Ptosis
- Usually bilateral and symmetrical
- In one series, up to 33% of patients with acquired ptosis had oculopharyngeal dystrophy.

Dysphagia
- Due to weakness of muscles in the pharynx and larynx
- May lead to aspiration and recurrent pneumonitis

External ophthalmoplegia, usually mild (pupillary reaction is spared)

Pathology

Pathologic examination reveals accumulation of autophagic vacuoles in non-necrotic myofibers and nuclear inclusions in striated muscles.

Workup

1. Evaluation of dysphagia

2. Creatine kinase level (five times higher than normal level)

3. Genetic testing

Treatment

1. Ptosis surgery

2. Cricopharyngeal myotomy or percutaneous feeding gastrostomy for dysphagia

---

14.3 Graves' Disease

Graves' disease is an autoimmune disease characterized by hyperthyroidism due to circulating autoantibodies. Thyroid-stimulating immunoglobulins bind to and activate thyrotropin receptors, causing continuous stimulation of the thyroid gland and synthesis of thyroid hormone. The disease affects predominantly young females (female-to-male ratio, 8:1; age range, 20–60 years).

Clinical Features of Graves' Disease

Tachycardia, palpitations, tremor, sleep disturbances, weight loss, heat intolerance, proximal muscle weakness, and easy fatigability.
Graves' ophthalmopathy may occur during hyperthyroid, euthyroid, or hypothyroid state:

- Proptosis, lid retraction, lacrimation, photophobia, and eye pain
- Extraocular muscle involvement causing diplopia and ophthalmoplegia
  Found in more than 80% of patients
  Involves the muscle tissue itself but spares the muscle tendons (this is in contrast to idiopathic inflammatory pseudotumor or orbital myositis, which involves both the muscles and tendons; see section 14.4.2)
  In the early stage, the muscles are swollen; in the later stage, infiltration and edema cause loss of muscle tissue, and the muscles become fibrotic.
- Exposure keratitis (caused by severe proptosis)
- Optic neuropathy (as a result of compression of the optic nerve by the swollen muscles in the orbital apex)

Differential Diagnosis of Extraocular Muscle Enlargement Causing Ophthalmoplegia

Graves' ophthalmopathy
Idiopathic inflammatory pseudotumor or orbital myositis (see section 14.4.2)
Infective myositis (see section 14.4.1)
Increased venous pressure in the orbit:

- High-flow carotid-cavernous fistula (see section 12.5.4)
- High-flow arteriovenous malformation
- Tumors or aneurysms in the anterior temporal fossa compressing the draining orbital veins

Tumor (e.g., rhabdomyosarcoma of extraocular muscles, metastasis, or lymphoma); it may also produce ocular motility disturbance by its mass effect within the muscle cone
Amyloidosis
Trauma causing intramuscular edema and hemorrhage; it may also produce ocular motility disturbance by causing muscle laceration, avulsion of the muscle origin or insertion, or muscle entrapment from orbital fracture (i.e., a restrictive ophthalmopathy)

Pathology

- Edema, lymphocytic and plasma cell infiltration, and accumulation of glycosamino-glycans within the endomysium of the extraocular muscles and in the orbital fat
- Primary autoimmune target appears to be orbital fibroblasts, rather than muscle cells

Workup

1. Ultrasound, computed tomography, or MRI of the orbit: extraocular muscle enlargement with sparing of tendons
2. Thyroid function tests: thyrotropin-receptor antibodies (diagnostic of Graves' diseases), free T3, free T4, thryoid-stimulating hormone, thyrotropin, antithyroglobulin or antithyroidal peroxidase antibodies
3. Radioactive iodine scanning and measurements of iodine uptake

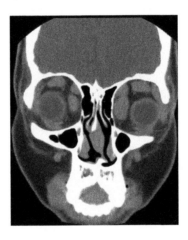

Coronal MRI of the orbit showing enlargement of the extraocular muscles in Grave's ophthalmopathy.

Treatment

1. For patients with hypothyroidism, replacement therapy
2. For patients with hyperthyroidism, radioablation therapy using radioiodine. Radioiodine may exacerbate preexisting ophthalmopathy, but this can be prevented by concurrent treatment with low-dose corticosteroids (beginning just before radioablation and continuing one month after). This treatment may prevent Graves' ophthalmopathy from developing or exacerbating.
3. For irritation and swelling, corticosteroids or low-dose orbital radiation (2000 cGy)
4. For proptosis, orbital decompression if severe (>3–4 mm of proptosis)
5. For strabismus, prisms or surgery
6. For exposure keratitis, lubrication, nocturnal taping of the eyes, or orbital decompression
7. For optic neuropathy, corticosteroids, radiation therapy, or orbital decompression

14.4 Myositis

14.4.1 Infective Myositis

Causes

1. Bacterial (e.g., *Staphylococcus aureus, Streptococcus pyogenes, Clostridium welchii*)
   - Ocular motility disturbances are usually indirectly caused by a generalized orbital inflammation with soft-tissue edema and rarely by direct muscle invasion.
   - Often occurs after trauma when the bacteria enter the orbit via infected paranasal sinuses
2. Viral (e.g., influenza virus, Coxsackie A and B viruses)
3. Parasitic induced (e.g., trichinosis)
4. Fungal (e.g., mucormycosis, aspergillosis)

14.4.2 Idiopathic Myositis

Acquired Brown's superior oblique tendon sheath syndrome

- Often intermittent (in contrast to congenital Brown's syndrome; see section 14.5.2)
- Associated with inflammation and scarring within the superior oblique tendon or next to the anterior sheath

Causes

1. Iatrogenic (e.g., following superior oblique surgery or retinal detachment surgery)
2. Trauma
3. Paranasal sinus disease
4. Rheumatoid arthritis

Some cases respond to local injections of corticosteroids.

Orbital myositis (myositic form of idiopathic inflammatory orbital pseudotumor)

- Sudden onset of diplopia with pain, conjunctival chemosis and edema, or proptosis
- Ultrasound, computed tomography, or MRI of the orbit shows enlargement of both the extraocular muscles and their tendons.
- Biopsy shows infiltration with chronic inflammatory cells.
- Occurs as an isolated phenomenon or in association with lupus, rheumatoid arthritis, sarcoidosis, or Wegener's granulomatosis
- Treatment: systemic corticosteroids

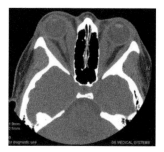

Axial MRI of the orbit showing enlargement of the extraocular muscles and their tendons in idiopathic inflammatory orbital pseudotumor.

14.5 Congenital and Developmental Disorders Affecting the Extraocular Muscles

14.5.1 Agenesis of Extraocular Muscles

- Most cases involve only a single muscle
- Often occurs in children with craniosynostoses

14.5.2 Anomalies of Extraocular Muscle Origin and Insertion

Anomalies of extraocular muscle origin often occur in children with craniosynostoses.

Brown's syndrome (congenital form) ▸▸

- Deficient elevation on adduction, improved elevation in the primary position, and normal or near-normal elevation on abduction
- Forced duction test shows mechanical restriction of upward and nasalward motion.

Causes

1. Congenital form: due to congenitally short or inelastic tendon or to abnormal tendon-trochlear complex (which may account for spontaneous resolution in some cases)
2. Acquired form: iatrogenic, trauma, inflammatory or infectious processes (see section 14.4.2)

Treatment

1. Superior oblique tendon tenotomy with inferior oblique recession (to prevent secondary superior oblique palsy)
2. Controlled weakening of the superior oblique using a silicone expander that is sewn between the cut ends of a tenotomized superior oblique tendon

14.5.3 Congenital Adherence of Extraocular Muscles

- Adhesion between the sheaths of the lateral rectus and inferior oblique muscles, causing deficient abduction (usually bilateral)
- Adhesion between the sheaths of the superior rectus and superior oblique muscles, causing deficient elevation

14.5.4 Congenital Myopathies

Congenital myopathies consist of a group of primarily nonprogressive myopathies that also affect the extraocular muscles, causing ptosis and ophthalmoplegia. This group includes:

1. Myotubular myopathy (centronuclear myopathy)
2. Nemaline myopathy
3. Central core myopathy
4. Multicore disease

Selected Bibliography

Chapter 1

Burde RM. The extraocular muscles. In: Adler FH, editor. Adler's Physiology of the Eye. 7th ed. St Louis: CV Mosby; 1981.

Demer JL, Miller JM, Poukens V, Vinters HV, Glasgow BJ. Evidence for fibromuscular pulleys of the recti extraocular muscles. Invest Ophthalmol Vis Sci. 1995;36:1125–36.

Donaldson IM. The functions of the proprioceptors of the eye muscles. Phil Trans R Soc Lond B. 2000;355:1685–754.

Niechwiej-Szwedo E, Gonzalez E, Bega S, Verrier MC, Wong AM, Steinbach MJ. Proprioceptive role for palisade endings in extraocular muscles: Evidence from the Jendrassik maneuver. Vision Res. 2006;46:2268–79

von Noorden GK. Binocular vision and ocular motility: Theory and management of strabismus. 5th ed. St. Louis: Mosby-Year Book, Inc.; 1996.

Porter JD, Baker RS, Ragusa RJ, Brueckner JK. Extraocular muscles: Basic and clinical aspects of structure and function. Surv Ophthalmol. 1995;39:451–84.

Simpson JI, Graf W. Eye-muscle geometry and compensatory eye movements in lateral-eyed and frontal-eyed animals. Ann NY Acad Sci. 1980;374:20–30.

Wolff E. Eugene Wolff's Anatomy of the Eye and Orbit: Including the Central Connexions, Development, and Comparative Anatomy of the Visual Apparatus. 7th ed. Philadelphia: Saunders; 1976.

Chapter 2

Hamstra SJ, Sinha T, Hallett PE. The joint contributions of saccades and ocular drift to repeated ocular fixations. Vision Res. 2001;41:1709–21.

Sharpe JA, Wong AM. Anatomy and physiology of ocular motor systems. In: Miller NR, Newman NJ, Biousse V, Kerrison JB, editors. Walsh and Hoyt's Clinical Neuro-Ophthalmology. 6th ed. Philadelphia: Lippincott Williams & Wilkins; 2005:809–85.

Steinman RM, Haddad GM, Skavenski AA, Wyman D. Miniature eye movements. Science. 1973;181:810–19.

Chapter 3

Angelaki DE. Eyes on target: what neurons must do for the vestibuloocular reflex during linear motion. J Neurophysiol 2004;92:20–35.

Blazquez P, Partsalis A, Gerrits NM, Highstein SM. Input of anterior and posterior semicircular canal interneurons encoding head-velocity to the dorsal Y group of the vestibular nuclei. J Neurophysiol 2000;83:2891–904.

Cohen B, Raphan T. The physiology of the vestibuloocular reflex (VOR). In: Highstein SM, Fay RR, Popper AN, editors. The Vestibular System. New York: Springer-Verlag; 2003:235–85.

Collewijn H, Van der Steen J, Ferman L, Jansen TC. Human ocular counterroll: assessment of static and dynamic properties from electromagnetic scleral coil recordings. Exp Brain Res 1985;59:185–96.

Leigh RJ, Zee DS. The Neurology of Eye Movements. 4th ed. New York: Oxford University Press; 2006.

LIVING without a balancing mechanism. N Engl J Med 1952;246(12):458–60.

Lysakowski A, Goldberg JM. Morphophysiology of the vestibular periphery. In: Highstein SM, Fay RR, Popper AN, editors. The Vestibular System. New York: Springer-Verlag; 2003:57–152.

McCrea RA, Strassman A, Highstein SM. Anatomical and physiological characteristics of vestibular neurons mediating the vertical vestibulo-ocular reflexes of the squirrel monkey. J Comp Neurol 1987;264:571–94.

McCrea RA, Strassman A, May E, Highstein SM. Anatomical and physiological characteristics of vestibular neurons mediating the horizontal vestibulo-ocular reflex of the squirrel monkey. J Comp Neurol 1987;264:547–70.

Miles FA. The sensing of rotational and translational optic flow by the primate optokinetic system. Rev Oculomotor Res 1993;5:393–403.

Rabbitt RD, Damiano ER, Grant JW, editors. Biomechanics of the semicircular canals and otolith organs. New York: Springer-Verlag; 2003.

Raphan T, Matsuo V, Cohen B. Velocity storage in the vestibulo-ocular reflex arc (VOR). Exp Brain Res 1979;35:229–48.

Sharpe JA, Wong AM. Anatomy and physiology of ocular motor systems. In: Miller NR, Newman NJ, Biousse V, Kerrison JB, editors. Walsh and Hoyt's Clinical Neuro-Ophthalmology. 6th ed. Philadelphia: Lippincott Williams & Wilkins; 2005:809–85.

Suzuki J-I, Tokumasu K, Goto K. Eye movements from single utricular nerve stimulation in the cat. Acta Otolaryngol (Stockh) 1969;68:350–62.

Uchino Y, Sasaki M, Sato H, Imagawa M, Suwa H, Isu N. Utriculoocular reflex arc of the cat. J Neurophysiol 1996;76:1896–1903.

Chapter 4

Bahill AT, Clark MR, Stark L. The main sequence: A tool for studying human eye movements. Math Biosci. 1975;24:191–204.

Baker R. The nucleus prepositus hypoglossi. In: Brooks BA, Bajandas FJ, editors. Eye Movements. New York: Plenum Press; 1977:145–78.

Baloh RW, Sills AW, Kumley WE, Honrubia V. Quantitative measurement of saccade amplitude, duration, and velocity. Neurology. 1975;25:1065–70.

Crawford JD, Cadera W, Vilis T. Generation of torsional and vertical eye position signals by the interstitial nucleus of Cajal. Science. 1991;252:1551–53.

Gomez CM, Thompson RM, Gammack JT, Perlman SL, Dobyns WB, Truwit CL, et al. Spinocerebellar ataxia type 6: Gaze-evoked and vertical nystagmus, Purkinje cell degeneration, and variable age of onset. Ann Neurol. 1997;42:933–50.

Leichnetz GR, Smith DJ, Spencer RF. Cortical projections to the paramedian tegmental and basilar pons in the monkey. J Comp Neurol. 1984;228:388–408.

Leigh RJ, Zee DS. The Neurology of Eye Movements. 4th ed. New York: Oxford University Press; 2006.

Moschovakis AK, Highstein SM. The anatomy and physiology of primate neurons that control rapid eye movements. Ann Rev Neurosci. 1994;17:465–88.

Moschovakis AK, Scudder CA, Highstein SM. Structure of the primate oculomotor burst generator. I. Medium-lead burst neurons with upward on-directions. J Neurophysiol. 1991;65:203–17.

Moschovakis AK, Scudder CA, Highstein SM, Warren JD. Structure of the primate oculomotor burst generator. II. Medium-lead burst neurons with downward on-directions. J Neurophysiol. 1991;65:218–29.

Optican LM, Robinson DA. Cerebellar-dependent adaptive control of primate saccadic system. J Neurophysiol. 1980;44:1058–76.

Optican LM, Zee DS, Miles FA. Floccular lesions abolish adaptive control of post-saccadic drift in primates. Exp Brain Res. 1986;64:596–98.

Robinson DA. The mechanics of human saccadic eye movement. J Physiol (Lond). 1964;174:245–64.

Robinson DA. Models of the saccadic eye movement control system. Kybernetik. 1973;14:71–83.

Robinson DA. Oculomotor unit behavior in the monkey. J Neurophysiol. 1970;33:393–404.

Robinson DA, Fuchs AF. Eye movements evoked by stimulation of frontal eye fields. J Neurophysiol. 1969;32:637–48.

Sharpe JA, Wong AM. Anatomy and physiology of ocular motor systems. In: Miller NR, Newman NJ, Biousse V, Kerrison JB, editors. Walsh and Hoyt's Clinical Neuro-Ophthalmology. 6th ed. Philadelphia: Lippincott Williams & Wilkins; 2005:809–85.

Strassman A, Highstein SM, McCrea RA. Anatomy and physiology of saccadic burst neurons in the alert squirrel monkey. I. Excitatory burst neurons. J Comp Neurol. 1986;249:337–57.

Strassman A, Highstein SM, McCrea RA. Anatomy and physiology of saccadic burst neurons in the alert squirrel monkey. II. Inhibitory burst neurons. J Comp Neurol. 1986;249:358–80.

Wadia NH, Swami RK. A new form of heredo-familial spinocerebellar degeneration with slow eye movements (nine families). Brain. 1971;94:359–74.

Chapter 5

Chubb MC, Fuchs AF. Contribution of y group of vestibular nuclei and dentate nucleus of cerebellum to generation of vertical smooth eye movements. J Neurophysiol. 1982;48:75–99.

Johnston JL, Sharpe JA, Morrow MJ. Paresis of contralateral smooth pursuit and normal vestibular smooth eye movements after unilateral brainstem lesions. Ann Neurol. 1992;31:495–502.

Keller EL, Heinen SJ. Generation of smooth-pursuit eye movements: Neuronal mechanisms and pathways. Neurosci Res. 1991;11:79–107.

Leigh RJ, Zee DS. The Neurology of Eye Movements. 4th ed. New York: Oxford University Press; 2006.

Lisberger SG, Morris EJ, Tychsen L. Visual motion processing and sensory-motor integration for smooth pursuit eye movements. Annu Rev Neurosci. 1987;10:97–129.

Mather JA, Lackner JR. The influence of efferent, proprioceptive, and timing factors on the accuracy of eye-hand tracking. Exp Brain Res. 1981;43:406–12.

Morrow M, Sharpe J. Retinotopic and directional deficits of smooth pursuit initiation after posterior cerebral hemispheric lesions. Neurology. 1993;43:595–603.

Robinson DA, Gordon JL, Gordon SE. A model of the smooth pursuit eye movement system. Biol Cybern. 1986;55:43–57.

Sharpe JA, Wong AM. Anatomy and physiology of ocular motor systems. In: Miller NR, Newman NJ, Biousse V, Kerrison JB, editors. Walsh and Hoyt's Clinical Neuro-Ophthalmology. 6th ed. Philadelphia: Lippincott Williams & Wilkins; 2005:809–85.

Steinbach MJ. Eye tracking of self-moved objects: The role of efference. J Exp Psychol. 1969;82:366–76.

Steinbach MJ. Pursuing the perceptual rather than the retinal stimulus. Vision Res. 1976;16:1371–76.

Tomlinson RD, Robinson DA. Signals in vestibular nucleus mediating vertical eye movements in the monkey. J Neurophysiol. 1984;51:1121–36.

Tusa RJ, Ungerleider LG. Fiber pathways of cortical areas mediating smooth pursuit eye movements in monkeys. Ann Neurol. 1988;23:174–83.

Westheimer G, Blair SM. Functional organization of primate oculomotor system revealed by cerebellectomy. Exp Brain Res. 1974;21:463–72.

Chapter 6

Buttner-Ennever JA, Horn AK, Graf W, Ugolini G. Modern concepts of brainstem anatomy: From extraocular motoneurons to proprioceptive pathways. Ann NY Acad Sci. 2002;956:75–84.

Eizenman M, Sapir-Pichhadze R, Westall CA, Wong AM, Lee H, Morad Y. Eye-movement responses to disparity vergence stimuli with artificial monocular scotomas. Curr Eye Res. 2006;31:471—80.

Leigh RJ, Zee DS. The Neurology of Eye Movements. 4th ed. New York: Oxford University Press; 2006.

MacInnis BJ. Ophthalmology Board Review: Optics and Refraction. St. Louis: Mosby; 1994.

Mays LE. Neural control of vergence eye movements: Convergence and divergence neurons in midbrain. J Neurophysiol. 1984;51:1091–108.

Mays LE, Porter JD. Neural control of vergence eye movements: Activity of abducens and oculomotor neurons. J Neurophysiol. 1984;52:743–61.

McLin LNJ, Schor CM, Kruger PB. Changing size (looming) as a stimulus to accommodation and vergence. Vision Res. 1988;28:883–98.

Owens DA, Leibowitz HW. Perceptual and motor consequences of tonic vergence. In: Schor CM, Ciuffreda KJ, editors. Vergence Eye Movements: Basic and Clinical Aspects. Boston: Butterworths; 1983:25–74.

Ringach DL, Hawken MJ, Shapley R. Binocular eye movements caused by the perception of three-dimensional structure from motion. Vision Res. 1996;36:1479–92.

Robinson DA. The mechanics of human vergence eye movement. J Ped Ophthalmol. 1966;3:31–7.

Semmlow JL. Oculomotor Responses to Near Stimuli: The Near Triad. Boca Raton, FL: CRC Press; 1981.

Sharpe JA, Wong AM. Anatomy and physiology of ocular motor systems. In: Miller NR, Newman NJ, Biousse V, Kerrison JB, editors. Walsh and Hoyt's Clinical Neuro-Ophthalmology. 6th ed. Philadelphia: Lippincott Williams & Wilkins; 2005:809–85.

Takagi M, Tamargo R, Zee DS. Effects of lesions of the cerebellar oculomotor vermis on eye movements in primate: Binocular control. Prog Brain Res. 2003;142:19–33.

Westheimer G, Mitchell AM. Eye movement responses to convergent stimuli. Arch Ophthalmol. 1956;55:848–56.

Wick B, Bedell HE. Magnitude and velocity of proximal vergence. Invest Ophthalmol Vis Sci. 1989 30:755–60.

Zee DS, Fitzgibbon EJ, Optican LM. Saccade-vergence interactions in humans. J Neurophysiol. 1992;68:1624–41.

Zhang H, Gamlin PD. Neurons in the posterior interposed nucleus of the cerebellum related to vergence and accommodation. I. Steady-state characteristics. J Neurophysiol. 1998;79:1255–69.

Chapter 7

Anteby I, Zhai HF, Tychsen L. Asymmetric MVEPs in infantile strabismus are not an artifact of latent nystagmus. J Am Assoc Pediatric Ophthalmol Strabismus. 1998;2:153–58.

Baloh RW, Spooner JW. Downbeat nystagmus: A type of central vestibular nystagmus. Neurology. 1981;31:304–10.

Baloh RW, Yee RD. Spontaneous vertical nystagmus. Rev Neurol (Paris). 1989;145:527–32.

Daroff RB. See-saw nystagmus. Neurology. 1965;15:874–77.

Dell'Osso L, Daroff R. Congenital nystagmus waveforms and foveation strategy. Doc Ophthalmol. 1975;39:155–82.

Dell'Osso LF, Schmidt D, Daroff RB. Latent, manifest latent, and congenital nystagmus. Arch Ophthalmol. 1979;97:1877–85.

Druckman R, Ellis P, Kleinfeld J, Waldman M. Seesaw nystagmus. Arch Ophthalmol. 1966;76:668–75.

Furman JM, Wall CD, Pang DL. Vestibular function in periodic alternating nystagmus. Brain. 1990;113:1425–39.

Gelbart SS, Hoyt CS. Congenital nystagmus: A clinical perspective in infancy. Graefes Arch Clin Exp Ophthalmol. 1988;226:178–80.

Gottlob I, Wizov SS, Reinecke RD. Spasmus nutans. A long-term follow-up. Invest Ophthalmol Vis Sci. 1995;36:2768–71.

Gresty MA, Ell JJ, Findley LJ. Acquired pendular nystagmus: Its characteristics, localising value and pathophysiology. J Neurol Neurosurg Psychiatry. 1982;45:431–39.

Gresty MA, Metcalfe T, Timms C, Elston J, Lee J, Liu C. Neurology of latent nystagmus. Brain. 1992;115:1303–21.

Halmagyi GM, Rudge P, Gresty MA, Sanders MD. Downbeating nystagmus. A review of 62 cases. Arch Neurol. 1983;40:777–84.

Hotson JR, Baloh RW. Acute vestibular syndrome. N Engl J Med. 1998;339:680–85.

Leigh RJ, Averbuch-Heller L, Tomsak RL, Remler BF, Yaniglos SS, Dell'Osso LF. Treatment of abnormal eye movements that impair vision: strategies based on current concepts of physiology and pharmacology. Ann Neurol. 1994;36:129–41.

Leigh RJ, Zee DS. The Neurology of Eye Movements. 4th ed. New York: Oxford University Press; 2006.

Lopez L, Bronstein AM, Gresty MA, Rudge P, du Boulay EP. Torsional nystagmus. A neuro-otological and MRI study of thirty-five cases. Brain. 1992;115:1107–24.

Nakada T, Remler MP. Primary position upbeat nystagmus. Another central vestibular nystagmus? J Clin Neuroophthalmol. 1981;1:185–89.

Newman SA, Hedges TRl, Wall M, Sedwick LA. Spasmus nutans—or is it? Surv Ophthalmol. 1990;34:453–56.

Waespe W, Cohen B, Raphan T. Dynamic modification of the vestibulo-ocular reflex by the nodulus and uvula. Science. 1985;228:199–202.

Yee R. Downbeat nystagmus: Characteristics and localization of lesions. Trans Am Ophthalmol Soc. 1989;87:984–1032.

Yee RD, Jelks GW, Baloh RW, Honrubia V. Uniocular nystagmus in monocular visual loss. Ophthalmology. 1979;86:511–22.

Yee R, Wong E, Baloh R, Honrubia V. A study of congenital nystagmus waveforms. Neurology. 1976;26:326–33.

Zee D, Yee R, Cogan D, Robinson DA, Engel WK. Ocular motor abnormalities in hereditary cerebellar ataxia. Brain. 1976;99:207–34.

Chapter 8

Altman A, Baehner R. Favorable prognosis for survival in children with coincident opsomyoclonus and neuroblastoma. Cancer. 1976;37:846–52.

Cogan D, Chu F, Reingold D. Ocular signs of cerebellar disease. Arch Ophthalmol. 1982;100:755–60.

Dell'Osso L, Troost B, Daroff R. Macro square-wave jerks. Neurology. 1975;25:975–79.

Digre KB. Opsoclonus in adults. Report of three cases and review of the literature. Arch Neurol. 1986; 43:1165–75.

Ellenberger CJ, Keltner JL, Stroud MH. Ocular dyskinesia in cerebellar diseases: Evidence for the similarity of opsoclonus, ocular dysmetria and flutter-like oscillations. Brain. 1972;95:685–92.

Fisher C. Some neuro-ophthalmologic observations. J Neurol Neurosurg Psychiatry. 1967;30:383–92.

Fisher CM. Ocular bobbing. Arch Neurol. 1964;11:543–46.

Hameroff SB, Garcia-Mullin R, Eckholdt J. Ocular bobbing. Arch Ophthalmol. 1969;82:774–80.

Herishanu Y, Sharpe J. Normal square wave jerks. Invest Ophthalmol Vis Sci. 1981;20:268–72.

Hoyt C, Mousel D, Weber A. Transient supranuclear disturbances of gaze in healthy neonates. Am J Ophthalmol. 1980;89:708–13.

Katz B, Hoyt WF, Townsend J. Ocular bobbing and unilateral pontine hemorrhage. Report of a case. J Clin Neuroophthalmol. 1982;2:193–95.

Keane J. Pretectal pseudobobbing. Five patients with 'V'-pattern convergence nystagmus. Arch Neurol. 1985;42:592–94.

Keane J, Rawlinson D, Lu A. Sustained downgaze deviation. Two cases without structural pretectal lesions. Neurology. 1976;26:594–95.

Knobler RL, Somasundaram M, Schutta HS. Inverse ocular bobbing. Ann Neurol. 1981;9:194–97.

Legge R, Weiss H, Hedges IT, Anderson M. Periodic alternating gaze deviation in infancy. Neurology. 1992;42:1740–43.

Lennox G. Reverse ocular bobbing due to combined phenothiazine and benzodiazepine poisoning. J Neurol Neurosurg Psychiatry. 1993;56:1136–37.

Masucci E, Fabara J, Saini N, Kurtzke J. Periodic alternating ping-pong gaze. Ann Ophthalmol. 1981;13:1123–27.

Ouvrier R, Billson F. Benign paroxysmal tonic upgaze of childhood. J Child Neurol. 1988;3:177–80.

Rascol O, Sabatini U, Simonetta-Moreau M, Montastruc J, Rascol A, Clanet M. Square wave jerks in parkinsonian syndromes. J Neurol Neurosurg Psychiatry. 1991;34:599–602.

Selhorst J, Stark L, Ochs A, Hoyt W. Disorder in cerebellar ocular motor control. Brain. 1976;99:509–22.

Sharpe J, Bondar R, Fletcher W. Contralateral gaze deviation after frontal lobe hemorrhage. J Neurol Neurosurg Psychiatry. 1985;48:86–88.

Shults W, Stark L, Hoyt W, Ochs A. Normal saccadic structure of voluntary nystagmus. Arch Ophthalmol. 1977;95:1399–404.

Tamura E, Hoyt C. Oculomotor consequences of intraventricular hemorrhages in premature infants. Arch Ophthalmol. 1987;105:533–35.

Tijssen C, van Gisbergen J, Schulte B. Conjugate eye deviation: side, site, and size of the hemispheric lesion. Neurology. 1991;41:846–50.

Titer EM, Laureno R. Inverse/reverse ocular bobbing. Ann Neurol. 1988;23:103–4.

Vignaendra V. Electro-oculographic analysis of opsoclonus: Its relationship to saccadic and non-saccadic eye movements. Neurology. 1977;27:1129–33.

Wong AM, Musallam S, Tomlinson RD, Shannon P, Sharpe JA. Opsoclonus in three dimensions: Oculographic, neuropathologic and modelling correlates. J Neurol Sci. 2001;189:71–81.

Yokochi K. Paroxysmal ocular downward deviation in neurologically impaired infants. Pediatr Neurol. 1991;7:426–28.

Zahn J. Incidence and characteristics of voluntary nystagmus. J Neurol Neurosurg Psychiatry. 1978;41:617–23.

Chapter 9

Baloh R, Yee R, Honrubia V. Internuclear ophthalmoplegia. I. Saccades and dissociated nystagmus. Arch Neurol. 1978;35:484–89.

Baloh R, Yee R, Honrubia V. Internuclear ophthalmoplegia. II. Pursuit, optokinetic nystagmus, and vestibulo-ocular reflex. Arch Neurol. 1978;35:490–93.

Blazquez P, Partsalis A, Gerrits NM, Highstein SM. Input of anterior and posterior semicircular canal interneurons encoding head-velocity to the dorsal Y group of the vestibular nuclei. J Neurophysiol. 2000;83:2891–904.

Brandt T, Dieterich M. Pathological eye-head coordination in roll: Tonic ocular tilt reaction in mesencephalic and medullary lesions. Brain. 1987;110:649–66.

Brandt T, Dieterich M. Skew deviation with ocular torsion: A vestibular brainstem sign of topographic diagnostic value. Ann Neurol. 1993;33:528–34.

Brodsky MC, Donahue SP, Vaphiades M, Brandt T. Skew deviation revisited. Surv Ophthalmol. 2006;51:105–28.

Büttner-Ennever J, Büttner U, Cohen B, Baumgartner G. Vertical gaze paralysis and the rostral interstitial nucleus of the medial longitudinal fasciculus. Brain. 1982;105:125–49.

Büttner-Ennever JA, Horn AKE. Pathways from cell groups of the paramedian tracts to the flocculus region. Ann NY Acad Sci. 1996;781:532–40.

Chokroverty S, Barron KD. Palatal myoclonus and rhythmic ocular movements: A polygraphic study. Neurology. 1969;19:975–82.

Cogan D, Chu F, Bachman D, Barranger J. The DAF syndrome. Neuro-ophthalmology. 1981;2:7–16.

Fletcher WA, Sharpe JA. Saccadic eye movement dysfunction in Alzheimer's disease. Ann Neurol. 1986;20:464–71.

Fletcher WA, Sharpe JA. Smooth pursuit dysfunction in Alzheimer's disease. Neurology. 1988;38:272–77.

Grant MP, Cohen M, Petersen RB, Halmagyi GM, McDougall A, Tusa RJ, et al. Abnormal eye movements in Creutzfeldt-Jakob disease. Ann Neurol. 1993;34:192–97.

Johnston J, Sharpe JA, Ranalli P, Morrow M. Oblique misdirection and slowing of vertical saccades after unilateral lesions of the pontine tegmentum. Neurology. 1993;43:2238–44.

Johnston JL, Miller JD, Nath A. Ocular motor dysfunction in HIV-1-infected subjects: A quantitative oculographic analysis. Neurology. 1996;46:451–57.

Keane J. The pretectal syndrome: 206 patients. Neurology. 1990;40:684–90.

Keane JR. Acute vertical ocular myoclonus. Neurology. 1986;36:86–89.

Kristensen M. Progressive supranuclear palsy — 20 years later. Acta Neurol Scand. 1985;71:177–89.

Leigh RJ, Zee DS. The Neurology of Eye Movements. 4th ed. New York: Oxford University Press; 2006.

Meienberg O, Büttner-Ennever J, Kraus-Ruppert R. Unilateral paralysis of conjugate gaze due to lesion of the abducens nucleus. Neuro-ophthalmology. 1981;2:47–52.

Sacco R, Freddo L, Bello J, Odel JG, Onesti ST, Mohr JP. Wallenberg's lateral medullary syndrome. Clinical-magnetic resonance imaging correlations. Arch Neurol. 1993;50:609–14.

Schwartz MA, Selhorst JB, Ochs AL, Beck RW, Campbell WW, Harris JK, et al. Oculomasticatory myorhythmia: a unique movement disorder occurring in Whipple's disease. Ann Neurol. 1986;20:677–83.

Wall M, Wray S. The one-and-a-half syndrome: A unilateral disorder of the pontine tegmentum: A study of twenty cases and a review of the literature. Neurology. 1983;33:971–80.

Westheimer G, Blair SM. The ocular tilt reaction—a brainstem oculomotor routine. Invest Ophthalmol. 1975;14:833–39.

Wong AM, Sharpe JA. Cerebellar skew deviation and the torsional vestibulo-ocular reflex. Neurology. 2005;65:412–19.

Ziffer A, Rosenbaum A, Demer J, Yee R. Congenital double elevator palsy: Vertical saccadic velocity utilizing the scleral search coil technique. J Pediatr Ophthalmol Strabismus. 1992;29:142–49.

Chapter 10

Benjamin EE, Zimmerman CF, Troost BT. Lateropulsion and upbeat nystagmus are manifestations of central vestibular dysfunction. Arch Neurol. 1986;43:962–64.

Bötzel K, Rottach K, Büttner U. Normal and pathological saccadic dysmetria. Brain. 1993;116:337–53.

Bürk K, Fetter M, Skalej M, Laccone F, Stevanin G, Dichgans J, et al. Saccade velocity in idiopathic and autosomal dominant cerebellar ataxia. J Neurol Neurosurg Psychiatry. 1997;62:662–64.

Cogan DG, Chu FC, Reingold D, Barranger J. Ocular motor signs in some metabolic diseases. Arch Ophthalmol. 1981;99:1802–8.

Dichgans J. Clinical symptoms of cerebellar dysfunction and their topodiagnostical significance. Human Neurobiol. 1984;2:269–79.

Duenas AM, Goold R, Giunti P. Molecular pathogenesis of spinocerebellar ataxias. Brain. 2006;129:1357–70.

Duncan GW, Parker SW, Fisher CM. Acute cerebellar infarction in the PICA territory. Arch Neurol. 1975;32:364–68.

Dyste G, Menezes A, VanGilder J. Symptomatic Chiari malformations. J Neurosurg. 1989;71:159–68.

Furman JM, Wall CD, Pang DL. Vestibular function in periodic alternating nystagmus. Brain. 1990;113:1425–39.

Giunti P, Sweeney M, Spadaro M, Jodice C, Novelletto A, Malaspina P, et al. The trinucleotide repeat expansion on chromosome 6p (SCA1) in autosomal dominant cerebellar ataxias. Brain. 1994;117:645–49.

Gordon N. Episodic ataxia and channelopathies. Brain Dev. 1998;20:9–13.

Kaseda Y, Kawakami H, Matsuyama Z, Kumagai R, Toji M, Komure O, et al. Spinocerebellar ataxia type 6 in relation to CAG repeat length. Acta Neurol Scand. 1999;99:209–12.

Monteagudo A, Alayon A, Mayberry P. Walker-Warburg syndrome: Case report and review of the literature. J Ultrasound Med. 2001;20:419–26.

Moschner C, Perlman S, Baloh R. Comparison of oculomotor findings in the progressive ataxia syndromes. Brain. 1994;117:15–25.

Niesen CE. Malformations of the posterior fossa: current perspectives. Semin Pediatr Neurol. 2002;9:320–34.

Saez R, Onofrio B, Yanagihara T. Experience with Arnold Chiari malformation, 1960 to 1970. J Neurosurg. 1976;45:416–22.

Straube A, Buttner U. Pathophysiology of saccadic contrapulsion in unilateral rostral cerebellar lesions. Neuroophthalmology. 1994;14:3–7.

Straube A, Scheurer W, Eggert T. Unilateral cerebellar lesions affect initiation of ipsilateral smooth pursuit eye movements in humans. Ann Neurol. 1997;42:891–98.

Wong AM, Heon E. Helicoid peripapillary chorioretinal degeneration in abetalipoproteinemia. Arch Ophthalmol. 1998;116:250–51.

Wong AM, Musallam S, Tomlinson RD, Shannon P, Sharpe JA. Opsoclonus in three dimensions: Oculographic, neuropathologic and modelling correlates. J Neurol Sci. 2001;189:71–81.

Wong AM, Sharpe JA. Cerebellar skew deviation and the torsional vestibulo-ocular reflex. Neurology. 2005;65:412–19.

Yee RD, Cogan DG, Zee DS. Ophthalmoplegia and dissociated nystagmus in abetalipoproteinemia. Arch Ophthalmol. 1976;94:571–75.

Zee DS. Considerations on the mechanisms of alternating skew deviation in patients with cerebellar lesions. J Vestib Res. 1996;6:395–401.

Zee DS, Yamazaki A, Butler PH, Gucer G. Effects of ablation of flocculus and paraflocculus on eye movements in primate. J Neurophysiol. 1981;46(4):878–99.

Chapter 11

Cogan DG. Congenital ocular motor apraxia. Can J Ophthalmol. 1966;1:253–60.

Cogan DG, Chu FC, Reingold D, Tychsen L. A long-term follow-up of congenital ocular motor apraxia. Neuroophthalmology. 1980;1:145–47.

Gaymard B, Rivaud S, Pierrot-Deseilligny C. Role of the left and right supplementary motor areas in memory-guided saccade sequences. Ann Neurol. 1993;34:404–6.

Hertle RW, Bienfang DC. Oculographic analysis of acute esotropia secondary to a thalamic hemorrhage. J Clin Neuro-ophthalmol. 1990;10:21–26.

Kristensen M. Progressive supranuclear palsy — 20 years later. Acta Neurol Scand. 1985;71:177–89.

Lasker AG, Zee DS, Hain TC, Folstein SE, Singer HS. Saccades in Huntington's disease: Slowing and dysmetria. Neurology. 1988;38:427–31.

Morrow M, Sharpe J. Retinotopic and directional deficits of smooth pursuit initiation after posterior cerebral hemispheric lesions. Neurology. 1993;43:595–603.

Pierrot-Deseilligny C, Gautier JC, Loron P. Acquired ocular motor apraxia due to bilateral frontoparietal infarcts. Ann Neurol. 1988;23:199–202.

Pierrot-Deseilligny C, Gray F, Brunet P. Infarcts of both inferior parietal lobules with impairment of visually guided eye movements, peripheral inattention and optic ataxia. Brain Cogn. 1986;109:81–97.

Pierrot-Deseilligny C, Israel I, Berthoz A, Rivaud S, Gaymard B. Role of the different frontal lobe areas in the control of the horizontal component of memory-guided saccades in man. Exp Brain Res. 1993;95:166–71.

Pierrot-Deseilligny C, Rivaud S, Gaymard B, Agid Y. Cortical control of reflexive visually-guided saccades. Brain. 1991;114:1473–85.

Pierrot-Deseilligny C, Rivaud S, Gaymard B, Muri R, Vermersch AI. Cortical control of saccades. Ann Neurol. 1995;37:557–67.

Rivaud S, Müri R, Gaymard B, Vermersch AI, Pierrot-Deseilligny C. Eye movement disorders after frontal eye field lesions in humans. Exp Brain Res. 1994;102:110–20.

Sharpe JA, Lo AW, Rabinovitch HE. Control of the saccadic and smooth pursuit systems after cerebral hemidecortication. Brain. 1979 102:387–403.

Sullivan HC, Kaminski HJ, Maas EF, Weissman JD, Leigh RJ. Lateral deviation of the eyes on forced lid closure in patients with cerebral lesions. Arch Neurol. 1991;48:310–11.

Thurston S, Leigh R, Crawford T, Thompson A, Kennard C. Two distinct deficits of visual tracking caused by unilateral lesions of cerebral cortex in humans. Ann Neurol. 1988;23:266–73.

Vidailhet M, Rivaud S, Gouider-Khouja N, Pillon B, Bonnet AM, Gaymard B, et al. Eye movements in parkinsonian syndromes. Ann Neurol. 1994;35:420–26.

Weiner WJ. A differential diagnosis of Parkinsonism. Rev Neurol Dis. 2005;2:124–31.

White OB, Saint-Cyr JA, Sharpe JA. Ocular motor deficits in Parkinson's disease. I. The horizontal vestibulo-ocular reflex and its regulation. Brain. 1983;106:555–70.

White OB, Saint-Cyr JA, Tomlinson RD, Sharpe JA. Ocular motor deficits in Parkinson's disease. II. Control of the saccadic and smooth pursuit systems. Brain. 1983;106:571–87.

Chapter 12

Asbury AK, Aldredge H, Hershberg R, Fisher CM. Oculomotor palsy in diabetes mellitus: A clinico-pathological study. Brain. 1970;93:555–66.

Barricks ME, Traviesa DB, Glaser JS, Levy IS. Ophthalmoplegia in cranial arteritis. Brain. 1977;100:209–21.

Barrow DL, Spector RH, Braun IF, Landman JA, Tindall SC, Tindall GT. Classification and treatment of spontaneous carotid-cavernous sinus fistulas. J Neurosurg. 1985;62:248–56.

Biousse V, Newman NJ. Intracranial vascular abnormalities. Ophthalmol Clin North Am 2001; 14:243–264.

Brazis PW, Miller NR, Henderer JD. The natural history and results of treatment of superior oblique myokymia. Arch Ophthalmol. 1994;112:1063–67.

Campbell RJ, Okazaki H. Painful ophthalmoplegis (Tolosa-Hunt variant): autopsy findings in a patient with necrotizing intracavernous carotid vasculitis and inflammartory disease of the orbit. Mayo Clin Proc. 1987;62:520–26.

Cox TA, Wurster JB, Godfrey WA. Primary aberrant oculomotor regeneration due to intracranial aneurysm. Arch Neurol. 1979;36:570–71.

Currie J, Lubin JH, Lessell S. Chronic isolated abducens paresis from tumors at the base of the brain. Arch Neurol. 1983;40:226–29.

DiNubile MJ. Septic thrombosis of the cavernous sinuses. Arch Neurol. 1988;45:567–72.

Guy JR, Day AL. Intracranial aneurysms with superior division paresis of the oculomotor nerve. Ophthalmology. 1989;96:1071–76.

Harley RD. Paralytic strabismus in children. Etiologic incidence and management of the third, fourth, and sixth nerve palsies. Ophthalmology. 1980;87:24–43.

Hughes RA, Cornblath DR. Guillain-Barre syndrome. Lancet 2005;366:1653–66.

Keane JR. Bilateral sixth nerve palsy. Analysis of 125 cases. Arch Neurol. 1976;33:681–83.

Keane JR. Fourth nerve palsy: historical review and study of 215 inpatients. Neurology. 1993;43:2439–43.

Kline LB. The Tolosa-Hunt syndrome. Surv Ophthalmol. 1982;27:79–95.

Ksiazek SM, Repka MX, Maguire A, Harbour RC, Savino PJ, Miller NR, Sergott RC, Bosley TM. Divisional oculomotor nerve paresis caused by intrinsic brainstem disease. Ann Neurol. 1989;26:714–18.

Lessell S, Lessell IM, Rizzo JFr. Ocular neuromyotonia after radiation therapy. Am J Ophthalmol. 1986;102:766–70.

Loewenfeld IE, Thompson HS. Oculomotor paresis with cyclic spasms. A critical review of the literature and a new case. Surv Ophthalmol. 1975;20:81–124.

Miller NR, Kiel SM, Green WR, Clark AW. Unilateral Duane's retraction syndrome (type 1). Arch Ophthalmol. 1982;100:1468–72.

Mori M, Kuwabara S, Fukutake T, Yuki N, Hattori T. Clinical features and prognosis of Miller Fisher syndrome. Neurology 2001;56:1104–6.

Richards BW, Jones FR, Younge BR. Causes and prognosis in 4,278 cases of paralysis of the oculomotor, trochlear, and abducens cranial nerves. Am J Ophthalmol. 1992;113:489–96.

Schatz NJ, Savino PJ, Corbett JJ. Primary aberrant oculomotor regeneration. A sign of intracavernous meningioma. Arch Neurol. 1977;34:29–32.

Shults WT, Hoyt WF, Behrens M, MacLean J, Saul RF, Corbett JJ. Ocular neuromyotonia. A clinical description of six patients. Arch Ophthalmol. 1986;104:1028–34.

Trobe JD. Managing oculomotor nerve palsy. Arch Ophthalmol. 1998;116:798.

Verzijl HT, van der Zwaag B, Cruysberg JR, Padberg GW. Möbius syndrome redefined: A syndrome of rhombencephalic maldevelopment. Neurology 2003;61:327–33.

Chapter 13

Caya JG. Clostridium botulinum and the ophthalmologist: A review of botulism, including biological warfare ramifications of botulinum toxin. Surv Ophthalmol. 2001;46:25–34.

Cherington M. Botulism. Ten-year experience. Arch Neurol. 1974;30:432–37.

Engel AG. Congenital myasthenic syndromes. Neurol Clin. 1994;12:401–37.

Engel AG. Myasthenia Gravis and Myasthenic Disorders. New York: Oxford University Press; 1999.

Kullmann DM, Hanna MG. Neurological disorders caused by inherited ion-channel mutations. Lancet Neurol. 2002;1:157–66.

Romi F, Gilhus NE, Aarli JA. Myasthenia gravis: Clinical, immunological, and therapeutic advances. Acta Neurol Scand. 2005;111:134–41.

Schmidt D, Dell'Osso L, Abel L, Daroff R. Myasthenia gravis: Saccadic eye movement waveforms. Exp Neurol. 1980;68:346–64.

Vincent A, Palace J, Hilton-Jones D. Myasthenia gravis. Lancet Neurol. 2001;357:2122–28.

Wirtz PW, Smallegange TM, Wintzen AR, Verschuuren JJ. Differences in clinical features between the Lambert-Eaton myasthenic syndrome with and without cancer: An analysis of 227 published cases. Clin Neurol Neurosurg. 2002;104:359–63.

Chapter 14

Bartley G, Gorman C. Diagnostic criteria for Graves' ophthalmopathy. Am J Ophthalmol. 1995;119:792–95.

Bau V, Zierz S. Update on chronic progressive external ophthalmoplegia. Strabismus. 2005;13:133–42.

ter Bruggen J, Bastiaensen L, Tyssen C, Gielen G. Disorders of eye movement in myotonic dystrophy. Brain. 1990;113:463–73.

Char DH, Miller T. Orbital pseudotumor. Fine-needle aspiration biopsy and response to therapy. Ophthalmology. 1993;100:1702–10.

Engle EC. The molecular basis of the congenital fibrosis syndromes. Strabismus. 2002;10:125–28.

Fang W, Huang CC, Lee CC, Cheng SY, Pang CY, Wei YH. Ophthalmologic manifestations in MELAS syndrome. Arch Neurol. 1993;50:977–80.

Van Goethem G, Martin JJ, Van Broeckhoven C. Progressive external ophthalmoplegia characterized by multiple deletions of mitochondrial DNA: Unraveling the pathogenesis of human mitochondrial DNA instability and the initiation of a genetic classification. Neuromolecular Med. 2003;3:129–46.

Hirano M, Silvestri G, Blake D, Lombes A, Minetti C, Bonilla E, et al. Mitochondrial neurogastrointestinal encephalomyopathy (MNGIE): Clinical, biochemical, and genetic features of an autosomal recessive mitochondrial disorder. Neurology. 1994;44:721–27.

Johnson C, Kuwabara T. Oculopharyngeal muscular dystrophy. Am J Ophthalmol. 1974;77:872–79.

Lee AG, Brazis PW. Chronic progressive external ophthalmoplegia. Curr Neurol Neurosci Rep. 2002; 2:413–17.

Siatkowski R, Capó H, Byrne S, Gendron EK, Flynn JT, Munoz M, et al. Clinical and echographic findings in idiopathic orbital myositis. Am J Ophthalmol. 1994;118:343–50.

Traboulsi EI. Congenital abnormalities of cranial nerve development: Overview, molecular mechanisms, and further evidence of heterogeneity and complexity of syndromes with congenital limitation of eye movements. Trans Am Ophthalmol Soc. 2004;102:373–89.

Wilson ME, Eustis HSJ, Parks MM. Brown's syndrome. Surv Ophthalmol. 1989;34:153–72.

Yazdani A, Traboulsi EI. Classification and surgical management of patients with familial and sporadic forms of congenital fibrosis of the extraocular muscles. Ophthalmology. 2004;111:1035–42.

Yeatts R. Graves' ophthalmopathy. Med Clin N Am. 1995;79:195–209.

Index

abducens nerve, 222
  anatomy, 222–223
  maldevelopment, 227
  nucleus, 40, 121, 130, 135
    contralateral, 32–33
    lesions of, 130–131, 224
    neurons in, 32–33, 64–65
    role in smooth pursuit, 76–77
    role in vergence, 86–87
  palsy
    congenital, 228–230
    diagnosis, 223–227
    workup and treatment, 231
  tumors, 225
abduction, 4–5
  effect of abducens nerve palsy on, 222
  limitation in Duane's syndrome, 228
  from stimulation of utricular nerve, 42–43
  in Wernicke's encelphalopathy, 154
abetalipoproteinemia, 156, 239
AC/A ratio, 88–89
accommodation, 85, 162
  accommodative-linked convergence and, 88–89
  in Guillain-Barré syndrome, 237
  loss in oculomotor nerve palsy, 201
  spasm, 140
  vergence and, 84
accommodative fibers, 142
accommodative vergence, testing, 88–89
acetazolamide, 173
  to treat nystagmus, 108
acetylcholine
  impaired release, 250
  release in Miller Fisher syndrome, 238
acetylcholine receptors
  deficiency of, 249
  in myasthenia gravis, 244–245
  transfer of antibodies to, 246
acetylcholinesterase deficiency, congenital, 248–249
achromatic neurons, 184
acquired ocular motor apraxia, 70, 186, 194
acquired pendular nystagmus, 103–104
acute peripheral vestibulopathy, 42, 149
adaptation, 46–47, 133, 166
adduction, 4–7
  deficient elevation on, 262
  deficits of, 134

limitation in Duane's syndrome, 228
palsy, 64–65, 209
from stimulation of utricular nerve, 42–43
adrenocorticotropic hormone, to treat opsoclonus, 117
AIDS-related dementia, 159–160
  as cause of acquired ocular motor apraxia, 194
akinetic-rigid syndrome, 186
alcohol, to treat nystagmus, 108
alcoholism, 154
Alexander's law, 97, 98, 100
α-tocopherol. See vitamin E
Alzheimer's disease, 147, 157
amantadine, 183
amblyopia, 104
aminoacidopathies, 155–156
4-aminopyridine, to treat nystagmus, 108
amphetamines, to treat saccadic intrusions, 112
ampulla, 28–29
amyloidosis, 259
amyotrophic lateral sclerosis, 147
aneurysms, 119, 201
  of carotid artery, 226
  as cause of subarachnoid space lesions, 218
  intracranial, 206, 212
angular acceleration, 28–29
anisometropia, 106
annulus of Zinn, 6–7, 202, 216, 222
anoxia, intrauterine, 115
anterior inferior cerebellar artery syndrome, 131, 176–177
anterior segment abnormalities, 200
anterior temporal fossa, tumors of, 259
antibiotics, to treat cavernous sinus thrombosis, 234
anticholinergic drugs, to treat oculogyric crisis, 183
anticipation, 257
antidepressants
  as cause of gaze-evoked nystagmus, 101
  to treat Huntington's disease, 186
antineuronal antibodies, 116
antiretroviral therapy, 162
antisaccades, 70–71, 144, 189
aplastic cerebellar vermis, 195
apnea, 195
aqueductal stenosis, congenital, 141

arachnoid cysts, retrocerebellar, 172
area 7a. *See* posterior parietal cortex
area V1. *See* striate cortex
area V5, 18–19. *See* middle temporal area
areflexia, 237
    in abetalipoproteinemia, 239
    in Miller Fisher syndrome, 238
Arnold-Chiari malformation, 98, 100 108, 162, 225
    as cause of convergence spasm, 162
    as cause of gaze deviation, 119
    as cause of internuclear ophthalmoplegia, 133
    eye movement abnormalities, 171
    types, 171
arteriovenous malformation, 259
arteritis, 218
ascending tract of Deiters, 32
Aspergillus, cavernous sinus thrombosis and, 234
aspiration pneumonia, 144
asthenopia, 162
astigmatism, in extraocular muscle fibrosis, 210
ataxia, 115, 150. *See also* spinocerebellar ataxias
    cerebellar, 238, 239, 255
    episodic, 173
    familial periodic, 218
    gait, 120, 176
    limb, 176
    in Miller Fisher syndrome, 238
    optic, 190
    recessive, 175
    truncal, 120
    in Wernicke's encephalopathy, 154
ataxia telangiectasia, 156, 175, 195
atherosclerosis, 225
auditory stimuli
    induction of vestibular symptoms, 149
    saccades in response to, 55
    smooth pursuit and, 73
auricular abnormalities, 228
autism spectrum disorder, 229
autoimmune responses, 116
autonomic dysfunction, in Lambert-Eaton
    myasthenic syndrome, 251
autophagic vacuoles, 258
Avonex, 153
axes of rotation, 3–5
axonal hyperexcitability, 242
azathioprine, to treat myasthenia gravis, 247

backup saccades, 78–79
baclofen, 108, 109, 153, 241
bacterial infections
    in cavernous sinus thrombosis, 234
    in infective myositis, 261
    in internuclear ophthalmoplegia, 133
    in opsoclonus, 115
balding, in myotonic dystrophy, 257

Balint's syndrome, 157, 158, 190
ballism, 186
Bardet-Biedl syndrome, 195
basal ganglia, 18–19
    diseases affecting, 124, 184, 187
    lesions of, 147, 181–187
    saccadic intrusions and, 112
    tumors, 225
basal meningitis
    in oculomotor nerve synkinesis, 212
    in subarachnoid space lesions, 218
basilar artery, 225
    stroke, 141
basilar insufficiency, 100
Bassen-Kornzweig syndrome. *See*
    abetalipoproteinemia
Battle's sign, 226
Bechterew nystagmus, 30
Bell's phenomenon, 140, 144
Benedikt's syndrome, 205
benign paroxysmal positioning vertigo, 97, 100
benign recurrent vertigo, 173
benzodiazepines
    intoxication, 119
    to treat Huntington's disease, 186
ß-interferon, to treat multiple sclerosis, 153
Betaseron, 153
Bickerstaff's brainstem encephalitis, 238
Bielschowsky's test, 220, 221
bihemispheric infarcts, as cause of acquired
    ocular motor apraxia, 194
bilateral superior oblique palsy, 221
biotin, 117
bismuth overdose, 158
blepharospasm, 144
    essential, 187
blink disorders, 144, 183
blood tests, for myasthenia gravis, 247
blurred vision, 26–27, 84, 162
Bosley-Salih-Alorainy syndrome, 229
botulinum injection, 214
botulism, 252
bradykinesia, 184
brainstem. *See also specific structures in the
    brainstem*
    abnormal feedback circuits, 103
    burst neurons in, 56–57
    damage to, 98, 103, 147, 230
    lesions of, 42, 121
    reflex, 46
    role in fixation, 18–19
    role in smooth pursuit, 76–77
    saccade generation, 62–67
    structures important in ocular motor control,
        124
    vergence commands, 86–87
branchial musculature, hypoplasia, 229

Brown's superior oblique tendon sheath
   syndrome, acquired, 261
Brown's syndrome, 197, 221, 262
Brudzinski sign, 234
Brun's nystagmus, 102
Burkitt's lymphoma, 226
burst neurons, 56, 132, 137
   lesions of, 70
   types and functions, 62–63

CA/C ratio, 88–89
calcium channel dysfunction, 251
caloric nystagmus, inability to suppress, 166
Campylobacter jejuni
   role in Guillain-Barré syndrome, 237
   role in Miller Fisher syndrome, 238
carbamazepine
   toxicity, 119
   to treat ocular neuromyotonia, 242
   to treat superior oblique myokymia, 241
carbidopa, to treat Parkinson's disease, 183
carbon monoxide poisoning, as cause of ocular
   bobbing, 119
cardiomyopathy
   in Leigh's syndrome, 256
   in Refsum's disease, 240
cardiovascular defects, 229, 254
   in myotonic dystrophy, 257
carotid artery, 232
   hypoplasia, 229
   ligation, 235
carotid-cavernous fistula, 235, 259
cataracts, 104
   Christmas tree, 257
   monocular, 106
   in Refsum's disease, 240
catch up saccades, 74, 78–79, 144, 194
catecholamines, urinary, 116
caudal fastigial nucleus, 68–69
caudate nucleus, 203
   lesions of, 181
   projections to, 68–69
cavernous sinus, 202, 216, 222. *See also*
   sphenocavernous syndrome
   anatomy, 232
   lesions of, 207, 218, 226
   thrombosis, 234
central core myopathy, 262
central mesencephalic reticular
   formation, 143
central pontine myelinosis, 131
centripetal nystagmus, 102, 158
cerebellopontine angle tumors, 102
cerebellum, 166. *See also specific structures within
   the cerebellum*
   abnormal feedback circuits, 103

ataxia, 238, 240, 255. *See also* spinocerebellar
   ataxias
   degeneration of, 98, 114
   effect of damage on saccades, 56, 58–59, 112
   gaze-evoked nystagmus and, 101
   hemorrhage, 119
   infarction, 176
   lesions of, 42, 122, 149, 161
   ocular motor disorders and, 122
   role in smooth pursuit, 73, 76–77, 78–79
   role in vertigo, 23
cerebral cortex
   role in saccades, 56–57
   saccadic intrusions and, 112
cerebrum. *See also* cerebral cortex; *specific
   structures within the cerebrum*
   areas involved in fixation, 18–19
   control of saccades, 68–69
   control of vergence, 86–87
   effect of damage on smooth pursuit, 78–79
   lesions of, 122, 162
   ocular motor disorders and, 122, 188–195
Charcot triad, 150
chemosis, 234
cholinesterase inhibitors, 157, 249, 252
chorea, 186
chronic progressive external ophthalmoplegia,
   156, 254–255
ciliary body, 201
ciliary nerves, 142
circularvection, 50–51
   abolishment of, 192
Claude's syndrome, 205
clonazepam
   to treat multiple sclerosis, 153
   to treat nystagmus, 108, 109
   to treat opsoclonus, 117
closed loop phase
   of smooth pursuit, 75
   of vergence movements, 84–85
Clostridium botulinum, 252
Clostridium welchii, 261
cochlear nerve, 28–29
Cockayne's syndrome, 96, 103
co-enzyme Q10, 255
Cogan's congenital ocular motor apraxia, 194–195
Cogan's lid-twitch sign, 244
Cogan's spasticity of conjugate gaze, 193
Collier's sign, 140
coloboma, 172
coma
   as cause of ocular bobbing, 119
   vergence oscillations during, 163
compensatory mechanisms, 30
completion phase, of vergence movements, 84–85
compression lesions, 206–207
congenital aqueductal stenosis, 141

dopaminergic neurons, 182
dorsal vermis
  lesions of, 114, 168
  role in saccade size, 68–69
  role in smooth pursuit, 76–79
  role in vergence, 86–87
  syndrome of, 122
dorsolateral pontine nucleus
  lesions of, 78–79, 136
  role in smooth pursuit, 76–77
dorsolateral prefrontal cortex, 18–19
  anatomy, 189
  lesions of, 189
  role in saccades, 68–69
double elevator palsy, 143–144
downbeat nystagmus, 34–35, 134, 140
  with floccular lesions, 166
  in multiple sclerosis, 151
  treatment of, 108
downgaze
  palsy, 138
  paralysis, 180
Down's syndrome, 106
drainage, in carotid-cavernous fistula, 235
DR syndrome. *See* Okihiro syndrome
drugs. *See also specific drugs*
  as cause of gaze-evoked nystagmus, 101
  as cause of internuclear
    ophthalmoplegia, 133
  as cause of ocular bobbing, 118–119
  as cause of opsoclonus, 115
  as cause of pretectal syndrome, 141
  intoxication, 147
Duane's syndrome, 131, 228–229
ductions, 4–5
  in extraocular muscle fibrosis, 210–211
dynamic imbalance, testing, 52–53
dysarthria, 150, 176
  in lateral medullary syndrome, 125
dyskinesia
  tardive, 187
  treatment, 183
dysmetric saccades, 191
  in Arnold-Chiari malformation, 171
  in Dandy-Walker malformation, 171
  with hemispheric lesions, 193
  in spinocerebellar ataxias, 174
dysphagia, 125, 247, 258
dystonia, 186, 187

edema
  intramuscular, 260
  periorbital, 234
Edinger-Westphal nucleus, 142, 203
edrophonium injection, 246
electromyography, for myasthenia gravis, 246

elevation, 4–7
  deficient, 262
  from stimulation of utricular nerve, 42–43
emboliform and globose nuclei, 86–87
encephalitis, 99, 162
  acute disseminated, 150
encephalopathy
  as cause of ocular bobbing, 118
  hepatic, 119, 133, 163
  in MELAS syndrome, 255
  mitochondrial, 156
  opsoclonus and, 115
  Wernicke's, 131, 133, 154, 156
endocrine dysfunction, in chronic progressive
    external ophthalmoplegia, 254
endolymph, 28–31, 38–39
ephaptic transmission, 241, 242
epibulbar dermoids, 228
episodic ataxias, 173
Epley procedure, 109
equal innervation, Hering's law, 8–9
esodeviation, 87, 136
esophoria, 12–13
  decompensated, 161
esotropia, 12–13
  in bilateral superior oblique palsy, 221
  caused by abducens nerve palsy, 222
  comitant, 161
  decompensated monofixation, 161
  due to thalamic lesions, 180
  in extraocular muscle fibrosis, 210
  infantile, 106
excitatory burst neurons, 62–63, 132
  inhibition of, 64–65
  role in saccades, 66–67
excyclodeviation, 12–13
excycloduction, 4–5
excyclotorsion, 4–7, 99, 220
  from stimulation of utricular nerve, 42–43
  in trochlear nerve palsy, 215
exodeviation, 87
exophoria, 12–13
exotropia, 12–13, 140, 161, 162
  in extraocular muscle fibrosis, 210, 211
  infantile constant, 106
  in oculomotor nerve palsy, 201
  paralytic pontine, 135
exposure keratitis, 259
  treatment, 260
express saccades, 58–59
extraocular muscles, 3. *See also names*
    of specific muscles
  actions of, 4–7
  connections to vestibular system, 32, 41
  desynchronized contraction, 241
  developmental and congenital
    disorders, 262

extraocular muscles (*continued*)
  differential diagnosis of enlargement, 259
  fibrosis, 195, 196, 210–211
  involuntary contractions, 244
  paresis of, 94, 95, 235
  structure and function of fibers, 10–11
  surgery, 105, 221
  tension changes in, 42
eye. *See also* eye movements
  geometry of, 3
  position and saccades, 55
  primary position, 6–9
  secondary position, 8–9
  torsional position, 44–45
  velocity commands, 60–62, 64, 65
eye-head coordination, 139
eye-head tracking. *See also* visual tracking
  impaired, 166
  in Parkinson's disease, 183
  use to shift gaze, 194
eyelids
  disorders
    closure paralysis, 158
    fatigue in myasthenia gravis, 245
    forced closure, 193
    nerve synkinesis, 212
    nystagmus, 126
    in Parkinson's disease, 183
    pathologic retraction, 140
    in progressive supranuclear palsy, 144
    spontaneous retraction, 244
  -eye coordination, 140
  fluttering, 117
eye movements
  abnormal, in neurodegenerative diseases,
    155–156, 174, 175, 184–185
  absence of horizontal conjugate, 230
  compensatory, 40
  division of systems, 16–17
  imbalance of slow, 91
  medullary structures for control, 121
  monocular, 4–5
  optokinetic, 22
  reasons for, 15
  during sleep, 82
  from stimulation of vestibular organs,
    36–37, 42–43
eyestrain, 84

Fabry's disease, 133
facial asymmetry, 215, 218
facial muscles
  contraction, 117
  weakness, 254
facial nerve palsy, 130, 177, 210, 224
facial pain, 226

facies
  dysmorphic, 229
  masklike in Parkinson's disease, 182
  in myotonic dystrophy, 257
failure to thrive, 256
familial periodic ataxia, 218
fastigial nucleus, 87, 122
  disinhibition of, 116
  lesions of, 169
  role in saccade size, 68–69
  role in smooth pursuit, 76–77
fatigue, 162
  eyelid, 244
  in Grave's disease, 259
  -induced nystagmus, 101
  in myasthenic syndromes, 250
  resistance of extraocular muscles, 3, 10
field of vision, versus visual acuity, 15
fixation, 16–19
  abnormal, 193
  disparity, 84–85
  maintenance of, 78–79
  removing, 52–53
  spasm of, 194
  target, 58–59
  unstable, 159
flocculus/paraflocculus
  convergence in, 46–47
  lesions of, 34–35, 48–49, 98, 166
  role in repair of saccades, 68–69
  role in smooth pursuit, 76–79
  role in vergence, 87
  syndrome of, 122
Flourens' law, 36
forced duction test, 262
fossa
  anterior temporal tumors, 259
  hemorrhage, 120
  posterior, 171–172, 225
fourth nerve
  anatomy, 216, 217
  involvement in sphenocavernous syndrome,
    232
fovea, 15
  smooth pursuit and, 73
foveal compromise, 15
foveation period, 105
Foville's fasciculus syndrome, 131, 224
fractures, as cause of petrous apex syndrome, 226
French-Canadians, oculopharyngeal dystrophy
    among, 258
Frenzel goggles, use to remove fixation, 52–53
Friedreich's ataxia, 112, 175
frontal eye field, 64–65, 136
  anatomy, 188
  damage of projections to, 112
  lesions of, 78–79, 188

role in saccades, 68–69
role in smooth pursuit, 76–77
role in vergence, 86–87
frontal lobe, lesions of, 188–189, 194
fungal infections, 234, 261
fusional maldevelopment nystagmus syndrome, 106
fusional vergence, 162
    testing, 88–89

gabapentin, 108, 109, 127, 241
gag reflex, 125
gain
    of smooth pursuit, 75
    testing for abnormalities in, 52–53
    of vestibulo-ocular reflex, 26–27, 193
gait disturbances, 120, 144, 176
γ-aminobutyric acid, defective, 112
gap paradigm, 58–59
gastrotomy, 258
Gaucher's disease, 131, 141, 155, 195
gaze. See also gaze palsy
    cardinal positions of, 8–9
    deviation, 118–120
        contralesional, 130, 132
        dissociated vertical, 107
        horizontal, 119
        with lesions, 168, 169, 180, 188, 190
        primary and secondary, 12–13
    holding
        impaired, 101, 139, 166
        lesions in system, 94
        loss of, 140
        medullary structures important in, 121
        role of neural integrator, 60–61, 64–65
    orientation, 44–45
    paresis, 143
    preference, 181
    shift, 82, 143, 198
    spasticity of, 193
gaze-evoked nystagmus, 60–61, 64–65, 101, 132
    in AIDS-related dementia, 159
    in cerebellar artery syndromes, 177
    in Leigh's syndrome, 256
    in multiple sclerosis, 151
    in myasthenia gravis, 245
    pathogenesis and causes, 101
gaze palsy, 138, 144. See also horizontal gaze palsy
        and progressive scoliosis
    in anterior inferior cerebellar artery syndrome, 177
    horizontal conjugate, 130–132, 135, 223
    in Leigh's syndrome, 256
    in Lewy body disease, 185
    vertical, 140–141
    in Wernicke's encelphalopathy, 154

glaucoma, 106
global layer, 10–11
glutaric aciduria, 156
GM1 gangliosidosis, 155, 195
Goldenhar syndrome, 228
gracile nucleus, damage to, 230
Gradenigo's syndrome, 226
Grave's disease, 259–260
gravitoinertial acceleration vector, 44–45
Guillain-Barré syndrome, 237

habituation, 46
    loss of, 167
hair cells, 30–31
    polarization, 39
    time constant, 48–49
hawks, vision of, 15
headache. See also migraine periocular, 84
head movement. See also head tilt
    acceleration, 28, 35
    nystagmus during, 97
    oscillopsia during, 92, 95
    semicircular canals and, 30–31, 35
    stabilization of eye position in, 73
    stabilization of images during, 22
    velocity storage and, 48
head nystagmus, 126
head position
    abnormal in spasmus nutans, 107
    in bilateral superior oblique palsy, 221
    in gaze deviations, 119–120
head-shaking visual acuity, 52–53
head thrust, 194
    -impulse test, 52–53
head tilt, 148, 167, 191. See also head
        movement
    compensatory eye movements during static,
        40–41
    in congenital trochlear nerve palsy, 220
    distinguishing between translation and, 48–49
    gravitoinerital acceleration vector and, 44–45
    ipsilesional, 149
    otolith organs and, 38–39
    pathologic, 42–43
head translation, 38–39
head velocity signal, 28–29
hearing. See auditory stimuli
hearing loss, 97, 229. See also deafness
    in MELAS syndrome, 255
heart block, 254
heat intolerance, 259
Heidenhain variant, 158
Heimann-Bielschowsky phenomenon, 104
hemifacial microsomia, 228
hemiplegia, contralateral, 224
hemispheric lesions, 193

hemorrhage
  as cause of third nerve palsy, 204
  cerebellar, 119
  intracranial, 115
  intraventricular, 122, 140
  thalamic, 120, 162
  vitreous, 145
hemotympanum, 226
Hering's law, 8–9, 32, 34, 134
heterodeviation, 12–13
heterophoria, 12–13
  method, 88–89
heterotropia, 12–13
hiccups, in lateral medullary syndrome, 125
hindbrain, developmental anomalies, 170–172
HIV, 159
hoarseness, in lateral medullary syndrome, 125
Holt-Oram syndrome, 229
horizontal conjugate gaze palsy, 130, 224
  differential diagnosis, 131
  in one-and-a-half syndrome, 135
horizontal gaze palsy and progressive scoliosis,
    210, 230
horizontal nystagmus, in paramedian medullary
    lesions, 128
horizontal saccadic palsy, 132
  conjugate, 64–65
Horner's syndrome, 125, 176, 217, 225, 226
Huntington's disease, 122, 141, 147, 186
  acquired ocular motor apraxia and, 194
Hutchinson pupil, 213
hydrocephalus, 171, 172
  as cause of internuclear ophthalmoplegia, 133
  as cause of pretectal syndrome, 141
  gaze deviations and, 120
hyperactivity, ocular motor nerve, 240–241
hyperalimentation, 154
hypermetric saccades, 60–61
  in ataxias, 175
  from dorsal vermis lesions, 68–69
  in myasthenia gravis, 245
  in spinocerebellar ataxias, 174
  with uncinate fascicular lesions, 169
hyperopia, 210
  effect on gain, 46
hyperphoria, 12–13
hyperpolarization, of hair cells, 30–31
hypertension, 208, 218
hyperthyroidism, 259, 260
hypertropia, 12–13
  determining increases, 220
  determining side of, 219
  in trochlear nerve palsy, 215
hyperuricemia, 187
hypometric saccades, 60–61, 134, 143, 144, 187
  with caudate nuclear lesions, 181
  with dorsal vermis lesions, 68–69, 168

  with frontal eye field lesions, 188
  in multiple system atrophy, 185
  in myasthenia gravis, 245
  nystagmus as correction for, 102
  in Parkinson's disease, 183
  with uncinate fascicular lesions, 169
hyponatremia, 131
hypophoria, 12–13
hyporeflexia, 250
hypotension, intracranial, 226
hypothyroidism, 260
hypotonia
  in Leigh's syndrome, 256
  in neonatal myasthenia gravis, 248
hypotropia, 12–13, 42
  ipsilesional, 149
hypoxia, neonatal, 201
hypoxic-ischemic insult, 120

ice test, for myasthenia gravis, 246
icthyosiform desquamation, in Refsum's
    disease, 240
idiopathic myositis, 261
image stability. *See* retinal image, stability
immunosuppression, to treat juvenile myasthenia
    gravis, 248
incyclodeviation, 12–13
incycloduction, 4–5
incyclotorsion, 4–7, 99, 220
  in oculomotor nerve palsy, 201
  from stimulation of utricular nerve, 42–43
inertia, 28, 30
  of otoconia, 39
infantile nystagmus, 96, 105–107
  differentiation from spasmus nutans, 107
infections
  role in cavernous sinus thrombosis, 234
  role in Guillain-Barré syndrome, 237
  role in Miller Fisher syndrome, 238
  role in sphenocavernous syndrome, 232
infective myositis, 259, 261
inferior cerebellar peduncle, 121
inferior oblique, 4–7, 9, 219
  adhesion with lateral rectus, 262
  innervation, 66–67
  overaction, 216, 221
  recession, 262
inferior olivary nucleus, 121
  lesions of, 127
inferior rectus, 4–7, 9, 219
  transposition, 230
inflammation
  role in cavernous sinus lesions, 226
  role in sphenocavernous syndrome, 232
  of superior oblique tendon, 261
  in Tolosa-Hunt syndrome, 236

information overload, 15
inhibitory burst neurons, 62–63, 132
initiation phase, of vergence movements, 84–85
initiation time, saccades,58–59
innervation
  abnormal, 200
  developmental errors in, 196, 210
  of eye muscle fibers, 3
  laws of, 8–9
  pulse-step, 60–62
insula, 192
internuclear ophthalmoplegia, 64–65, 121,
    133–134, 144, 147, 170
  dissociated nystagmus in, 102
  in multiple sclerosis, 150
interstitial nucleus of Cajal, 66–67, 101, 124
  interruption of pathways, 134
  lesions of, 139, 149
  as neural integrator, 60–61
  role in smooth pursuit, 76–77
intestinal dysmotility
  in MNGIE syndrome, 255
  in myotonic dystrophy, 257
intracranial hemorrhage, 115
intracranial hypotension, 226
intracranial pressure, 149, 161
  as cause of subarachnoid lesions, 218, 225
intraocular pressure, in cavernous sinus
    thrombosis, 234
intravenous immunoglobulin, 117, 247, 251
intraventricular hemorrhage, 120, 140
ipsilesional adduction palsy, 64–65
ipsipulsion of saccades, 126, 169
iris sphincter, 201
ischemia, 204–207
  as cause of cavernous sinus lesions, 226
  as cause of nerve palsy, 204, 218
  as cause of ophthalmoplegia, 213
  as cause of sphenocavernous syndrome, 207, 233
  vertebrobasilar, 162

jerk nystagmus, 94, 97
  congenital, 105
Joubert's syndrome, 195
jugular vein ligation, 226

Kearns-Sayre syndrome, 254–255
keratitis, 145, 259–260
kernicterus, 156
Kernig sign, 234
Kestenbaum procedure, 105
kinocilium, 30–31
Klippel-Feil anomaly, 228
Korsakoff psychosis, 154
Krabbe's leukodystrophy, 155, 195

Kugelberg-Welander disease, 204
kyphoscoliosis, 230

labyrinthine lesion, 46
lacrimation, in Grave's disease, 259
Lambert-Eaton myasthenic syndrome, 250–251
latency
  saccadic, 58–59
  vergence response, 84–87
latent fixation nystagmus. See fusional
    maldevelopment nystagmus syndrome
lateral geniculate nucleus, role in smooth pursuit,
    76–77
lateral medullary syndrome, 121, 125–126, 149,
    169, 176
lateral rectus, 4–7, 9
  adhesion with inferior oblique, 262
  innervation of, 76–77
  maldevelopment of, 228
  recession, 162
  resection, 161, 230
lateral vestibular nucleus, 32
  damage to, 230
lateropulsion, 125
  in lateral medullary syndrome, 126
Leigh's syndrome, 131, 156, 255–256
lens gradient method, of calculating AC/A ratio,
    88–89
lentiform nucleus, bilateral lesions of, 187
Lesch-Nyhan disease, 187, 195
lesions. See also under names of specific structures
  functional recovery, 30
  localizing, 16–17
leukemia, 207
leukodystrophy, 155
leukoencephalopathy, in MNGIE syndrome, 255
leukomalacia, periventricular, 120
levadopa, 186
  to treat gaze deviations, 120
  to treat Parkinson's disease, 183
levator palpebrae, 10, 203
levocycloversion, 4–5
levoversion, 4–5
Lewy bodies, 182, 184–185
Lewy body disease, 141, 185
Lhermitte's sign, 150
limb malformations, 229
limbus, 6–7
linear acceleration input, 38
lipid storage diseases, 147
lissenchephaly, 172
Listing's law, 136
lithium
  overdose, 158
  role in Guillain-Barré syndrome, 237
  toxicity, 119

looming, 84–85
Louis-Bar syndrome. *See* ataxia telangiectasia
lumbar puncture, 226
lungs, small-cell cancer, 250
lupus erythematosus, 261
lymphadenopathy, 145
lymphoma, 207, 226
lysosomal disorders, 155
Lytico-Bodig, 184

macrosaccadic oscillations, 114
macro-square wave jerks, 112
macula, 28–29
  otolith, 38–39
Maddox rod, 220
main sequence relationship, 58–59
malnutrition, 154
maple syrup urine disease, 133, 141, 155
mastoiditis, 226
mechanical restriction, 200
medial longitudinal fasciculus, 32–34, 64–65,
    121–122
  effect of damage on ocular tilt, 42–43
  lesions of, 66–67, 133–134, 149
  rostral interstitial nucleus, 66–67,
    137–138
medial orbital floor, 6
medial rectus, 4–7, 9
  hypometric saccades and, 102
  innervation of, 64–65, 76–77, 86
  internuclear pathway to, 32
  recession, 230
  subnuclei, 204
medial superior temporal area, 18–19
  anatomy, 192
  lesions of, 192
medial vestibular nucleus, 32–34,
    101, 121
  interruption of fibers, 130
  lesions of, 125
  as neural integrator, 60–61, 64–65
  role in smooth pursuit, 76–77
medulla. *See also specific medullary structures*
  effect of lesions on nystagmus, 60
  ocular motor syndromes caused by lesions of,
    125–129
  structures important in ocular motor control,
    121, 125
medulloblastoma, 119
mega cisterna magna, 172
MELAS syndrome, 156, 255
memantine, 109
memory-guided saccades, 70–71
meningeal signs, in cavernous sinus
    thrombosis, 234
meningioma, intracavernous, 212

meningitis
  basal, 212, 218
  as cause of subarachnoid lesions, 225
mental retardation, 229
mesencephalic reticular formation, 143
  role in vergence control, 86–87
mestinon, 247
metal metabolism, disorders of, 156
methylphenidate, to treat saccadic intrusions, 112
methylprednisolone, to treat multiple sclerosis, 152
methysergide, to treat progressive supranuclear
    palsy, 145
M ganglion cells, 76
M-group, 143
microdrift, 18–19
micrognathia, 229
micrographia, 182
microphthalmia, 172
microsaccades, 18–19
microtremor, 18–19, 241
microtubule binding protein τ, 145
midbrain. *See also specific midbrain structures*
  effect of damage on ocular tilt, 42–43
  involvement in ocular motor syndromes,
    137–146
  lesions of, 120, 143–146, 147
  role in saccades, 56
  stroke, 162
  structures important in ocular motor control, 124
  tumors of, 161
middle temporal area, 18–19
  anatomy, 191
  effect of damage on pursuit, 78–79
  lesions of, 191
  role in smooth pursuit, 76–77
migraine, 173, 206, 218, 227
  as cause of oculomotor palsy, 201
Millard-Gubler syndrome, 224
Miller Fisher syndrome, 161, 238
mitochondrial dysfunction, 255
mitochondrial encephalopathies, 156
mitochondrial myopathies, 254
mitoxantrone, 153
mixed horizontal-torsional nystagmus, 36–37
MNGIE syndrome, 156, 255
Ménière's disease, 97
Möbius syndrome, 131, 210, 229
molar tooth sign, 195
monoamine oxidase-ß inhibitor, 183
monoclonal gammopathy, 207
monocular elevator palsy. *See* double elevator palsy
monocular movements, 4–5
monocular occlusion, 161
motion
  monocular clues from, 84–85
  perception, 78
  speed and direction signals, 76

motor commands, for vergence, 86–87
motor learning, 46
motor weakness, in Guillain-Barré syndrome, 237
multicore disease, 262
multiple ocular nerve palsies, 231–236
multiple sclerosis, 96, 98, 99, 100, 150
  acquired pendular nystagmus and, 103
  convergence spasm and, 162
  internuclear ophthalmoplegia and, 133
  one-and-a-half syndrome and, 135
  opsoclonus and, 115
  pathogenesis and pathology, 151
  pretectal syndrome and, 141
  relapsing-remitting, 153
  saccadic pulses in, 113
multiple system atrophy, 185
multiply innervated fibers, 10–11
muscle atrophy
  in Grave's disease, 259
  in slow-channel syndrome, 249
muscles. *See also* extraocular muscles
  damage of peripheral, 229
  skeletal, 257
  tension changes during stimulation, 42
  weakness
    in botulism, 252
    in Grave's disease, 259
    in myasthenia gravis, 244
muscle-specific kinase, in myasthenia
    gravis, 246
muscular dystrophy, 172, 257–258
myasthenia gravis, 244–247
  pediatric, 248–249
myasthenic syndromes
  congenital, 248–249
  Lambert-Eaton, 250–251
myelin. *See also names of demyelinating diseases*
  central pontine myelinosis, 131
  disorders and acquired pendular nystagmus, 103
Myerson's sign, 144
myoclonic jerks, in Creutzfeld-Jakob disease, 158
myopathies. *See also* cardiomyopathy
  congenital, 262
  mitochondrial, 254
myopia, 104
  effect on gain, 46
myositis, 259, 261
myotonic dystrophy, 257–258
myotonin-protein kinase, 257
myotubular myopathies, 262

nasal retinal fibers, 142
nasopharyngeal carcinoma, 226
nausea, in botulism, 252
near point of convergence, 88–89
near triad, spasm of, 162

neck
  dystonia, 144
  flexion, 150
  retroflexion, 139
  surgery, 226
nemaline myopathy, 262
neostigmine, 248
neural integrator, 60–61, 139
  damage of, 113
  leaky, 64–67, 101
  for smooth pursuit, 76
neurodegenerative disease, 155–156. *See also*
    specific neurodegenerative diseases
neurofibrillary tangles, 145, 157, 184
neuroleptic drugs, 187
  as cause of oculogyric crisis, 183
  use in Huntington's disease, 186
neuronal transmission, changes in patterns, 242
neuropathies, causing ophthalmoplegia, 237–240
Niemann-Pick disease, 141, 155
night blindness, 254
N-methyl-D-aspartate, antagonists to treat
    Alzheimer's disease, 157
nodulus
  dysfunction, 120
  lesions of, 48–49, 167
  syndrome of, 122
Nothnagel's syndrome, 205
Novantrone, 153
nucal rigidity, 234
nucleus incertus, 129
nucleus interpositus, role in vergence, 86–87
nucleus paragigantocellularis dorsalis, 62–63, 132
nucleus paraphales, 129
nucleus prepositus hypoglossi, 101, 121
  lesions of, 128
  as neural integrator, 60–61, 64–65, 76
nucleus raphe interpositus, 64–65, 136
  omnipause neurons in, 66–67
  role in vertical pursuit, 76–77
nucleus reticularis pontis caudalis, 132
nucleus reticularis tegmenti pontis, 68–69
  lesions of, 78–79, 136
  role in vergence, 86–87
nucleus solitarius, 225
nucleus substantia nigra pars reticulata, 68–69
null zone, 105
nystagmus, 18–19
  abducting, 134
  in Arnold-Chiari malformation, 171
  Bechterew, 30
  Brun's, 102
  caloric, 166
  centripetal and rebound, 102, 158
  classification, 96
  convergence-retraction, 140
  in Dandy-Walker malformation, 171

ophthalmopathy, thyroid-related, 222
ophthalmoplegia, 64–65
  in botulism, 252
  in cavernous sinus thrombosis, 234
  chronic progressive external, 156, 254–255
  differential diagnosis of acquired, 231
  in Grave's disease, 259
  internuclear, 64–65, 102, 121, 133–134, 144,
     147, 150, 170
  in Leigh's syndrome, 257
  in MELAS syndrome, 255
  in neonatal myasthenia gravis, 248
  neuropathies causing, 237–240
  in oculomotor nerve palsy, 213
  in oculopharyngeal dystrophy, 258
  progressive, 175
  in Refsum's disease, 240
  in sphenocavernous syndrome, 232
  supranuclear, 144
  in Tolosa-Hunt syndrome, 236
  in Wernicke's encephalopathy, 154
ophthalmoscope, use to remove fixation,
    52–53
ophthalmoscopy, of optic disk to detect fusional
    nystagmus, 106
opsoclonus, 115, 169
  pathogenesis, 116
  testing, 116
  treatment, 117
optical infinity, 82
optic ataxia, 190
optic atrophy
  in Leigh's syndrome, 256
  in MELAS syndrome, 255
optic chiasma, 142
  lesion of, 99
optic nerve, 142
  disease, 104
  head, 52
  pallor, 174
optic neuritis, in multiple sclerosis, 150
Optic Neuritis Treatment Trail, 152
optic neuropathy
  in Grave's disease, 259
  treatment, 260
optic tract
  lesions of, 78–79, 142
  nucleus, 76–77
optokinetic after-nystagmus, 48–51
  impaired, 193
optokinetic drum
  use in saccade testing, 70
  use in smooth pursuit testing, 78–79
optokinetic nystagmus, 22–23, 50–51. *See also*
    optokinetic after-nystagmus
  in Arnold-Chiari malformation, 171
  asymmetry, 107

  cancellation, 75
  eliciting, 70
  with frontal eye field lesions, 188
  reversed, 105
optokinetic reflex, 22
optokinetic system, 15–17, 50–51
orbicularis weakness, 244
  in neonatal myasthenia gravis, 248
orbit, 202, 216, 222
  decompression, 260
  layer, 10–11
  lesions of, 208, 218, 227
orbital myositis, 259, 261
orthophoria, 12–13
orthoptic exercises, 162
orthotropia, 12–13
  in extraocular muscle fibrosis, 210
oscillopsia, 18–19, 22, 26–27, 92, 118
  constant, 103
  differential diagnosis, 95
  in superior oblique myokymia, 241
ossicular chain, abnormalities of, 149
otoconia, 28–29
  specific gravity of, 38–39
otolith-ocular pathway, 40–41
  disruption of, 42, 148
otolith-ocular reflex, 38–39, 44
otolith organs, 24–25
  abnormal projections of, 99
  lesions of, 44–45
  physiology and organization, 28–29,
    38–39
  role in posture and eye orientation, 44–45
otorrhea, 226
overlap paradigm, 58–59

pacemakers, 257
pain
  impairment of sensation, 125
  loss of sensation, 176
palinopsia, 200
palisade tendon organs, 10–11
pallidotomy, to treat Parkinson's disease, 183
palpebral fissure, narrowing in Duane's
    syndrome, 228
palsy, definition, 12
papilledema, in Guillain-Barré
    syndrome, 237
paracrystalline inclusions, 254
paralysis, definition, 12
paramedian medulla, lesions of, 128
paramedian midbrain, 143
paramedian nuclei, lesions of, 114
paramedian pontine reticular formation,
    64–65, 121
  lesions of, 132

paramedian tracts
    cell groups of, 129
    interruption of, 102, 130, 134
    lesions of, 128
    role in gaze holding, 60–61
paranasal sinus disease, 261
paraneoplastic syndrome, 114, 147, 250
    in children, 116
    internuclear ophthalmoplegia and, 133
    opsoclonus and, 115
parasellar tumors, 99
parasitic infections, as cause of infective myositis,
    261
parasympathetic fibers, 142
paresis, definition, 12
paresthesia, in multiple sclerosis, 150
parietal cortex, role in smooth pursuit, 76–77
parietal eye field, 18–19
    anatomy, 190
    role in saccades, 68–69
parietal lobe, lesions of, 190
Parkinsonism, 186
    eye movement abnormalities in, 184–185
Parkinson's disease, 122, 147, 162, 182–183
    clinical features and pathophysiology, 182
    convergence insufficiency, 84
    defects of saccadic control in, 70–71
    square-wave oscillations in, 114
    treatment, 183
paroxysmal tonic upgaze, 120
pause neurons. See ominpause neurons
peek sign, 244
Pelizaeus-Merzbacher disease, 96, 103, 156, 195
pendular nystagmus, 94, 95, 96, 195
    acquired, 103
    congenital, 105
    in oculopalatal tremor, 127
    in spasmus nutans, 107
periaqueductal gray matter, 202
    lesions of, 120, 143
perilymph fistula, 97, 149
periodic alternating nystagmus, 48–49, 100, 109,
    158, 167
peripheral muscles, damage in Möbius syndrome,
    229
peripheral nerve palsy, 147
peripheral neuropathy
    in MNGIE syndrome, 255
    in Refsum's disease, 240
peripheral vestibular disorders, 32, 42, 149
    nystagmus in, 36–37, 52–53, 97, 108
pernicious anemia, 250
peroxisomal assembly disorders, 103, 156, 195
petrous apex syndrome, 226
phase difference, 26–27
phenobarbital, 255
    to treat saccadic intrusions, 112

phenothiazine intoxication, 118
phenytoin
    intoxication, 162
    to treat myotonic dystrophy, 257
phlebitis, 226
photophobia, in Grave's disease, 259
physiological end-point nystagmus, 101
phytanic acid metabolism, 240
pigmentary retinopathy
    in abetalipoproteinemia, 239
    in chronic progressive external
        ophthalmoplegia, 254–255
    in MELAS syndrome, 255
    in myotonic dystrophy, 257
    in Refsum's disease, 240
pill-rolling motion, 182
pineal gland tumors, 141, 162
ping-pong gaze, 119
plasmapheresis, 117, 237, 238, 247, 251
pleocytosis, 236
pneumonia, aspiration, 144
Poland anomaly, 229
poliomyelitis, as cause of opsoclonus, 115
polyarthralgia, 145
polyopia, 200
polysynaptic pathway, 40
pons. See also specific pontine structures
    compression, 119
    lesions of, 119, 147, 224
    maldevelopment of dorsomedial
        structures, 230
    role in saccades, 56
    role in smooth pursuit, 76–77
    role of damage in ocular motor syndromes,
        130–136
    structures important in ocular motor control,
        121, 124
pontomedullary junction, lesions of, 98, 99
positional nystagmus, 97, 100
    in multiple sclerosis, 151
posterior commissure, 121
    lesions of, 140–142
posterior cortex, lesions of, 191–192
posterior fossa
    differential diagnosis of malformations, 172
    enlargement, 171
    lesions of, 225
posterior inferior cerebellar artery
        syndrome, 176
posterior parietal cortex
    anatomy, 190
    role in saccades, 68–69
posterior temporal lobe, anatomy and lesions of,
        192
posterior thalamosubthalamic paramedian artery,
        137
post-rotary nystagmus, 48–51

postsaccadic drift, 68, 102, 166
postural stability, 44–45, 182
potassium channel dysfunction, 242
preauricular appendages, 228
predictive saccades, 70–71
prednisone, to treat multiple sclerosis, 152
prefrontal cortex, effect of lesions on antisaccades,
    70–71
prematurity, gaze deviation and, 120, 140
pretectal pseudo-bobbing, 163
pretectal syndrome, 140–142
primary deviation, 12–13
primary position, 8–9
primary visual cortex, lesions of, 191
prion diseases, 157
prisms, 222, 230, 247
    base-in, 162
    base-out, 105, 161
    for diplopia, 257
    reversing, 46
progressive supranuclear palsy, 114, 133,
    144–145, 162, 184
    as cause of pretectal syndrome, 141
    convergence insufficiency in, 82
    neuropathology, 145
promethazine, to treat nystagmus, 108
propanolol
    to treat opsoclonus, 117
    to treat superior oblique myokymia, 241
propioception, 10–11
    loss in abetalipoproteinemia, 239
    smooth pursuit and, 73
propionic acidemia, 195
proptosis
    in carotid-cavernous fistula, 235
    in cavernous sinus thrombosis, 234
    in Grave's disease, 259
    in orbital apex lesions, 233
    treatment of, 260
pseudo-abducens palsy, 140
pseudo-Argyll Robertson pupil, 212
pseudobulbar palsy, 144
pseudo-divergence excess, 161
pseudo-Graefe sign, 212
pseudotumors, 259
psychic paralysis of gaze. See Balint's syndrome
ptosis, 201
    bilateral, 202
    in botulism, 252
    in chronic progressive external
        ophthalmoplegia, 254–255
    congenital, 210
    in extraocular muscle fibrosis, 210–211
    in Guillain-Barré syndrome, 237
    in myasthenia gravis, 244, 248
    in myotonic dystrophy, 257
    in oculomotor nerve palsy, 209, 213

    in oculopharyngeal dystrophy, 258
    in slow-channel syndrome, 249
    surgery, 214, 257, 258
    in Tolosa-Hunt syndrome, 236
pulse, of innervation, 60–61
pupillary constriction, 82, 118, 142
pupillary disorders, 142, 162
    in botulism, 252
    light-near dissociation, 140
    in myotonic dystrophy, 257
    in oculomotor nerve palsy, 201, 208, 213
    in sphenocavernous syndrome, 207, 233
    in third nerve palsy, 206
    in Tolosa-Hunt syndrome, 236
    in trochlear nerve palsy, 218
pupillary distance, 88–89
pupillomotor fibers, 142
Purkinje cells, 48
    malfunction of, 116
pursuit. See smooth pursuit
putative pathway, smooth pursuit, 76–77

quick phases, of smooth pursuit, 78–79

rabbits, vision of, 15
radial ray anomalies, 229
radioablation therapy, 260
radioactive iodine scanning, 260
ragged-red fibers, 254
Raymond-Cestan syndrome, 224
Rebif, 153
reciprocal inhibition, 34
reciprocal innervation, 8–9
recruitment, of muscle fibers, 10–11
rectus muscles, 3–5. See also specific rectus muscles
    position, 6–7
reflexive saccades, 70–71
refraction, cycloplegic for infantile nystagmus,
    105
Refsum's disease, 240
relative afferent pupillary defect, 217
renal failure, 154
resolution, 15
respiratory failure, in Leigh's syndrome, 256
resting tremor, 182
retina, 56
    abnormalities, 200
    dysplasia, 172
    veins, 235
retinal disparity, 82
    as stimulus for vergence, 84–85
retinal image
    blur, 82, 84–85
    slip, 46
    stability, 22, 24–25, 50–51, 75, 86–87

defects of, 78–79, 144, 192
in disease states, 126, 151, 157, 183, 186, 194
effect of lesions on, 94, 166, 168, 169, 188, 190
functions and characteristics, 75
gain, 75, 193
in horizontal conjugate saccadic palsy, 132
inverted, 105
latency, 75
nerve pathways, 76–77
phases, 75, 77–78
predictive properties, 75
testing, 78–79
spasmodic torticollis, 187
spasmus nutans, 96, 103, 107
sphenocavernous syndrome, 207–208, 232–233
spinal trigeminal nucleus, 10–11
spinocerebellar ataxias, 147, 161
saccades in, 58–59, 174
spinocerebellar degeneration, 101, 103
as cause of saccadic intrusions, 112
spontaneous drift, 70–71
square-wave jerks, 112, 140, 144, 175
in hemispheric lesions, 193
in Parkinson's disease, 183
in spinocerebellar ataxias, 174
square-wave oscillations, 114
Staphylococcus aureus, 234, 261
static imbalance, testing, 52–53
steatorrhea, in abetalipoproteinemia, 239
Steele-Richardson-Olszewski syndrome. *See*
progressive supranuclear palsy
step, of innervation, 60–61
stereocilia, 30–31, 40
stereopsis, 86–87
impaired, 162
steroacuity, loss with thalamic lesions, 180
stimulus, frequency content, 39
strabismus, 260
acquired vertical, 215
in Arnold-Chiari malformation, 171
binocular diplopia and, 200
comitant and incomitant, 12–13
in Dandy-Walker malformation, 171–172
relation to skew deviation, 42
surgery, 214
terminology, 12–13
vertical or torsional, 82
strabismus fixus, 211
striate cortex, 56, 73
disparity neurons in, 86–87
lesions of, 191
striola, 39, 40
strokelike episodes, 255
subacute necrotizing encephalomyelopathy,
255–256
subarachnoid space, 206–207, 216, 222
aneurysm, 216

hemorrhage, 119
lesions of, 206–209, 218, 225
suboccipital craniotomy, to treat nystagmus, 108
substantia nigra pars reticulata, 18–19
inhibition of superior colliculus, 112
lesions of, 181
subthalamotomy, to treat Parkinson's disease, 183
superior cerebellar artery syndrome, 176
superior colliculus, 18–19, 64–65, 136
damage to, 230
inhibition of, 112
projections to, 68–69
role in saccades, 55–56
superior oblique, 4–7, 9, 219–221
myokymia, 241
palsy, 221
tendon sheath syndrome, 261
tenotomy, 241, 262
superior olivary nucleus, deafness and, 225
superior orbital fissure, lesions of, 207, 218, 226
superior rectus, 4–7, 9, 203, 220
innervation, 66–67
subnucleus, 204
transposition, 230
superior vestibular nucleus, 34–35
supplementary eye field, 18–19
anatomy and lesions of, 189
role in saccades, 68–69
role in smooth pursuit, 76–77
supranuclear lesions, 42
supratenorial masses, 206
surgery. *See also specific procedures*
cataract, 257
neck, 226
to treat abducens nerve palsy, 230
to treat carotid-cavernous fistula, 235
to treat congenital trochlear nerve palsy, 221
to treat superior oblique myokymia, 241
sursumversion. *See* elevation
Sydenham's chorea, 187
sympathetic paralysis, 207, 233
sympathetic plexus, 232
synaptic organization, changes in, 116
synkinesis, oculomotor nerve, 212
syphilis, 212

tachycardia, 259
tachypnea, 195
tactile stimuli
saccades in response to, 56
smooth pursuit and, 73
tardive dyskinesia, 187
targets, proximity of, 84–85
target velocity, 75
taste, loss of, 224
Tay-Sachs disease, 141, 155

velocity
 saccadic, 58–59
 smooth pursuit, 75
velocity storage, 48–51
 abnormal, 167
 gain of, 100
 integrator, 38–39
venous pressure, orbital, 259
ventriculomegaly, 172
verapamil, to treat opsoclonus, 117
vergence, 15
 accommodation and, 84
 cerebral control of, 86–87
 disorders, 161–163
 eye rotations, 4–5
 functions and characteristics, 84–85
 fusional, 88–89
 interaction with saccades, 84–85
 oscillations, 163
 in pretectal syndrome, 140
 sparing in gaze palsy, 130
 testing, 88–89
vermis. See also dorsal vermis
 agenesis of, 171
 hypoplasia, 172
versions, 4–5
vertebral anomalies, 228
vertical gaze palsy, 140–141, 144, 145
vertical retraction syndrome, 209
vertigo, 23, 30, 176
 benign, 97, 100, 173
 in lateral medullary syndrome, 125
vestibular atelectasis, 97
vestibular nucleus, 32–34, 40
 central, 230
 lateral, 32, 228
 lesions of, 128, 149
 medial, 32–34, 101, 121
  interruption of fibers, 130
  as neural integrator, 60–61, 64–65
  role in smooth pursuit, 76–77
 superior, 34–35
 velocity storage and, 48–49
vestibular nystagmus, 33, 50–53, 96–100
 central, 98–100
 eliciting, 70
 peripheral, 36–37, 97, 108
vestibular system, 15–17. See also vestibular
  nucleus
 connections to extraocular muscles, 32, 41
 ganglion, 28–29
 lesions of, 23, 34, 36–37, 94, 149,
  166–167
 peripheral disorders, 32, 42, 149
 testing functions, 52–53
 vestibular cortex, 192
vestibulo-collic reflex, 44

vestibulo-ocular reflex, 16–17, 22, 24–25
 abnormal in Arnold-Chiari
  malformation, 171
 adaptation, 46–47, 129, 166
 cancellation, 75, 78–79
 characteristics of, 26–27
 in disease states, 155, 183, 186, 187
 gain, 193
 horizontal pathway, 32–33
 role of optokinetic system in, 50–51
 stabilization of eye position, 73
 vertical and torsional pathway, 34–35
vestibulopathy, 95
 acute peripheral, 42, 149
vibration sense, decreased, 150
viral infections, 133, 261
viscous drag, 60–61
visual acuity
 versus field of vision, 15
 head-shaking, 52–53
visual attention
 in Alzheimer's disease, 157
 impaired with parietal lobe lesions, 190
 importance in antisaccades, 70
visual axes, 12–13
 direction of, 6–7
 misalignment, 148
visual blur, 26–27, 82, 84–85
visual cortex, 82
visual dumping, 50
visual enhancement, 26
visual feedback, duration of, 82
visual field, constriction in Refsum's
  disease, 240
visual fixation, 18–19
visual glabellar sign, 144
visual loss, 96
 acquired pendular nystagmus with, 103–104
 with orbital apex lesions, 233
visual processing, structures involved in,
  10–11
visual stimuli, reaction to novel, 58
visual tracking, 50, 73, 75
vitamin B_1. See thiamine
vitamin E deficiency, hereditary, 175
vitreous hemorrhage, 145
vitritis, 145
volitional saccades, 70–71
voluntary flutter, 163
voluntary nystagmus, 118

Walker-Warburg syndrome, 172
Wallenberg's syndrome. See lateral medullary
  syndrome
waveform and trajectory, of vergence
  movements, 84–85

Instructions for Using the CD-ROM

The CD-ROM that accompanies this book contains all 14 chapters, including figures, tables, and associated video clips. The CD-ROM is presented in HTML format, and is viewable with any standard Web browser. To view the videos, you will need Windows Media Player or Apple QuickTime, both of which are available for free.

Inserting the CD-ROM will automatically start up and display the table of contents page on your web browser. If the CD-ROM does not automatically start, point your browser at the file index.html on the CD-ROM.

System Requirement

CD-ROM drive

Internet Explorer, Mozilla Firefox, or any standard Web browser

Windows Media Player or Apple QuickTiyme

Video Legends

Filename: Video 4.2 - Hypermetric saccades v2
Video Legend: Hypermetric saccades

A young woman with progressive cerebellar ataxia and myoclonic seizure since 13 year of age. On looking to the left, the saccade overshot the target, which was followed by a corrective rightward saccade. Similarly, rightward saccades were hypermetric and were followed by corrective saccades in the opposite direction.

Filename: Video 7.5.1 - Downbeat nystagmus v2
Video Legend: Downbeat nystagmus

A teenager on carbamazepine for seizure disorder presented with downbeat nystagmus. The nystagmus was present in primary position, and its intensity increased on lateral gaze. The nystagmus resolved once carbamazepine was discontinued.

Filename: Video 7.5.2 - Upbeat nystagmus v2
Video Legend: Upbeat nystagmus

A middle-aged woman with cerebellar degeneration and upbeat nystagmus.

Filename: Video 7.5.3 - Torsional nystagmus v2
Video Legend: Torsional nystagmus

An elderly woman with lateral medullary syndrome and torsional nystagmus. The nystagmus was present in primary position and beat clockwise from the patient's point of view (i.e., counterclockwise from the examiner's point of view). It was more prominent on lateral gaze, especially on looking to the right.

Filename: Video 7.5.4 - Seesaw nystagmus v2
Video Legend: Seesaw nystagmus

A teenager with a peri-chiasmal lesion presented with seesaw nystagmus. Half-cycle of the nystagmus consisted of depression and excyclotorsion of one eye, and synchronous elevation and incyclotorsion of the fellow eye; during the next half-cycle, the movements reversed in direction in each eye. Note that the nystagmus waveform consisted by slow eye movement in both phases (i.e., pendular) and hence the name seesaw nystagmus.

Filename: Video 7.5.5 - Periodic alternating nystagmus v2
Video Legend: Periodic alternating nystagmus

A teenager with periodic alternating nystagmus. Initially, there was a left-beating nystagmus in the primary position with intensity that varied in a crescendo-decrescendo fashion for about 90s. During this period, when he rotated his head to the left to put his eyes in the right orbital position (i.e., head turn toward the direction of the quick phase), the nystagmus intensity decreased, in accordance with Alexander's law. This was followed by a null period of about 20s when there was no nystagmus. After that, a right-beating nystagmus occurred in the primary position with intensity that again varied in a crescendo-decrescendo fashion for about 90s. This right-beating nystagmus also followed Alexander's law; its intensity decreased when the patient rotated his head to the right. In fact, this patient adopted a periodic alternating head turn to minimize the oscillopsia caused by the changing nystagmus. Video courtesy of Dr. Lawrence Tychsen.

Filename: Video 7.6.2 - Gaze evoked & rebound nystagmus v2
Video Legend: Gaze-evoked and rebound nystagmus

A young woman with ataxia-oculomotor apraxia type 2 presented with gaze-evoked and rebound nystagmus. On primary gaze, there was no nystagmus. On right gaze, there was a right-beating nystagmus (i.e., gaze-evoked nystagmus) with a small downbeat component. After sustained right gaze, when the eyes returned to the primary position, a left-beating nystagmus was present (i.e., rebound nystagmus).

Filename: Video 7.6.4 - Dissociated nystagmus in internuclear ophthalmoplegia v2
Video Legend: Dissociated nystagmus in internuclear ophthalmoplegia

A young woman with bilateral internuclear ophthalmoplegia secondary to Arnold-Chiari malformation type 2. On left gaze, adduction of the right eye was limited, and there was a dissociated left-beating nystagmus in the abducting left eye. Similarly, on right gaze, adduction of the left eye was limited, with a dissociated right-beating nystagmus in the abducting right eye.

Filename: Video 7.7 - Acquired pendular nystagmus v2
Video Legend: Acquired pendular nystagmus

A middle-aged man with multiple sclerosis and acquired vertical pendular nystagmus. The nystagmus caused severe oscillopsia.

Filename: Video 7.8.1 - Infantile nystagmus syndrome v2
Video Legend: Infantile nystagmus syndrome

A child with infantile nystagmus who habitually adopted a left face turn to put his eyes in the null zone where the nystagmus intensity was minimum. When he rotated his head to the straight ahead position, a left-beating nystagmus was present, the intensity of which increased when he turned his head further to the right. Video courtesy of Dr. Lawrence Tychsen.

Filename: Video 7.8.2 - A. Fusional maldevelopment nystagmus syndrome (latent fixation nystagmus) v2
Video Legend: Fusional maldevelopment nystagmus syndrome (latent nystagmus)

A child with Down's syndrome and infantile esotropia. On covering the right eye, the left eye and the covered right eye beat to the left (i.e., away from the covered eye). On covering the left eye, the quick phases changed direction immediately, such that both eyes beat to the right (i.e., also away from the covered eye). Video courtesy of Dr. Lawrence Tychsen.

Filename: Video 7.8.2 - B. Fusional maldevelopment nystagmus syndrome (DVD & pursuit asymmetry) v2
Video Legend: Dissociated vertical deviation and smooth pursuit asymmetry

A child with a history of infantile esotropia who had undergone strabismus surgery. Despite successful realignment of the eyes, a left dissociated vertical deviation persisted. When the left eye was covered, it moved upward while the viewing right eye maintained fixation. When the covered left eye was then uncovered, it moved downward to primary position, without any corresponding downward movement of the previously fixating right eye, in violation of Herring's law. In addition, smooth pursuit asymmetry also persisted. During monocular viewing, when the target moved toward the nose with respect to the viewing eye, pursuit was normal and smooth. However, when the target moved away from the nose, pursuit was abnormal and saccadic. Video courtesy of Dr. Lawrence Tychsen.

Filename: Video 7.8.3 - Spasmus nutans v2
Video Legend: Spasmus nutans

A child with spasmus nutans presented with the classic triad of head nodding, left head turn, and nystagmus. The nystagmus was highly variable; the left eye had a dissociated horizontal nystagmus for a short period of time, which was followed by a horizontal conjugate nystagmus in both eyes. Video courtesy of Dr. Lawrence Tychsen.

Filename: Video 8.1.1 - Square wave jerks v2
Video Legend: Square wave jerks

A young man presented with blurry vision and square wave jerks following a closed-head injury from a motor vehicle accident. Small saccades took the eyes off fixation (mostly to the right). After an intersaccadic interval of about 200ms, small corrective saccades brought the eyes back to fixation.

Filename: Video 8.2.2 - Macrosaccadic oscillation v2
Video Legend: Macrosaccadic oscillations
A young woman with progressive cerebellar ataxia and myoclonic seizure since 13 years of age. Note the involuntary large saccades that straddled fixation that were highly characteristic of macrosaccadic oscillations.

Filename: Video 8.2.3 - Opsoclonus v2
Video Legend: Opsoclonus
An elderly woman with oscillopsia and small cell carcinoma of the lung presented with multidirectional, high-frequency saccadic oscillations that were highly characteristic of opsoclonus.

Filename: Video 8.2.4 - Voluntary flutter v3
Video Legend: Voluntary flutter
A young girl who could generate voluntary flutter at will. The saccadic oscillations were confined to the horizontal plane and lasted no longer than 20-30s at a time. Video courtesy of Dr. Lawrence Tychsen.

Filename: Video 9.2.1 - A. Lesions in the lateral medulla - lateral medullary syndrome (ipsipulsion of saccades) v2
Video Legend: Ipsipulsion of saccades
A middle-aged man with left lateral medullary syndrome and ipsipulsion of vertical saccades. During upward saccades, the eyes veered toward the left, which were followed by small, rightward corrective saccades to bring the eyes back on target.

Filename: Video 9.2.1 - A. Lesions in the lateral medulla - lateral medullary syndrome (torsional nystagmus) v2
Video Legend: Torsional nystagmus
An elderly woman with lateral medullary syndrome and torsional nystagmus. The nystagmus was present in primary position and beat clockwise from the patient's point of view (i.e., counterclockwise from the examiner's point of view). It was more prominent on lateral gaze, especially on looking to the right.

Filename: Video 9.2.2 - Lesions in the inferior olivary nucleus - oculopalatal tremor v2
Video Legend: Oculopalatal tremor
A middle-aged woman with a hemorrhagic cavernoma in the cerebellum presented with oculopalatal tremor. A vertical pendular nystagmus with a torsional component was present in primary position. Synchronous rhythmic movements of the palate were also evident.

Filename: Video 9.3.3 - Lesions in the medial longitudinal fasciculus - internuclear ophthalmoplegia v2
Video Legend: Internuclear ophthalmoplegia
A young woman with schwannoma of the vestibulocochlear nerves presented with a bilateral internuclear ophthalmoplegia after resection of the tumors. On right

gaze, adduction of the left eye was limited, and a dissociated left-beating nystagmus in the abducting right eye was evident. Similarly, on left gaze, adduction of the right eye was limited, with a dissociated right-beating nystagmus in the abducting left eye.

Filename: Video 9.4.3 - Lesions in the posterior commissure...
vertical gaze palsy and pretectal syndrome v3
Video Legend: Pretectal syndrome

A teenaged boy with a pineal germinoma presented with upgaze palsy that affected upward pursuit and saccades. Convergence-retraction nystagmus was evident during attempted upward saccades and when the optokinetic drum rotated downward. The pupils did not respond to light but constricted when a near target was presented (i.e., light-near dissociation of the pupils). Convergence was preserved. Video courtesy of Dr. Lawrence Tychsen.

Filename: Video 9.4.4 - F. Whipple disease (oculomasticatory myorhythmia) v2
Video Legend: Oculomasticatory myorhythmia in Whipple's disease

A middle-aged man presented with Whipple's disease and oculomasticatory myorhythmia. The abnormal eye movements consisted of pendular, horizontal convergent-divergent oscillations. Video courtesy of Dr. Edsel Ing.

Filename: Video 9.5.3 - Multiple sclerosis (internuclear
ophthalmoplegia and adduction lag)
Video Legend: Adduction lag in internuclear ophthalmoplegia

A young man with multiple sclerosis and internuclear ophthalmoplegia. The first segment shows limited adduction in the adducting eye and dissociated nystagmus in the abducting eye. The second segment shows that during horizontal saccades, the ipsilesional adducting eye exhibited slow adducting saccades, giving the appearance of an "adduction lag".

Filename: Video 9.5.7 - D. Convergence spasm v2
Video Legend: Convergence spasm

A middle-aged woman presented with intermittent convergence spasm. Note the involuntary convergence of the left eye.

Filename: Video 11.1 - Ocular motor syndromes caused by lesions
in the thalamus (thalamic esotropia) v2
Video Legend: Thalamic esotropia

A middle-aged man with glioblastoma multiforme in the thalamus, which resulted in a thalamic esotropia and defective horizontal eye movements.

Filename: Video 11.3.5 - Ocular motor apraxia (congenital ocular motor apraxia) v3
Video Legend: Congenital ocular motor apraxia

A young girl with ataxia-oculomotor ataxia type 2. Both voluntary horizontal and vertical saccades were impaired, with compensatory head thrust. This is in contrast to idiopathic congenital oculomotor ataxia (Cogan's type) which usually affects horizontal saccades only.

Filename: Video 12.2.2 - Congenital oculomotor nerve palsy
(oculomotor paresis with cyclic spasms) v2
Video Legend: Oculomotor paresis with cyclic spasms

A teenager presented with right congenital oculomotor paresis with cyclic spasm since age two. The paretic phase lasted for about 2 min and was characterized by a right ptosis, right exotropia, and dilated right pupil. The paretic phase alternated with the spastic phase. During the spastic phase which lasted for about 10-20s, the right upper eyelid elevated, the right exotropia resolved, and the right pupil constricted.

Filename: Video 12.4.2 - Congenital abducens palsy (Duane's syndrome) v2
Video Legend: Duane's syndrome

A young boy with left Duane's syndrome Type I. The left eye had limited abduction when looking to the left. On looking to the right, the left eye showed narrowing of the palpebral fissure and retraction of the globe on adduction. Video courtesy of Dr. Lawrence Tychsen.

Filename: Video 12.4.2 - Congenital abducens palsy (horizontal
gaze palsy and progressive scoliosis) v2
Video Legend: Horizontal gaze palsy and progressive scoliosis

A teenaged girl with horizontal gaze palsy and progressive scoliosis. Horizontal eye movements were absent, but vertical movements were preserved.

Filename: Video 14.1.1 - Chronic progressive external ophthalmoplegia
and Kearns-Sayre syndrome v2
Video Legend: Chronic progressive external ophthalmoplegia

A teenager presented with chronic progressive external ophthalmoplegia. He had bilateral ptosis, as well as severely limited horizontal and upward eye movements, with preservation of some downward movements.

Filename: Video 14.5.2 - Anomalies of extraocular muscle origin
and insertion (Brown's syndrome) v2
Video Legend: Brown's syndrome

A child with bilateral Brown's syndrome. On looking to the left, the right eye fully adducted, but it was not able to elevate in the adducted position. Similarly, on looking to the right, the left eye fully adducted, but it again was not able to elevate in the adducted position. Video courtesy of Dr. Lawrence Tychsen.